Hot Topics in Acute Care Surgery and Trauma

This series covers the most debated issues in acute care and trauma surgery, from perioperative management to organizational and health policy issues. Since 2011, the founder members of the World Society of Emergency Surgery's (WSES) Acute Care and Trauma Surgeons group, who endorse the series, realized the need to provide more educational tools for young surgeons in training and for general physicians and other specialists new to this discipline: WSES is currently developing a systematic scientific and educational program founded on evidence-based medicine and objective experience. Covering the complex management of acute trauma and non-trauma surgical patients, this series makes a significant contribution to this program and is a valuable resource for both trainees and practitioners in acute care surgery.

More information about this series at http://www.springer.com/series/15718

Nicola de'Angelis • Salomone Di Saverio
Francesco Brunetti
Editors

Emergency Surgical Management of Colorectal Cancer

Springer

Editors
Nicola de'Angelis
Department of General Surgery
Unit of Digestive, Minimally Invasive
and Robotic Surgery,
Henri Mondor Hospital
Créteil
France

Salomone Di Saverio
Cambridge Colorectal Unit, Cambridge
Biomedical Campus
Cambridge University Hospitals NHS
Foundation Trust, Addenbrooke's Hospital
Cambridge
UK

Francesco Brunetti
Department of General Surgery
Unit of Digestive, Minimally Invasive
and Robotic Surgery,
Henri Mondor Hospital
Créteil
France

ISSN 2520-8284 ISSN 2520-8292 (electronic)
Hot Topics in Acute Care Surgery and Trauma
ISBN 978-3-030-06224-8 ISBN 978-3-030-06225-5 (eBook)
https://doi.org/10.1007/978-3-030-06225-5

This Springer imprint is published by the registered company Springer Nature Switzerland AG
The registered company address is: Gewerbestrasse 11, 6330 Cham, Switzerland

To my family, who makes my dreams real by supporting me every single day of my life.

Nicola de' Angelis

To the memory of my Dad "Paito," to my mother Gabriella who is inspiring and missing me, and to the patience and dedication of my beloved wife Omeshnie

Salomone Di Saverio

To my mother Anna and my hometown Napoli

Francesco Brunetti

Preface

This book is part of the series "Hot Topics in Acute Care Surgery," as a result of a successful collaboration between Springer and the World Society of Emergency Surgery (WSES). The WSES is an "open access" society funded in 2009. In less than 10 years, WSES has expanded worldwide, accounting delegates in every continent who share and endorse its aim: promoting emergency surgery training and education through scientific communications, international consensus, academic exchanges, and surgical fellowship.

In the same perspective, this book is addressed to general surgeons, emergency specialists, fellow surgeons, and residents to provide them an extensive and updated overview on the emergency surgical management of colorectal cancer. The increasing prevalence of colorectal cancer, especially in industrialized countries, makes this malignant pathology as one of the most commonly encountered in daily practice and more and more often in the emergency setting. Indeed, the whole book is dedicated to develop the multiple aspects related to the challenging management of colorectal cancer as an emergency, including imaging and interventional radiology strategies, endoscopy, and surgery for both primary tumor and metastases. Novel strategies and techniques, such as the implementation of enhanced recovery program or minimally invasive surgery, are discussed in detail. Particular interest is assigned to specific categories of patients presenting with colorectal cancer emergencies, such as elderly patients, transplanted patients, or patients with hemostatic disorders or receiving immunotherapy or chemoradiation therapy. The postoperative cares and the difficult decision-making process in emergency settings are discussed in dedicated chapters with the aim of providing the reader with detailed descriptions of these important issues. Finally, three chapters focusing on surgical training curriculum, technical aspects, and documented clinical cases have been written specifically for residents and trainees who can find a rapid source of practical and technical information to improve their knowledge and skills in the field.

As editors, we are very satisfied of this work, which emphasizes the international and multidisciplinary collaboration of more than 50 authors from all over the world. Their scientific contribution allowed treating an exhaustive range of pertinent topics and has ensured a perceptive and balanced approach to the complex field of colorectal cancer emergencies.

In this rapidly evolving medical and surgical domain, there remains a shortage of specialists specifically trained to deal with colorectal cancer emergencies.

Those learning more about this field will discover that a successful management is dependent on a consolidated multidisciplinary approach and a straightforward decision-making process in the emergency setting, which relies upon evidence-based knowledge, experience, and pragmatism.

Créteil, France Nicola de'Angelis
Cambridge, UK Salomone Di Saverio
Créteil, France Francesco Brunetti

Contents

Colorectal Cancer Research: A State of the Art

1

Nicola de'Angelis

1.1 Introduction

Research in colorectal cancer is vast and multitudinous, spreading from genetics to surgical techniques. The increasing amount of publications in the last two decades discloses the enormous progress made in the screening, diagnosis, and treatment of this common malignant pathology. Nowadays, colorectal cancer (CRC) is the third most commonly diagnosed cancer in males and the second in females [1]. The worldwide CRC incidence varies over a tenfold extent; in developing countries, the incidence amounts to 1–5 patients per 100,000 inhabitants, while it can increase to 20–60 patients per 100,000 inhabitants in industrialized regions, a difference that is likely attributable to lifestyle habits, socioeconomic status, and environmental exposures over distinct genetic susceptibility. Overall, CRC incidence has been steadily decreasing in the last 15 years, thanks to the improvements in diagnostic techniques and the implementation of screening programs. Conversely, the incidence rates of CRC in adolescents and young adults have been progressively increasing; this may be partially explained by a lack of routine screening and emerging lifestyle issues such as obesity, poor physical exercise, and dietary factors, but it seems to have a distinctive molecular profile in this specific young patient population, very different to late-onset CRC cases [2]. Thus, the overall global burden of CRC is expected to rise, with 2.2 million predicted new cases and 1.1 million deaths by 2030 [3], and an estimated global economic burden approaching $100 billion [4].

Although it remains strictly dependent upon the stage of disease at diagnosis, CRC prognosis and related survival have significantly improved. An early-detected localized CRC is associated with a 90% survival at 5 years, whereas a distant metastatic cancer has a much lower chance of survival (10%) [1, 5]. Thus, despite the

N. de'Angelis (✉)
Unit of Digestive, Hepato-Pancreato-Biliary Surgery and Liver Transplantation,
Henri Mondor Hospital, AP-HP, University of Paris Est, UPEC, Créteil, France

N. de'Angelis et al. (eds.), *Emergency Surgical Management of Colorectal Cancer*,
Hot Topics in Acute Care Surgery and Trauma,
https://doi.org/10.1007/978-3-030-06225-5_1

great progress made, researchers must continue to search for enhancing the accuracy of the available screening methods and the implementation of prevention programs, as well as identifying the best treatment protocols for CRC in order to impact on cancer incidence and mortality. What should not exist in 2019 is a considerable variation in CRC prognosis that is attributable to global and regional disparities in access to diagnostic and treatment services. Unfortunately, mortality rates are still higher in countries with more limited resources and health infrastructures [6], as well as for socioeconomically deprived neighborhoods in developed countries [7–9]. Moreover, due the growth and aging of the population and the adoption of westernized lifestyle worldwide, the global burden of CRC is expecting to further increase supporting any single effort in CRC research.

1.2 Colorectal Cancer Research: A State of the Art

1.2.1 Advances in Colorectal Cancer Research

In the timeline of colorectal cancer research, several milestones can be found [10] concerning the identification of causes and risk factors, the development of diagnostic and screening tools, the discovery of effective drugs. and the advancements in surgical techniques.

Understanding the basic biology of colorectal cancer development, growth and spread, as well as the environmental risk factors and genetic alterations that contribute to CRC occurrence has been essential for the advancements in CRC prevention and treatments [11]. Indeed, it is well established nowadays that the most important risk factors are age, gender, race, and positive family history, which are related to the genetic component in CRC etiology. Other acquired risk factors include lifestyle (e.g., smoking, lack of physical exercise), dietary habits, and geographic areas [12]. Primary and tertiary preventions of CRC focus on these acquired risk factors, whose modification can contribute to lower the risk of cancer development and recurrence [13–15].

Since the first publication in 1927 by Lockhart-Mummery JP and Dukes C in surgery, gynecology, and obstetrics, research has clearly demonstrated that CRC does not arise de novo from the colon mucosa but from a preexisting lesion that can be early detected and treated to the benefit of the patient's cure and survival. This raised the important issue of screening tests with a high sensitivity for detecting early-stage CRC, but even more importantly, for advanced adenomas and high-grade dysplasia, which are the bridge to invasive cancers [16].

Thus, the screening paradigm has shifted; in 2017, the American Cancer Society recommends to screen for CRC in people at average risk aged between 50 and 75 years with a screening strategy that is able to identify polyps and cancer (i.e., by sigmoidoscopy every 5 years, colonoscopy every 10 years, or CT colonoscopy every 5 years). This is preferred over alternative tools that mainly find cancer (i.e., take-home gFOBT yearly, take-home FIT yearly, or a stool-DNA test every 3 years) [17]. It is noteworthy that the widespread implementation of those screening methods that can accurately identify premalignant polyps or early-stage cancers allowing for the treatment of curable lesions led to an up to 50% reduction in cancer-related mortality [16, 18, 19].

The twenty-first century has been characterized by the introduction of new agents for CRC chemotherapy, modified therapeutic protocols (adjuvant vs. neoadjuvant chemotherapy), and targeted therapies [10, 20–23], which all contributed to improve survival outcomes also in advanced stages of disease. From the sole active agent available until the year 2000, namely, the fluorouracil, molecules such as irinotecan, oxaliplatin, and humanized monoclonal antibodies (bevacizumab, ramucirumab, cetuximab, and panitumumab) were approved for the treatment of CRC. Moreover, the introduction of an orally active drug, the capecitabine, signed another milestone in the CRC chemotherapeutic protocol.

In the era of personalized medicine and with the effort of predicting or improving drug responses in CRC patients, gene expression-based subtyping and molecular CRC classifications were developed as valuable approaches for patient stratification [24, 25]. Most of the molecular mechanisms involved in colorectal carcinogenesis have been characterized, and 16% of CRCs were found to be hypermutated: three-quarters of these had the expected high microsatellite instability, which is known as predictor of a favorable response to immunotherapy in patients with advanced-stage CRC [26, 27].

In the particular case of locally advanced rectal cancer, the administration of neoadjuvant radiotherapy in combination with total mesorectal excision was proved to decrease the local recurrence rate, and it is nowadays considered as the gold standard protocol [28–30]. Going forward, some authors suggested a true paradigm shift in 2004 in case of a complete response to neoadjuvant chemoradiation therapy: the "wait and watch" approach aiming at sparing organs and tissues and avoiding radical, invasive, and morbid surgery with a tremendous impact on the patient's quality of life [31–35]. Although promising, the oncological safety of this treatment strategy in rectal cancer is currently under investigations.

1.2.2 Critical Issues and Research Gaps in Colorectal Cancer Research

Many critical issues remain unsolved or under investigation in the field of CRC biology, prevention, and treatment [36]. A better understanding of the molecular and cellular interplay between CRC and its macro- and microenvironment would represent a key step forward. In the near future, we expect to have deciphered the roles of gut microbiome in the regulation of the host immune-inflammatory responses and the genesis of neoplastic lesions and, consequently, the possibility of using colorectal microbiota biomarkers to improve treatment outcomes in CRC patients [37].

Definitely, we are still facing an incomplete picture in the etiology of CRC; the absolute risk attributable to inherited, environmental, or lifestyle factors and their synergic interactions remain unclear. To apply precision medicine and tailored interventions, the risk assessment and patient stratification must become as precise as possible, and this represents the main pathway to undermine the global burden of CRC [38].

Improvements are awaited at any step of CRC cares: in the prevention and screening processes, at the diagnostic level, in the prognostic evaluation, and finally in the application of curative treatments. In general, research advancement should aim to optimize current strategies, fill the gaps, and correct inadequacy while searching for new treatments and novel technologies. Most importantly, there is a real need for more studies focusing on strategies to improve health-related quality of life in patients living with and beyond CRC [36]. Prolonging patient's survival could not be the only objective of modern CRC therapies; research must find a way to weight and counteract the psychological, emotional, and social impact of CRC treatment sequelae, which may include disabling and embarrassing symptoms such as fecal incontinence or sexual dysfunction (observed in up to 35% of patients with rectal cancer) [39–41].

Finally, CRC research in the last decades emphasized the importance of a multidisciplinary team approach to CRC cares, which promoted the creation of national and international networks of colorectal cancer centers of excellence that apply evidenced-based medicine for the standardization of best practices [42]. However, this must be implemented involving not only clinicians and surgeons but also biologists and physical scientists whose expertise is highly required to further advance in CRC research. Moreover, the widespread formation of CRC research networks will assure effective communications between healthcare professionals and optimal knowledge transfer toward healthcare policy-makers, research funders, and CRC patients [36].

1.3 Colorectal Cancer Surgery

1.3.1 Milestones in Colorectal Cancer Surgery

Among all therapeutic options, surgery remains the best chance of cure for CRC when a curative-intent surgery is still possible.

Colon cancer can be safely and efficacy treated by surgery. During the last two centuries, extensive debates have followed about the best technique of colon cancer resection. These concerned the critical issue of high ligation of the lymphovascular pedicle before or after manipulating the tumor, wide or restricted excisions, and the interest of no-touch isolation technique (i.e., early isolation of the lymphovascular pedicle with minimal manipulation).

In general, the type of colectomy is based on tumor location and vascular lymphatic drainage. Although it remains controversial, the high ligation of the lymphovascular pedicle and the no-touch technique seem to confer no additional oncological benefit; however, recent evidence supports the principle of complete mesocolic excision (CME) as the optimal approach that should be applied to all colon cancer. CME includes three essential components: firstly, the dissection between the mesenteric plane and parietal fascia and the removal of the mesentery within a complete envelope of mesenteric fascia and visceral peritoneum that contains all lymph nodes draining the tumor area. The second component is the central vascular ligation that potentially removes lymph node metastases, vascular and neural invasion in the whole regional draining area. Then, the third component is represented by the resection of an adequate length of bowel to remove all the involved pericolic lymph nodes [43, 44].

Supported by several randomized clinical trials and in order to preserve at best patient's quality of life, the general tendency today is to opt for more conservative and organ-sparing surgical techniques rather than extended resection. Indeed, segmental resections appear as safe as extended ones in case of colon cancer, even located in the transverse colon or at the splenic flexure [45–47].

Rectal cancer was considered incurable until the eighteenth century, when surgery was applied to remove the rectum. However, prior to the introduction of anesthesia, asepsis, and blood transfusions, rectal surgery was highly invasive, aggressive, disabling, and associated with extremely high mortality rates [48]. Early in the twentieth century, Sir Miles described the radical abdominoperineal resection (APR) with permanent colostomy recommending an extensive mesenteric lymphadenectomy to prevent recurrence. To counteract the extreme invasiveness of the radical APR, some surgeons proposed an anastomosis between the rectum and sigmoid colon, which, however, was associated with poor oncological outcomes at that time. The introduction of the Hartmann's procedure with the construction of an end colostomy leaving the distal rectum in place signed a real milestone in rectal cancer management. Since then, the tendency has shifted toward less radical and more sphincter-sparing surgical procedures including anterior resection, low anterior resection (LAR), and pouch reconstructions. The cornerstone in rectal cancer surgery is definitely represented by the concept of total mesorectal excision (TME), proposed by Richard Heald in 1982 [49]. Heald's TME was based on the embryologic development of the hindgut, and it included the excision of the rectal cancer together with the en bloc excision of the mesorectum. By applying this technique, he decreased the rates of positive lateral margins and local recurrence as low as 3.6% and improved the disease-free survival up to 80% at 5 years and 78% at 10 years [49]. Over the years, TME was proved to improve oncologic outcomes and patients' survival over non-TME approaches, and thus, it is currently considered as the gold standard approach in rectal cancer surgery [50, 51].

Parallel to the evolution of surgical principles and surgical techniques, the introduction of new surgical materials and devices allowed for fatal advancements. Particularly, the routinely use of mechanical staplers since the 1970s has revolutionized colorectal surgery and made many challenging or tedious procedures much easier and expeditious [48].

The current debate in CRC surgery concerns the application of minimally invasive approaches, such as laparoscopy, robotics, and transanal endoscopic microsurgery [52]. Laparoscopy in general has refashioned surgery of the last three decades transforming completely the operative and postoperative courses of the operated patients.

Laparoscopic colectomy was first introduced in 1991, and it becomes successively the gold standard approach. Indeed, patients operated on by laparoscopy show faster recovery, shorter hospital stay, lesser pain, and improved cosmetic outcomes compared to open surgery [53–55]. The short-term advantages of laparoscopy are doubtless in both colon and rectal cancer resection, but its oncological safety in case of rectal cancer has been recently questioned [56–59]. Indeed, the adaption of laparoscopy for colon cancer has improved recovery outcomes and patient's acceptation of surgery at no expense to survival [55, 60], whereas laparoscopic rectal cancer surgery has been associated with significantly lower rates of complete mesorectal excision with free resection margins, threating the oncological principles of TME [57]. However, long-term results are lacking, and they will be necessary to finally assess the role of laparoscopy in rectal cancer treatment.

Despite the widespread enthusiasm toward laparoscopy and the encouraging results of randomized controlled trials, especially for colon cancer, it must be noted that the adaption of laparoscopy for CRC surgery remains relatively low. In the USA, a bit more than one patient over two with colon cancer undergoes elective laparoscopic colectomy, whereas only 10% of rectal cancer surgeries are performed by laparoscopy, with significant disparity between urban and rural areas and in high-volume compared with low-volume centers [61, 62]. In France, up to 29% of patients with CRC receive an elective laparoscopic resection [63], with higher rates in high-volume, tertiary, referral hospitals. The hesitation toward laparoscopy, which after more than 20 years from its introduction is still reserved to a minority of patients, may be explained by its complex use in CRC surgery compared to other abdominal operations, leading to long operative times, high conversion rates, steep learning curve, and thus necessary specialized training periods.

To overcome laparoscopic pitfalls, robotic surgery was proposed as high technological approach that allows for a three-dimensional view of the operating field, a 7-degree-of-freedom motion with wristed instruments, and a great surgical ergonomics. The literature is expanding, and several studies have been published on the comparison between robotic and laparoscopic colorectal surgery [45, 64–66]. Despite good surgical outcomes that are most of time comparable to those obtained by laparoscopy, the main drawback of robotic surgery appears to be the costs/benefits ratio that is still unfavorable limiting the indications and spreading of robotics at approximately 1–3% of CRC surgeries [67, 68].

Alternative techniques include natural-orifice transluminal endoscopic surgery (NOTES) and transanal TME (TaTME), which are seen as promising approaches to treat rectal especially located in the low rectum, or in male patients, narrow pelvis or in case of obesity. Still, there is a need for well-designed and executed randomized, controlled trials to define the safety and indications of NOTES or TaTME, as well as their superiority over laparoscopy [52].

Overall, the evolution of CRC surgery is characterized by the progressive shift from radical to organ-sparing procedures and from aggressive to minimally invasive approaches. The pattern of this evolutionary process has definitely accelerated in the last decades reflecting the accelerated rate of technology development in general as in the medical fields. The development and application of minimally invasive surgical techniques in CRC management must continue because it is supported by a huge clinical impact on patient-centered outcomes as well as on the healthcare systems. In the modern era, it is imperative to optimize the standard of cares in order to reduce the costs of colorectal surgery; this may be pursued by applying the surgical approach with the highest efficiency, the less morbidity rate, and the best oncological outcomes.

1.3.2 The Body of Evidence in Emergency Colorectal Cancer Surgery

Despite increased screening efforts, it is estimated that up to 33% of patients with CRC will present with symptoms requiring acute or emergent surgical interventions. While treating in an emergency setting, the rate of associated morbidity, mortality, and stoma formation is significantly higher compared to elective CRC management. Thus, specific considerations should be made for emergency CRC management and particularly emergency CRC surgery.

The present book is entirely dedicated to the current knowledge and actual issues in the emergency surgical management of colorectal cancer. Each chapter has been written by clinicians and surgeons highly expert in the field with the objective of summarizing the up-to-date literature and merging it with their personal experience. This is one of the fundamental principles of evidence-based medicine, for which any therapeutic choice should be based upon the best available scientific evidence combined with the surgeon's clinical experience and the patient's demand. However, it must be noted that in the specific domain of emergency colorectal cancer surgery, the amount and quality of evidence is limited and mainly supported by retrospective studies. Obviously, practical and ethical issues curtail the feasibility of randomized controlled trails (RCTs), and due to the heterogeneous presentation of CRC in emergency, this latter type of cancer has often represented an exclusion criterion.

It is worth noting that the surgical field in general is not awarded by a high amount of well-conducted RCTs. Indeed, RCTs account for less than 4% of all publications in the leading surgical journals, and their number showed a tendency to decline over time. Hence, most of the available evidence surgery, in both elective and emergency settings, may be considered of poor quality on the evidence-based medicine scale whether it comes from non-RCTs (case-control or cohort studies), retrospective case series, or qualitative reviews [69].

Despite this, systematic reviews and meta-analyses were conducted to summarize the results of emergency vs. elective surgery in CRC patients and compare the outcomes of different surgical approaches [70–73].

In general, a worse prognosis is associated with CRC presenting as a surgical emergency; worse outcomes are related on one side to the patient's specific conditions when admitted in emergency settings (e.g., dehydration, poor nutrition, neglected comorbidities) and, on the other side, to the characteristics of tumors resected emergently. Indeed, CRC requiring an emergency surgery is typically of a more advanced T stage, of higher histologic grade, or already involving regional lymph nodes or adjacent organs.

Laparoscopy for the emergency surgical management of CRC is gaining popularity, although there is little guidance in the literature about the preoperative evaluation and risk stratification upon which select the type of the operative approach. Moreover, the surgeon's experience and proficiency in laparoscopy play a major role in the adoption of this minimally invasive technique into emergency clinical practice [71].

Finally, in the emergency setting, the individualization of surgical management is even of a greater importance than in elective surgery. However, the emergency colorectal surgeon will face several problems, such as incomplete or unavailable information about diagnosis and staging, complex risk assessment and stratification, and sometimes even the impossibility to gather the patient's consent for surgery. Thus, the decision-making process may be challenging. The available international guidelines and consensus agree that the literature concerning the emergency surgical management of CRC is relatively poor and the existing RCTs are often not sufficiently robust in design and sample size to the point that only few recommendations may be considered as having a strong evidence base (i.e., Grade A). Despite this, the oncologic principles that should be met even in case of CRC requiring an emergency surgery are clear. The Clinical Practice Guidelines Committee of the American Society of Colon and Rectal Surgeons listed the following goals in the treatment of CRC-related emergencies: (1) avert the immediate negative impact of the complication, (2) achieve the best possible tumor control, and (3) ensure timely recovery to permit initiation of appropriate adjuvant or systemic treatment [73]. Surgical principles include wide radial, proximal, and distal margins and a high ligation of the lymphovascular pedicle to obtain an extended lymphadenectomy (>12 lymph nodes) as for CRC resection performed in elective settings.

1.4 Conclusion: Being an Emergency Colorectal Surgeon

With wide disparities among countries and regions, most of colorectal emergencies are still managed by general surgeons, but a greater body of evidence highlights the impact of specialization to reduce morbidity and mortality [74, 75]. Indeed, being a specialized colorectal surgeon seems to be associated with improved surgical outcomes and increased chances for the patient of receiving the best treatment option. Thus, Chap. 26 of this book will discuss the importance of advanced surgical training, revised curriculum, and specialization in colorectal surgery. In parallel, there is a need to progressively shift, especially in tertiary referral hospitals, toward clinical and surgical units that are organized on specialized clinical interest or professional activity to the benefit of the patients' cares and management.

References

1. Global Burden of Disease Cancer, C, Fitzmaurice C, Allen C, Barber RM, Barregard L, Bhutta ZA, Brenner H, Dicker DJ, Chimed-Orchir O, Dandona R, Dandona L, Fleming T, Forouzanfar MH, Hancock J, Hay RJ, Hunter-Merrill R, Huynh C, Hosgood HD, Johnson CO, Jonas JB, Khubchandani J, Kumar GA, Kutz M, Lan Q, Larson HJ, Liang X, Lim SS, Lopez AD, MF MI, Marczak L, Marquez N, Mokdad AH, Pinho C, Pourmalek F, Salomon JA, Sanabria JR, Sandar L, Sartorius B, Schwartz SM, Shackelford KA, Shibuya K, Stanaway J, Steiner C, Sun J, Takahashi K, Vollset SE, Vos T, Wagner JA, Wang H, Westerman R, Zeeb H, Zoeckler L, Abd-Allah F, Ahmed MB, Alabed S, Alam NK, Aldhahri SF, Alem G, Alemayohu MA, Ali R, Al-Raddadi R, Amare A, Amoako Y, Artaman A, Asayesh H, Atnafu N, Awasthi A, Saleem HB, Barac A, Bedi N, Bensenor I, Berhane A, Bernabe E, Betsu B, Binagwaho A, Boneya D, Campos-Nonato I, Castaneda-Orjuela C, Catala-Lopez F, Chiang P, Chibueze C, Chitheer A, Choi JY, Cowie B, Damtew S, das Neves J, Dey S, Dharmaratne S, Dhillon P, Ding E, Driscoll T, Ekwueme D, Endries AY, Farvid M, Farzadfar F, Fernandes J, Fischer F, GH TT, Gebru A, Gopalani S, Hailu A, Horino M, Horita N, Husseini A, Huybrechts I, Inoue M, Islami F, Jakovljevic M, James S, Javanbakht M, Jee SH, Kasaeian A, Kedir MS, Khader YS, Khang YH, Kim D, Leigh J, Linn S, Lunevicius R, HMA ER, Malekzadeh R, Malta DC, Marcenes W, Markos D, Melaku YA, Meles KG, Mendoza W, Mengiste DT, Meretoja TJ, Miller TR, Mohammad KA, Mohammadi A, Mohammed S, Moradi-Lakeh M, Nagel G, Nand D, Le Nguyen Q, Nolte S, Ogbo FA, Oladimeji KE, Oren E, Pa M, Park EK, Pereira DM, Plass D, Qorbani M, Radfar A, Rafay A, Rahman M, Rana SM, Soreide K, Satpathy M, Sawhney M, Sepanlou SG, Shaikh MA, She J, Shiue I, Shore HR, Shrime MG, So S, Soneji S, Stathopoulou V, Stroumpoulis K, Sufiyan MB, Sykes BL, Tabares-Seisdedos R, Tadese F, Tedla BA, Tessema GA, Thakur JS, Tran BX, Ukwaja KN, BSC U, Vlassov VV, Weiderpass E, Wubshet Terefe M, Yebyo HG, Yimam HH, Yonemoto N, Younis MZ, Yu C, Zaidi Z, MES Z, Zenebe ZM, CJL M, Naghavi M. Global, regional, and national cancer incidence, mortality, years of life lost, years lived with disability, and disability-adjusted life-years for 32 cancer groups, 1990 to 2015: a systematic analysis for the global burden of disease study. JAMA Oncol. 2017;3(4):524–48.
2. Connell LC, Mota JM, Braghiroli MI, Hoff PM. The rising incidence of younger patients with colorectal cancer: questions about screening, biology, and treatment. Curr Treat Options Oncol. 2017;18(4):23.
3. Arnold M, Sierra MS, Laversanne M, Soerjomataram I, Jemal A, Bray F. Global patterns and trends in colorectal cancer incidence and mortality. Gut. 2017;66(4):683–91.
4. TAC Society. Global cancer control work. 2018. Accessed 8 May, 2018.
5. Heinemann V, von Weikersthal LF, Decker T, Kiani A, Vehling-Kaiser U, Al-Batran SE, Heintges T, Lerchenmuller C, Kahl C, Seipelt G, Kullmann F, Stauch M, Scheithauer W, Hielscher J, Scholz M, Muller S, Link H, Niederle N, Rost A, Hoffkes HG, Moehler M, Lindig RU, Modest DP, Rossius L, Kirchner T, Jung A, Stintzing S. FOLFIRI plus cetuximab versus FOLFIRI plus bevacizumab as first-line treatment for patients with metastatic colorectal cancer (FIRE-3): a randomised, open-label, phase 3 trial. Lancet Oncol. 2014;15(10):1065–75.
6. Center MM, Jemal A, Smith RA, Ward E. Worldwide variations in colorectal cancer. CA Cancer J Clin. 2009;59(6):366–78.
7. Henry KA, Niu X, Boscoe FP. Geographic disparities in colorectal cancer survival. Int J Health Geogr. 2009;8:48.
8. Lian M, Schootman M, Doubeni CA, Park Y, Major JM, Stone RA, Laiyemo AO, Hollenbeck AR, Graubard BI, Schatzkin A. Geographic variation in colorectal cancer survival and the role of small-area socioeconomic deprivation: a multilevel survival analysis of the NIH-AARP diet and health study cohort. Am J Epidemiol. 2011;174(7):828–38.
9. Favoriti P, Carbone G, Greco M, Pirozzi F, Pirozzi RE, Corcione F. Worldwide burden of colorectal cancer: a review. Updates Surg. 2016;68(1):7–11.

10. ASoC Oncology. Cancer progress timeline. 2018.
11. Vogelstein B, Fearon ER, Hamilton SR, Kern SE, Preisinger AC, Leppert M, Nakamura Y, White R, Smits AM, Bos JL. Genetic alterations during colorectal-tumor development. N Engl J Med. 1988;319(9):525–32.
12. Huxley RR, Ansary-Moghaddam A, Clifton P, Czernichow S, Parr CL, Woodward M. The impact of dietary and lifestyle risk factors on risk of colorectal cancer: a quantitative overview of the epidemiological evidence. Int J Cancer. 2009;125(1):171–80.
13. Crosara Teixeira M, Braghiroli MI, Sabbaga J, Hoff PM. Primary prevention of colorectal cancer: myth or reality? World J Gastroenterol. 2014;20(41):15060–9.
14. Massat NJ, Moss SM, Halloran SP, Duffy SW. Screening and primary prevention of colorectal cancer: a review of sex-specific and site-specific differences. J Med Screen. 2013;20(3):125–48.
15. Schoenberg MH. Physical activity and nutrition in primary and tertiary prevention of colorectal cancer. Visc Med. 2016;32(3):199–204.
16. Winawer SJ. The history of colorectal cancer screening: a personal perspective. Dig Dis Sci. 2015;60(3):596–608.
17. ACS Reccomandations. Colorectal cancer early detection 2017.
18. Mandel JS, Bond JH, Church TR, Snover DC, Bradley GM, Schuman LM, Ederer F. Reducing mortality from colorectal cancer by screening for fecal occult blood. Minnesota Colon Cancer Control Study. N Engl J Med. 1993;328(19):1365–71.
19. Yang DX, Gross CP, Soulos PR, Yu JB. Estimating the magnitude of colorectal cancers prevented during the era of screening: 1976 to 2009. Cancer. 2014;120(18):2893–901.
20. Andre T, Boni C, Navarro M, Tabernero J, Hickish T, Topham C, Bonetti A, Clingan P, Bridgewater J, Rivera F, de Gramont A. Improved overall survival with oxaliplatin, fluorouracil, and leucovorin as adjuvant treatment in stage II or III colon cancer in the MOSAIC trial. J Clin Oncol. 2009;27(19):3109–16.
21. Grothey A, Van Cutsem E, Sobrero A, Siena S, Falcone A, Ychou M, Humblet Y, Bouche O, Mineur L, Barone C, Adenis A, Tabernero J, Yoshino T, Lenz HJ, Goldberg RM, Sargent DJ, Cihon F, Cupit L, Wagner A, Laurent D, Group, CS. Regorafenib monotherapy for previously treated metastatic colorectal cancer (CORRECT): an international, multicentre, randomised, placebo-controlled, phase 3 trial. Lancet. 2013;381(9863):303–12.
22. Karapetis CS, Khambata-Ford S, Jonker DJ, O'Callaghan CJ, Tu D, Tebbutt NC, Simes RJ, Chalchal H, Shapiro JD, Robitaille S, Price TJ, Shepherd L, Au HJ, Langer C, Moore MJ, Zalcberg JR. K-ras mutations and benefit from cetuximab in advanced colorectal cancer. N Engl J Med. 2008;359(17):1757–65.
23. G Foxtrot Collaborative. Feasibility of preoperative chemotherapy for locally advanced, operable colon cancer: the pilot phase of a randomised controlled trial. Lancet Oncol. 2012;13(11):1152–60.
24. Dragani TA, Castells A, Kulasingam V, Diamandis EP, Earl H, Iams WT, Lovly CM, Sedelaar JP, Schalken JA. Major milestones in translational oncology. BMC Med. 2016;14(1):110.
25. Guinney J, Dienstmann R, Wang X, de Reynies A, Schlicker A, Soneson C, Marisa L, Roepman P, Nyamundanda G, Angelino P, Bot BM, Morris JS, Simon IM, Gerster S, Fessler E, De Sousa EMF, Missiaglia E, Ramay H, Barras D, Homicsko K, Maru D, Manyam GC, Broom B, Boige V, Perez-Villamil B, Laderas T, Salazar R, Gray JW, Hanahan D, Tabernero J, Bernards R, Friend SH, Laurent-Puig P, Medema JP, Sadanandam A, Wessels L, Delorenzi M, Kopetz S, Vermeulen L, Tejpar S. The consensus molecular subtypes of colorectal cancer. Nat Med. 2015;21(11):1350–6.
26. N Cancer Genome Atlas. Comprehensive molecular characterization of human colon and rectal cancer. Nature. 2012;487(7407):330–7.
27. Le DT, Uram JN, Wang H, Bartlett BR, Kemberling H, Eyring AD, Skora AD, Luber BS, Azad NS, Laheru D, Biedrzycki B, Donehower RC, Zaheer A, Fisher GA, Crocenzi TS, Lee JJ, Duffy SM, Goldberg RM, de la Chapelle A, Koshiji M, Bhaijee F, Huebner T, Hruban RH, Wood LD, Cuka N, Pardoll DM, Papadopoulos N, Kinzler KW, Zhou S, Cornish TC, Taube JM, Anders RA, Eshleman JR, Vogelstein B, Diaz LA Jr. PD-1 blockade in tumors with mismatch-repair deficiency. N Engl J Med. 2015;372(26):2509–20.

28. Initial report from a Swedish multicentre study examining the role of preoperative irradiation in the treatment of patients with resectable rectal carcinoma. Swedish Rectal Cancer Trial. Br J Surg. 1993;80(10):1333–6.
29. Kye BH, Cho HM. Overview of radiation therapy for treating rectal cancer. Ann Coloproctol. 2014;30(4):165–74.
30. Dahlberg M, Glimelius B, Graf W, Pahlman L. Preoperative irradiation affects functional results after surgery for rectal cancer: results from a randomized study. Dis Colon Rectum. 1998;41(5):543–9. discussion 549–551.
31. Kong JC, Guerra GR, Warrier SK, Ramsay RG, Heriot AG. Outcome and salvage surgery following "watch and wait" for rectal cancer after neoadjuvant therapy: a systematic review. Dis Colon Rectum. 2017;60(3):335–45.
32. Nakagawa WT, Rossi BM, de OFF, Ferrigno R, David Filho WJ, Nishimoto IN, Vieira RA, Lopes A. Chemoradiation instead of surgery to treat mid and low rectal tumors: is it safe? Ann Surg Oncol. 2002;9(6):568–73.
33. Habr-Gama A, Perez RO, Nadalin W, Sabbaga J, Ribeiro U Jr, Silva e Sousa AH Jr, Campos FG, Kiss DR, Gama-Rodrigues J. Operative versus nonoperative treatment for stage 0 distal rectal cancer following chemoradiation therapy: long-term results. Ann Surg. 2004;240(4):711–7. discussion 717–718.
34. Hendren SK, O'Connor BI, Liu M, Asano T, Cohen Z, Swallow CJ, Macrae HM, Gryfe R, McLeod RS. Prevalence of male and female sexual dysfunction is high following surgery for rectal cancer. Ann Surg. 2005;242(2):212–23.
35. Chen TY, Wiltink LM, Nout RA, Meershoek-Klein Kranenbarg E, Laurberg S, Marijnen CA, van de Velde CJ. Bowel function 14 years after preoperative short-course radiotherapy and total mesorectal excision for rectal cancer: report of a multicenter randomized trial. Clin Colorectal Cancer. 2015;14(2):106–14.
36. Lawler M, Alsina D, Adams RA, Anderson AS, Brown G, Fearnhead NS, Fenwick SW, Halloran SP, Hochhauser D, Hull MA, Koelzer VH, McNair AGK, Monahan KJ, Nathke I, Norton C, Novelli MR, Steele RJC, Thomas AL, Wilde LM, Wilson RH, Tomlinson I, Bowel Cancer, UKCRGiCCI. Critical research gaps and recommendations to inform research prioritisation for more effective prevention and improved outcomes in colorectal cancer. Gut. 2018;67(1):179–93.
37. Raskov H, Burcharth J, Pommergaard HC. Linking gut microbiota to colorectal cancer. J Cancer. 2017;8(17):3378–95.
38. Weinberg DS, Myers RE, Keenan E, Ruth K, Sifri R, Ziring B, Ross E, Manne SL. Genetic and environmental risk assessment and colorectal cancer screening in an average-risk population: a randomized trial. Ann Intern Med. 2014;161(8):537–45.
39. Andreyev J. Gastrointestinal symptoms after pelvic radiotherapy: a new understanding to improve management of symptomatic patients. Lancet Oncol. 2007;8(11):1007–17.
40. Battersby NJ, Juul T, Christensen P, Janjua AZ, Branagan G, Emmertsen KJ, Norton C, Hughes R, Laurberg S, Moran BJ, United Kingdom Low Anterior Resection Syndrome Study, G. Predicting the risk of bowel-related quality-of-life impairment after restorative resection for rectal cancer: a multicenter cross-sectional study. Dis Colon Rectum. 2016;59(4):270–80.
41. Scheer AS, Boushey RP, Liang S, Doucette S, O'Connor AM, Moher D. The long-term gastrointestinal functional outcomes following curative anterior resection in adults with rectal cancer: a systematic review and meta-analysis. Dis Colon Rectum. 2011;54(12):1589–97.
42. Dietz DW, Consortium for Optimizing Surgical Treatment of Rectal, C. Multidisciplinary management of rectal cancer: the OSTRICH. J Gastrointest Surg. 2013;17(10):1863–8.
43. Sondenaa K, Quirke P, Hohenberger W, Sugihara K, Kobayashi H, Kessler H, Brown G, Tudyka V, D'Hoore A, Kennedy RH, West NP, Kim SH, Heald R, Storli KE, Nesbakken A, Moran B. The rationale behind complete mesocolic excision (CME) and a central vascular ligation for colon cancer in open and laparoscopic surgery: proceedings of a consensus conference. Int J Colorectal Dis. 2014;29(4):419–28.
44. West NP, Hohenberger W, Weber K, Perrakis A, Finan PJ, Quirke P. Complete mesocolic excision with central vascular ligation produces an oncologically superior specimen compared with standard surgery for carcinoma of the colon. J Clin Oncol. 2010;28(2):272–8.

45. de'Angelis N, Alghamdi S, Renda A, Azoulay D, Brunetti F. Initial experience of robotic versus laparoscopic colectomy for transverse colon cancer: a matched case-control study. World J Surg Oncol. 2015;13:295.
46. de'Angelis N, Hain E, Disabato M, Cordun C, Carra MC, Azoulay D, Brunetti F. Laparoscopic extended right colectomy versus laparoscopic left colectomy for carcinoma of the splenic flexure: a matched case-control study. Int J Colorectal Dis. 2016;31(3):623–30.
47. Martinez-Perez A, Brunetti F, Vitali GC, Abdalla S, Ris F, de'Angelis N. Surgical treatment of colon cancer of the splenic flexure: a systematic review and meta-analysis. Surg Laparosc Endosc Percutan Tech. 2017;27(5):318–27.
48. Galler AS, Petrelli NJ, Shakamuri SP. Rectal cancer surgery: a brief history. Surg Oncol. 2011;20(4):223–30.
49. Heald RJ, Moran BJ, Ryall RD, Sexton R, MacFarlane JK. Rectal cancer: the Basingstoke experience of total mesorectal excision, 1978-1997. Arch Surg. 1998;133(8):894–9.
50. Carlsen E, Schlichting E, Guldvog I, Johnson E, Heald RJ. Effect of the introduction of total mesorectal excision for the treatment of rectal cancer. Br J Surg. 1998;85(4):526–9.
51. Stewart DB, Dietz DW. Total mesorectal excision: what are we doing? Clin Colon Rectal Surg. 2007;20(3):190–202.
52. Abu Gazala M, Wexner SD. Re-appraisal and consideration of minimally invasive surgery in colorectal cancer. Gastroenterol Rep (Oxf). 2017;5(1):1–10.
53. Martinez-Perez A, Carra MC, Brunetti F, de'Angelis N. Short-term clinical outcomes of laparoscopic vs open rectal excision for rectal cancer: a systematic review and meta-analysis. World J Gastroenterol. 2017;23(44):7906–16.
54. Vennix S, Pelzers L, Bouvy N, Beets GL, Pierie JP, Wiggers T, Breukink S. Laparoscopic versus open total mesorectal excision for rectal cancer. Cochrane Database Syst Rev. 2014;(4):CD005200.
55. Veldkamp R, Kuhry E, Hop WC, Jeekel J, Kazemier G, Bonjer HJ, Haglind E, Pahlman L, Cuesta MA, Msika S, Morino M, Lacy AM, Group, COcLoORS. Laparoscopic surgery versus open surgery for colon cancer: short-term outcomes of a randomised trial. Lancet Oncol. 2005;6(7):477–84.
56. Fleshman J, Branda M, Sargent DJ, Boller AM, George V, Abbas M, Peters WR Jr, Maun D, Chang G, Herline A, Fichera A, Mutch M, Wexner S, Whiteford M, Marks J, Birnbaum E, Margolin D, Larson D, Marcello P, Posner M, Read T, Monson J, Wren SM, Pisters PW, Nelson H. Effect of laparoscopic-assisted resection vs open resection of stage II or III rectal cancer on pathologic outcomes: the ACOSOG Z6051 randomized clinical trial. JAMA. 2015;314(13):1346–55.
57. Martinez-Perez A, Carra MC, Brunetti F, de'Angelis N. Pathologic outcomes of laparoscopic vs open mesorectal excision for rectal cancer: a systematic review and meta-analysis. JAMA Surg. 2017;152(4):e165665.
58. Petrucciani N, Martinez-Perez A, Bianchi G, Memeo R, Brunetti F, De' Angelis N. The use of laparoscopy for locally advanced rectal cancer. Minerva Chir. 2018;73(1):77–92.
59. Stevenson AR, Solomon MJ, Lumley JW, Hewett P, Clouston AD, Gebski VJ, Davies L, Wilson K, Hague W, Simes J, Investigators AL. Effect of laparoscopic-assisted resection vs open resection on pathological outcomes in rectal cancer: the ALaCaRT randomized clinical trial. JAMA. 2015;314(13):1356–63.
60. Guillou PJ, Quirke P, Thorpe H, Walker J, Jayne DG, Smith AM, Heath RM, Brown JM, Group, MCt. Short-term endpoints of conventional versus laparoscopic-assisted surgery in patients with colorectal cancer (MRC CLASICC trial): multicentre, randomised controlled trial. Lancet. 2005;365(9472):1718–26.
61. Carmichael JC, Masoomi H, Mills S, Stamos MJ, Nguyen NT. Utilization of laparoscopy in colorectal surgery for cancer at academic medical centers: does site of surgery affect rate of laparoscopy? Am Surg. 2011;77(10):1300–4.
62. Moghadamyeghaneh Z, Carmichael JC, Mills S, Pigazzi A, Nguyen NT, Stamos MJ. Variations in laparoscopic colectomy utilization in the united states. Dis Colon Rectum. 2015;58(10):950–6.

63. Panis Y, Maggiori L, Caranhac G, Bretagnol F, Vicaut E. Mortality after colorectal cancer surgery: a French survey of more than 84,000 patients. Ann Surg. 2011;254(5):738–43. discussion 743–734.
64. de'Angelis N, Felli E, Azoulay D, Brunetti F. Robotic-assisted reversal of Hartmann's procedure for diverticulitis. J Robot Surg. 2014;8(4):381–3.
65. de'Angelis N, Lizzi V, Azoulay D, Brunetti F. Robotic versus laparoscopic right colectomy for colon cancer: analysis of the initial simultaneous learning curve of a surgical fellow. J Laparoendosc Adv Surg Tech A. 2016;26(11):882–92.
66. Jayne D, Pigazzi A, Marshall H, Croft J, Corrigan N, Copeland J, Quirke P, West N, Rautio T, Thomassen N, Tilney H, Gudgeon M, Bianchi PP, Edlin R, Hulme C, Brown J. Effect of robotic-assisted vs conventional laparoscopic surgery on risk of conversion to open laparotomy among patients undergoing resection for rectal cancer: the ROLARR randomized clinical trial. JAMA. 2017;318(16):1569–80.
67. de'Angelis N, Portigliotti L, Azoulay D, Brunetti F. Robotic surgery: a step forward in the wide spread of minimally invasive colorectal surgery. J Minim Access Surg. 2015;11(4):285–6.
68. Yeo HL, Isaacs AJ, Abelson JS, Milsom JW, Sedrakyan A. Comparison of open, laparoscopic, and robotic colectomies using a large national database: outcomes and trends related to surgery center volume. Dis Colon Rectum. 2016;59(6):535–42.
69. Meshikhes AW. Evidence-based surgery: the obstacles and solutions. Int J Surg. 2015;18:159–62.
70. Felli E, Brunetti F, Disabato M, Salloum C, Azoulay D, De'angelis N. Robotic right colectomy for hemorrhagic right colon cancer: a case report and review of the literature of minimally invasive urgent colectomy. World J Emerg Surg. 2014;9:32.
71. Harji DP, Griffiths B, Burke D, Sagar PM. Systematic review of emergency laparoscopic colorectal resection. Br J Surg. 2014;101(1):e126–33.
72. Ansaloni L, Andersson RE, Bazzoli F, Catena F, Cennamo V, Di Saverio S, Fuccio L, Jeekel H, Leppaniemi A, Moore E, Pinna AD, Pisano M, Repici A, Sugarbaker PH, Tuech JJ. Guidelines in the management of obstructing cancer of the left colon: consensus conference of the world society of emergency surgery (WSES) and peritoneum and surgery (PnS) society. World J Emerg Surg. 2010;5:29.
73. Chang GJ, Kaiser AM, Mills S, Rafferty JF, Buie WD, Standards Practice Task Force of the American Society of, C, and Rectal, S. Practice parameters for the management of colon cancer. Dis Colon Rectum. 2012;55(8):831–43.
74. Biondo S, Kreisler E, Millan M, Fraccalvieri D, Golda T, Frago R, Miguel B. Impact of surgical specialization on emergency colorectal surgery outcomes. Arch Surg. 2010;145(1):79–86.
75. Zorcolo L, Covotta L, Carlomagno N, Bartolo DC. Toward lowering morbidity, mortality, and stoma formation in emergency colorectal surgery: the role of specialization. Dis Colon Rectum. 2003;46(11):1461–7. discussion 1467–1468.

2 Epidemiology of Colorectal Cancer: Incidence, Survival, and Risk Factors

Florence Canouï-Poitrine, Claudia Martinez-Tapia, Lydia Guittet, and Anne-Marie Bouvier

2.1 Introduction

Colorectal cancer is still a major challenge in oncology. Population-based studies, which accurately record all cases diagnosed in a well-defined population and thus provide unbiased measurements, are the best way to assess changes in colorectal cancer frequency or survival. Worldwide incidence data are available from cancer registries, in particular through the successive volumes of Cancer Incidence in Five Continents covering registration up to 2012 [1–3]. For meaningful survival

F. Canouï-Poitrine (✉)
Public Health Department, University Henri-Mondor Hospital, Créteil, France

Paris Est Creteil University (UPEC), A-TVB DHU, CEpiA (Clinical Epidemiology And Ageing) Unit EA4393, Créteil, France
e-mail: florence.canoui-poitrine@aphp.fr

C. Martinez-Tapia
Paris Est Creteil University (UPEC), A-TVB DHU, CEpiA (Clinical Epidemiology And Ageing) Unit EA4393, Créteil, France
e-mail: claudia.tapia@aphp.fr

L. Guittet
U1086 INSERM-UCBN, ANTICIPE, Caen, France

University Hospital of Caen, Caen, France
e-mail: guittet-l@chu-caen.fr

A.-M. Bouvier
Digestive Cancer Registry of Burgundy, Dijon, France

EPICAD INSERM LNC-UMR 1231, Dijon, France

University Bourgogne Franche-Comté, Dijon, France

Dijon University Hospital, Dijon, France
e-mail: anne-marie.bouvier@u-bourgogne.fr

N. de'Angelis et al. (eds.), *Emergency Surgical Management of Colorectal Cancer*, Hot Topics in Acute Care Surgery and Trauma,
https://doi.org/10.1007/978-3-030-06225-5_2

comparisons between countries or time periods, net survival is used. Net survival from cancer is the survival that would be observed if cancer were the only cause of death. This major epidemiological indicator allows thus comparisons without interference from other causes of death. Reliable survival rates are regularly published through international (CONCORD) [4–6] and European (EUROCARE) [7, 8] programs and using the French population-based cancer registries network (FRANCIM) [9–11] data. The aim of the present study was to provide updated temporal trends in colorectal cancer incidence and prognosis over the past decades.

2.2 Incidence

Last available worldwide data showed that colorectal cancer was the third most common cancer in men (746,000 cases, 10.0% of the total) and the second in women (614,000 cases, 9.2% of the total) in 2012 [12]. Differences in the incidence of colorectal cancers over the world are striking, with a tenfold variation between highest and lowest area, and geographical patterns are very similar in men and women (Fig. 2.1). Historically, the highest incidence rates have been reported in more developed countries. North America; Australia; New Zealand; Western Europe, including France; and Japan were considered high-risk incidence countries. Colorectal cancer was scarce in South America, China, or Africa. Other countries, mainly Northern, Southern, and Eastern Europe, were considered as middle-risk area. Starting from the mid-1990s, incidence rates declined for both sexes (Fig. 2.2) in the high-risk countries whereas slightly increased in most middle-risk ones (Denmark, Italy, Spain, or the Netherlands) and remained relatively stable in

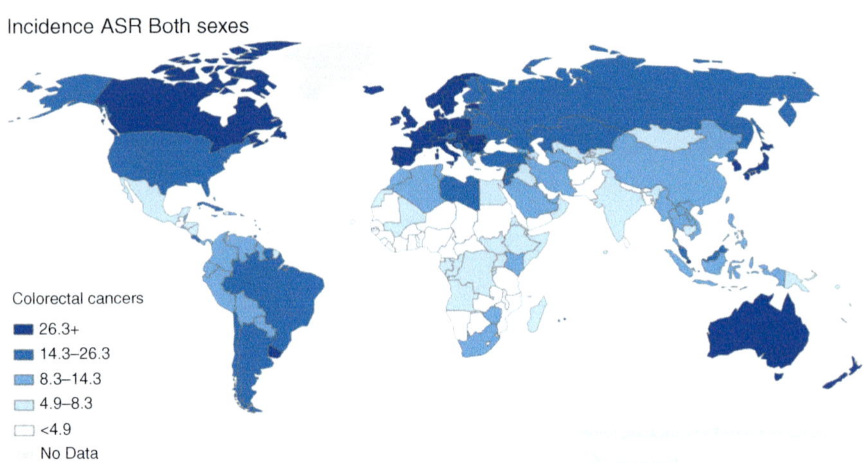

Fig. 2.1 Worldwide colorectal cancer incidence—*GLOBOCAN 2012, International Agency for Research on Cancer IARC*

Switzerland and the UK. In contrast, increasing trends have been seen in developing countries. In the last worldwide published monography covering the 2008–2012 time period, European countries exhibited similar incidence rates as the USA and North America, whereas Eastern Europe and Japan had the highest rates. In France, incidence slightly decreased from the early 2000s with a mean annual decreased of −0.3% in men and in women between 2005 and 2012. The cumulative risk decreased from 2.0% for men born around 1920 to 0.9% for those born around 1950, a more than twofold increase. The corresponding values in women were 0.1% and 0.2%.

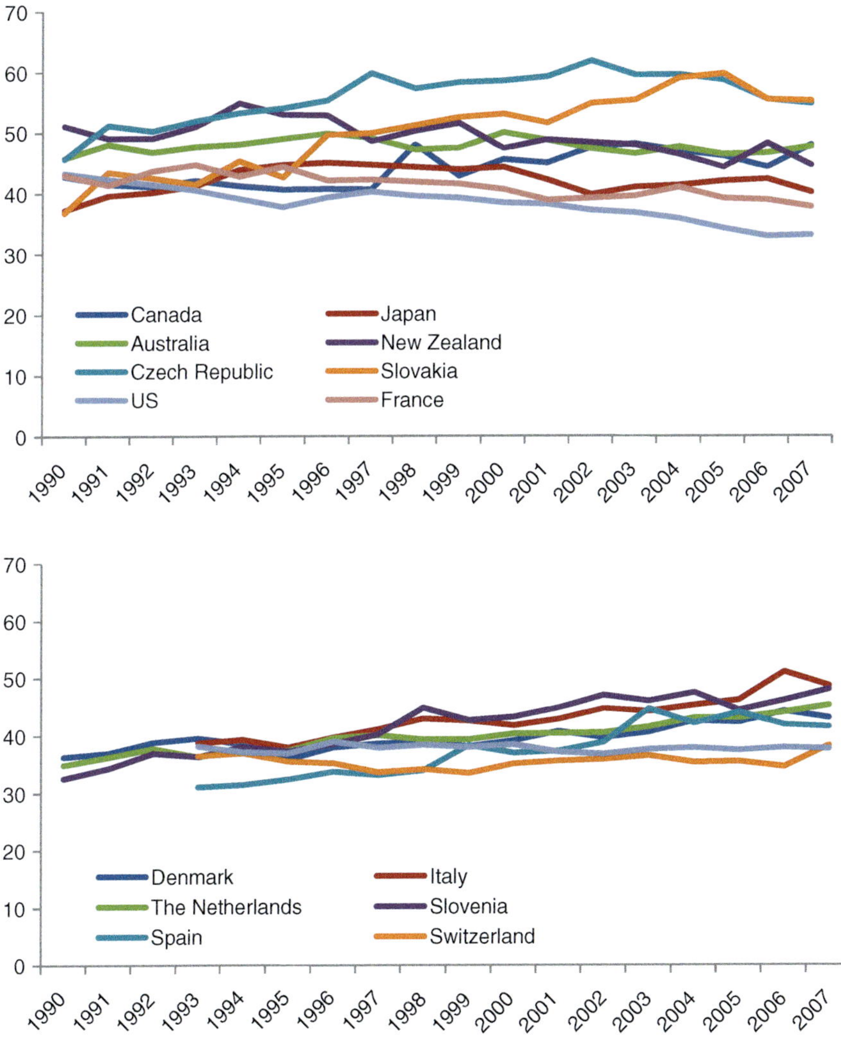

Fig. 2.2 Time trends in incidence of colorectal cancer *(International Agency for Research on Cancer (IARC). Cancer Incidence in Five Continents monographies)*

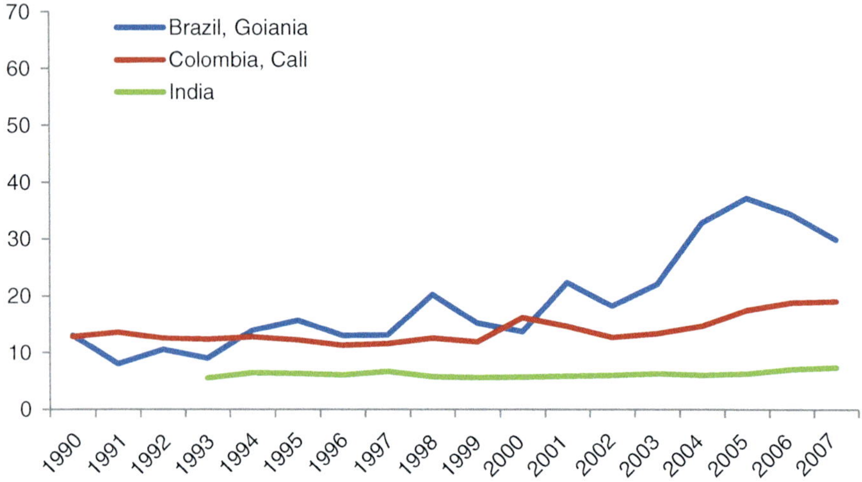

Fig. 2.2 (continued)

Estimated world standardized incidence rates in 2015 are 37.0 per 100,000 inhabitants in men 23.6 per 100,000 in women. Through the GLOBOCAN database, the effects of demographic changes on the expected number of new cancer cases in different regions can be estimated (Fig. 2.3). Overall, nearly 1,700,000 new cases are predicted worldwide in 2020.

In contrast to this overall decreasing trend, the incidence of colorectal cancer has appeared to be increasing in male and female young adults under age 50 years in the USA, Canada, Australia, and New Zealand [13–16]. This trend is not described in European data. Reasons for explaining this trend are unclear or speculative. The measure of the role of established risk factors such as smoking, sedentary lifestyle, and diet in this population required dedicated epidemiologic research.

2.3 Survival

Results from the 65 countries involved in the CONCORD program comparing data from population-based registries show wide variations in survival from colorectal cancer (Fig. 2.4). For patients diagnosed with colon or rectal cancer during 2010–2014, 5-year net survival was higher than 60% in Australia, Canada, the USA, Japan, and New Zealand. In Europe, survival was as high in Northern (Denmark, Finland, Iceland, Ireland, Norway, Sweden, the UK), Southern (Italy, Portugal, Slovenia, Spain), and Western countries (Belgium, France, Germany, the Netherlands, Switzerland). For colon cancer, survival ranged from 50% to 60% in Central and South America, in China, and in Eastern Europe such as Estonia, Lithuania, the Czech Republic, Poland, and Slovakia. Survival was less than 50% in Colombia and India. For rectal cancer, survival ranged from 50% to 60% in Central

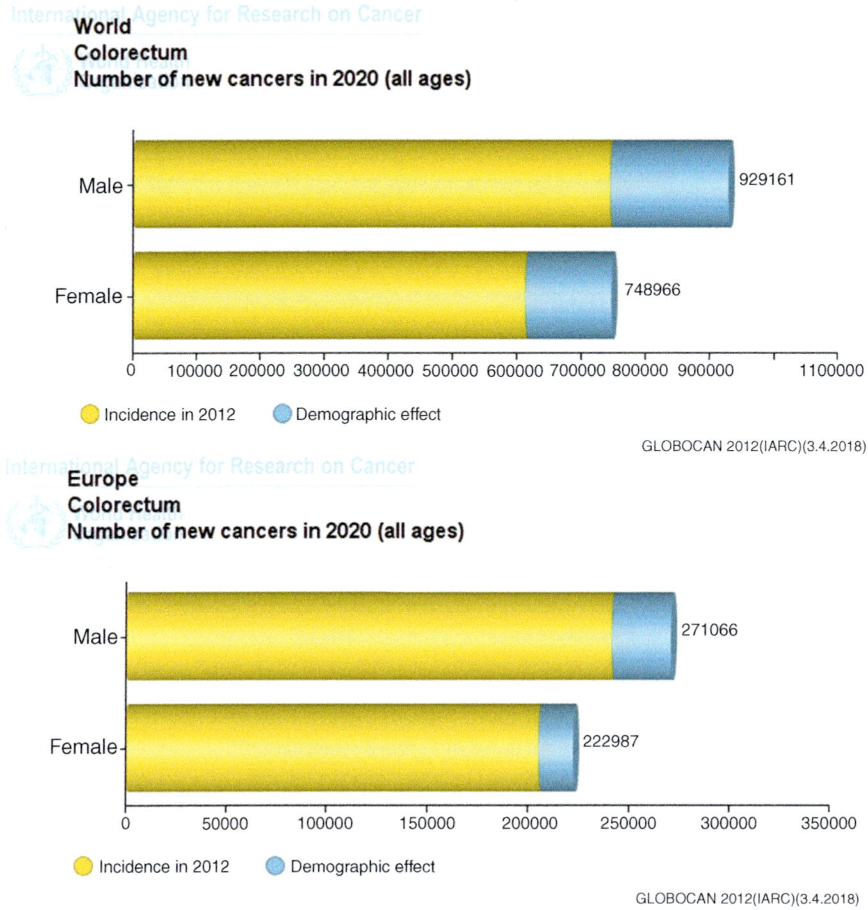

Fig. 2.3 Expected changes in incidence of colorectal cancer between 2012 and 2020, due to demographic changes in Europe and in the World. *GLOBOCAN 2012, International Agency for Research on Cancer IARC. Numbers are computed using age-specific rates and corresponding populations for ten age-groups*

and South America, in China, in Estonia, and in the Czech Republic and was less than 50% in Slovakia, Poland, Croatia, and India.

Through the CONCORD program, a high-resolution study was set up among colorectal cancer cases diagnosed during 1996–1998, in order to explain the difference in 5-year net survival observed between the USA and Europe [4]. Age-standardized survival was quite similar in the USA and Northern and Western Europe (around 54–58%) while lowest in Southern Europe (49%) and in Eastern Europe (42%). The transatlantic difference in survival was attributed to an earlier stage at diagnosis, a higher frequency of surgery, and use of adjuvant treatments in the USA.

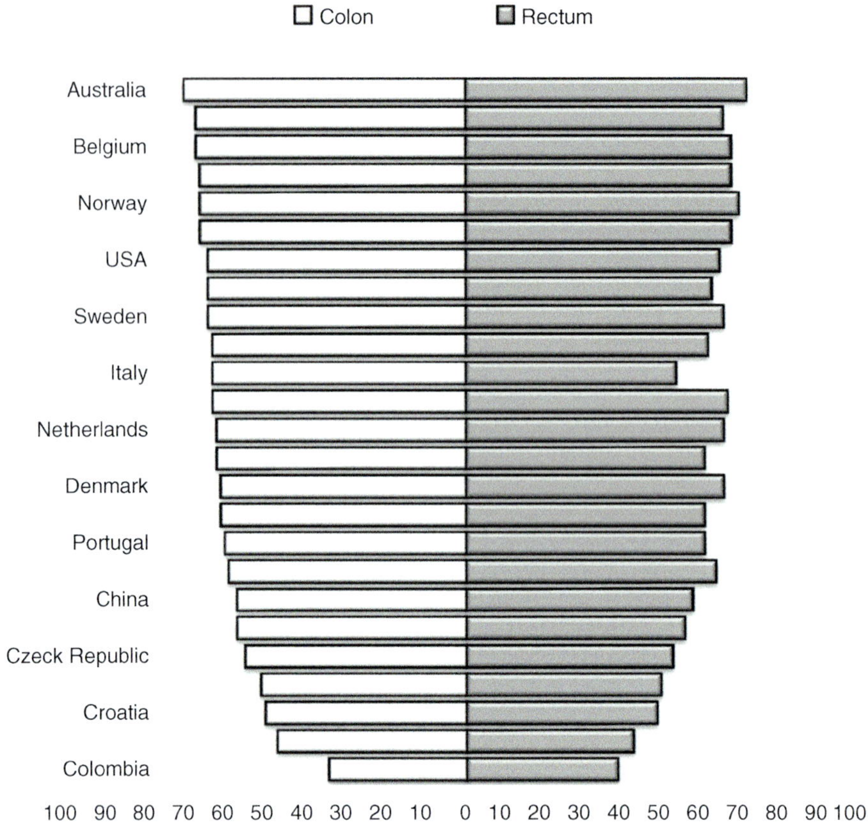

Fig. 2.4 Five-year net survival of colorectal cancer. *Cancer survival 2000–2014, CONCORD-3 program*

Taking into account bowel location, European mean age-standardized 5-year relative survival was 57% after colon cancer and 56% after rectal cancer [8]. There were negligible differences between the sexes for colon cancer, but survival was higher for women than for men for rectal cancer. In all European regions, survival was best for patients aged 15–44 years, roughly constant for those aged 45–64 years, and decreased thereafter for colon cancer, whereas there were smooth age differences up to 74 years with a substantial drop thereafter in rectal cancer.

According to time period, survival varied little between 1995 and 1999 and 2000–2014 [6]. For colon cancer, it mostly flatted, with an increase less than 10% in Canada, Australia, Japan, Estonia, Finland, Lithuania, Sweden, Italy, France, and the Netherlands. It was more than 10% in China, Denmark, Norway, the UK, Portugal, Slovenia, Spain, the Czech Republic, Poland, and Switzerland. For rectal cancer, time trend did not vary in Japan, France, Italy, and New Zealand, whereas it was more marked, with a 10–20% increase in Australia, Canada, Denmark, Estonia, the UK, Portugal, Spain, the Czech Republic, Poland, the Netherlands, and Switzerland. Increase in 5-year relative survival was about 20% or more in China and Slovenia.

2.4 Risk Factors for Colorectal Cancer

Three risk's levels are identified for colorectal cancer according to personal or familial past history:

- *Individuals with middle risk*: men and women aged 50 and more. More than 90% of colorectal cancer cases are diagnosed after this age [17]. The median age at diagnosis for colon cancer, 69 in men and 73 in women, is older than that of rectal cancer, which is 63 in men and 65 in women [18].
- *Individuals with high risk*:
    1. First-degree relatives of patients with common colorectal cancer or with a large adenoma (>1 cm) have an increased risk of colorectal cancer when occurred before 60 years, or two first-degree relatives of patients with common colorectal cancer or with a large adenoma (>1 cm) have an increased risk of colorectal cancer irrespective of age.
    2. Personal past history of colorectal cancer or large adenoma.
    3. Personal history of chronic gastrointestinal inflammatory bowel disease (ulcerative colitis and Crohn's disease).
- *Individuals with very high risk*: familial adenomatosis polyposis and hereditary nonpolyposis colorectal cancer (Lynch syndrome).

2.4.1 Environmental Risk Factors

Based on solid evidence from the published literature, these factors include excessive alcohol intake, smoking, and excess body weight. A sedentary behavior has been also associated with an increased risk of colorectal cancer [19, 20]. Conversely, high levels of physical activity are associated with a lower risk of colon cancer with a reported risk reduction of approximately 25% [21]. Such a relationship has not been established for rectal cancer [21]. Other modifiable risk factors that have been convincingly associated with higher colorectal cancer risk are the consumption of red and processed meat [22]. The findings for some risk factors suggest sex differences and/or sub-site variations. Additionally, some studies show a dose-response association. Table 2.1 summarizes the results of each environmental risk factor mentioned above from recent and large meta-analyses.

Table 2.1 Environmental and lifestyle risk factors for colorectal cancer

Risk factor	Meta-analyses	No. of studies	Study population	Measure	Relative risk (RR) or hazard ratio (HR) [95% CI]
Overweight/ obesity	Xue et al. [23]	CRC: 12 CC: 17 RC: 13	Systematic review of prospective cohort studies from databases inception to April 2015 (the USA, Asia, Europe, and Australia) CRC, 3,574,422 participants; follow-up, 5.5–49 years, 15,958 cases CC, 5,731,240 participants; follow-up, 5.5–23 years, 14,637 cases RC, 5,500,069 participants; follow-up, 5.5–23 years, 8000 cases	Body mass index (BMI): obesity (BMI ≥ 30) vs. normal (18 < BMI < 25)	RRs or CRC: – Among males: 1.38 [1.32–1.44] – Among females: 1.17 [1.06–1.30] RRs for CC: – Among males: 1.48 [1.40–1.57] – Among females: 1.12 [1.01–1.25] RRs for RC: – Among males: 1.25 [1.17–1.35] – Among females: 1.05 [0.99–1.12]
Tobacco (smoking)	Cheng J et al. [24]	24	Systematic review of prospective studies from databases MEDLINE (from 1966) and EMBASE (from 1974) through April 2013 14,186 colon cases; 6814 rectal cases (the USA, Europe, Canada, and Asia)	Smoking status Daily cigarette consumption Pack-years (p-y) Duration (years)	Summary RRs for current vs. never smokers: – CC: 1.09 [1.01–1.18] – RC: 1.24 [1.16–1.39] Summary RRs for former vs. never smokers: – CC: 1.16 [1.11–1.28] – RC: 1.20 [1.11–1.30] RR for an increase of 10 cigarettes/day – CC: 1.05 [1.02–1.09] – RC: 1.11 [1.02–1.21] RR for every additional 10 p-y: – CC: 1.08 [1.04–1.11] – RC: 1.10 [1.01–1.20] RR for an increase of 10 years: – CC: 1.02 [1.00–1.04] – RC: 1.06 [1.03–1.10]

Alcohol intake	Bagnardi V et al. [25]	66	Systematic review using MEDLINE, ISI Web of Science and EMBASE databases before September 2012 41,715 CRC cases (North America, Europe, Asia, other areas)	Grams (g) per day (1 drink = 12.5 g)	Pooled RRs compared with nondrinkers: – Light drinkers (12.5 g/d): 0.99 [0.95–1.04] – Moderate drinkers (12.6–50 g/d): 1.17 [1.11–1.24] – Heavy drinkers (>50 g/d): 1.44 [1.25–1.65]
Sedentary behavior	Ma P et al. [20]	28	Systematic review from PubMed and EMBASE databases through February 2017 4,784,339 participants with 46,071 CRC cases (North America, Europe, Asia, and Australia)	Prolonged television viewing time per day (12 studies) Prolonged total sitting time per day (6 studies)	Pooled RR compared with the lowest time: – CC: 1.23 [1.08–1.39] – RC: 1.15 [1.07–1.23] Summary RR for an increase of 2 h per day: 1.07 [1.05–1.10] Pooled RR compared with the lowest time: – CC: 1.03 [1.01–1.06] – RC: 1.42 [1.04–1.79] Summary RR for an increase of 2 h per day: 1.04 [1.01–1.06]
	Cong YJ et al. [19]	23	Systematic review from PubMed, EMBASE, and Google Scholar databases through May 2013 4,324,756 participants with 27,231 CC cases and 13,813 RC cases (North America, Europe, Australia, Asia)	Sedentary behavior (sedentary work, total sitting time, TV viewing time)	Pooled RRs for sedentary vs. non-sedentary behavior: – CC: 1.30 [1.22–1.39] – RC: 1.05 [0.98–1.13]

(continued)

Table 2.1 (continued)

Processed meat	Zhao Z et al. [26]	34	Systematic review using PubMed and EMBASE databases from inception through September 2016 1,892,692 participants and 35,165 CRC cases (America, Europe, Asia, and Australia)	Highest vs. lowest consumption (12 cohort studies) grams per day (g/d) (8 cohort studies)	Pooled RRs: – CRC: 1.15 [1.07–1.24] – CC: 1.21 [1.13–1.31] – RC: 1.17 [0.99–1.38] ->10 studies Pooled RRs for 50 g/d increase: – CRC: 1.22 [1.12–1.33] – CC: 1.23 [1.11–1.37] – RC: 1.22 [0.99–1.28] ->7 studies
Red Meat	Zhao Z et al. [26]	34	Systematic review using PubMed and EMBASE databases from inception through September 2016 1,892,692 participants and 35,165 CRC cases (America, Europe, Asia, and Australia)	Highest vs. lowest consumption (15 cohort studies) Grams per day (g/d) (9 cohort studies)	Pooled RRs: – CRC: 1.12 [1.03–1.21] – CC: 1.12 [1.04–1.20] ->11 studies – RC: 1.12 [0.89–1.40] -> 8 studies Pooled RRs for 100 g/d increase: – CRC: 1.16 [1.05–1.29] – CC: 1.10 [0.96–1.26] -> 8 studies – RC: 1.22 [1.01–1.47] -> 6 studies

CRC colorectal cancer, *CC* colon cancer, *RC* rectal cancer, *RR* relative risk, *HR* hazard ratio, *95% CI* 95% confidence interval, *BMI* body mass index, *p-y* pack-years, *g/d* grams per day

2.4.2 Personal or Familial History of Adenoma or Colorectal Cancer

Results from population-based studies and meta-analyses showed that the risk of developing colorectal cancer is about two times higher in persons with at least one affected first-degree relative than in those without family history. The risk of colorectal cancer is more than threefold higher among persons with a first-degree relative diagnosed under age 50 (pooled relative risk (RR) from meta-analysis = 3.55; 95% confidence interval = 1.84–6.83) and between two- and threefold higher if a first-degree relative is diagnosed under the age of 60 (RR range = 1.81–3.30). The risk of colorectal cancer associated with having a first-degree relative with an adenoma is less than 2 (RR range = 1.3–51.99). The risk of colorectal cancer is higher if the adenoma was 'large' (>10 mm; RR = 1.68; 1.29–2.18) or 'advanced' (with villous histology; RR = 3.90; 0.89–17.01) and if the first-degree relative is diagnosed with an adenoma under age 60 (RR range: 1.41–1.54) [27].

2.4.3 Inflammatory Bowel Diseases: Ulcerative Colitis and Crohn's Disease

Several meta-analyses of population-based studies quantified the over-risk of colorectal cancer associated with ulcerative colitis and Crohn's disease (RR from 1.7 to 21.6). The variation of over-risk is attributable to the age of onset of the disease, extent of the disease (pancolitis is associated with a 10–15-fold excess risk), intensity of inflammation, concomitant primary sclerosing management, and familial history of colorectal cancer. The incidence of colorectal cancer, in this population with inflammatory bowel diseases, is from 0.5 to 12.4/100,000 persons-years between 0 and 10 years of follow-up, from 1.4 to 11.5 between 10 and 20 years, and between 2.4 and 44.9 after 20 years [28].

2.4.4 Genetic Mutation

High-risk mutations in known colorectal cancer susceptibility genes are involved in 5–10% of colorectal cancer cases [29]. Two dominantly inheritant syndromes are described: the familial adenomatosis polyposis (APC adenomatous polyposis coli gene; <1% of colorectal cancer cases) and the hereditary nonpolyposis colorectal cancer (Lynch syndrome with several mutations in mismatch repair genes; roughly 5% of colorectal cancer cases). In both of these syndromes, the mean age of onset of colorectal cancer is much smaller (less than 50 years old) than in sporadic colorectal cancers, and extracolonic malignancies are also observed. The prevalence of Lynch syndrome varies according to studies. Recently, using data from the international Colon Cancer Family Registry, the prevalence of Lynch syndrome was estimated at 1 in 279 of the population [30]. The overall hazard ratio for colorectal cancer in carriers of Lynch syndrome decreased with each additional decade of life, from 135 (95%CI, 112–165) for men and 99 (95%CI, 79–125) for women when in their 30s to 4.0 (95%CI, 2.8–5.7), respectively, when in their 70s [31].

2.5 Emergency Presentation with Colorectal Cancer: Frequency and Risk Factors

Studies examining risk factors and circumstances surrounding emergency colorectal cancer diagnosis are limited. Incidence of obstructing and perforated colorectal cancers is variously estimated in the literature, from 8% to 40% due to varying definition, from sub-occlusion to the necessity of emergency surgery. Using a strict definition of obstruction through population-based studies, approximately, 10% will occur in an emergency context because of obstruction, and less than 5% because of perforation [32–34].

Two large database studies [34, 35] have found that patients with advanced age (adjusted odds ratios, $aOR_{\text{per 10 years increment}} = 1.19$; 95% confidence interval, 1.16–1.22 [34], and $aOR_{\text{80 years vs. 70 years}} = 1.49$; 1.47–1.52 [35]), women (aOR = 1.08; 1.01–1.14 and 1.12; 1.08–1.16, respectively), and patients with lower income ($aOR_{\text{lowest vs. highest}} = 1.28$; 1.18–1.39) [34] or higher socioeconomic deprivation ($aOR_{\text{most vs. least deprived}} = 1.54$; 1.45–1.64) [35] and comorbidities are significantly associated with emergency presentation. In the Canadian population-based study, which included 41,356 patients (7739 emergency presentations), Rabeneck et al. [34] reported that lack of a regular source of a family physician (aOR = 1.43; 1.30–1.54) and not having a previous bowel evaluation (aOR = 1.45; 1.33–1.59) were additionally associated with colorectal cancer emergencies and consistent with other studies [36–38]. In their large study of over 90,000 patients, Wallace and colleagues found that ethnicity had an impact on the risk of an emergency admission for colorectal cancer, with higher risk for nonwhite patients (aOR = 1.13; 1.02–1.24) [35]. *The most recent systematic review by Mitchell et al.* [39] identified 19 studies that considered factors associated with diagnosis of colorectal cancer in the context of an emergency presentation and found older age to be a strong significant factor in the majority of the studies analyzed, with aOR varying from 1.19 to 5.85. Results for the other risk factors were less conclusive. Evidence regarding symptoms before emergency cancer diagnosis is still limited. Abdominal pain, constipation, weight loss, and diarrhea are the preceding symptoms more generally associated with an increased risk of emergency presentation [39–42].

2.6 Conclusion

Colorectal cancer is the third most common cancer in men and the second in women worldwide (2012). Starting from the mid-1990s, incidence rates decline for both sexes in the high-risk countries (mostly developed countries) whereas increase in most middle-risk ones (mostly developing countries). Five-year net colorectal cancer survival varies from 35% to 75%. Survival varies little between 1995 and 1999 and

2000–2014. The main risk factors for colorectal cancer are environmental factors (obesity, tobacco use, alcohol intake, sedentary behavior, and consumption of red and processed meat), inflammatory bowel disease (ulcerative colitis and Crohn's disease), family or personal history of colorectal cancer or large adenoma, and inherited genetic factors (familial adenomatosis polyposis and hereditary nonpolyposis colorectal cancer). Colorectal cancer diagnosis occurs in an emergency context in about 10% because of obstruction and less than 5% because of perforation particularly in older patients, women, and patients with socioeconomic deprivation and comorbidities.

References

1. Foman D, Bray F, Brewster D, Gombe Mbalawa C, Kholer B, Pinreros M, et al. Cancer incidence in five continents, vol. X. Lyon: International Agency for Research on Cancer; 2013.
2. Curado MP, Edwards B, Shin HR, Storm H, Ferlay J, Heanue M, et al. Cancer incidence in five continents, vol. IX. Lyon: IARC; 2007.
3. Bray F, Colombet M, Mery L, Piñero M, Znaor A, Zanetti R, et al. Cancer incidence in five continents, vol. XI. Lyon: International Agency for Research on Cancer; 2017.
4. Allemani C, Rachet B, Weir HK, Richardson LC, Lepage C, Faivre J, et al. Colorectal cancer survival in the USA and Europe: a CONCORD high-resolution study. BMJ Open. 2013;3(9):e003055. https://doi.org/10.1136/bmjopen-2013-003055.
5. Allemani C, Weir HK, Carreira H, Harewood R, Spika D, Wang XS, et al. Global surveillance of cancer survival 1995-2009: analysis of individual data for 25,676,887 patients from 279 population-based registries in 67 countries (CONCORD-2). Lancet. 2015;385(9972):977–1010. https://doi.org/10.1016/S0140-6736(14)62038-9.
6. Allemani C, Matsuda T, Di Carlo V, Harewood R, Matz M, Niksic M, et al. Global surveillance of trends in cancer survival 2000-14 (CONCORD-3): analysis of individual records for 37 513 025 patients diagnosed with one of 18 cancers from 322 population-based registries in 71 countries. Lancet. 2018;391(10125):1023–75. https://doi.org/10.1016/S0140-6736(17)33326-3.
7. Holleczek B, Rossi S, Domenic A, Innos K, Minicozzi P, Francisci S, et al. On-going improvement and persistent differences in the survival for patients with colon and rectum cancer across Europe 1999-2007 - results from the EUROCARE-5 study. Eur J Cancer. 2015;51(15):2158–68. https://doi.org/10.1016/j.ejca.2015.07.024.
8. De Angelis R, Sant M, Coleman MP, Francisci S, Baili P, Pierannunzio D, et al. Cancer survival in Europe 1999-2007 by country and age: results of EUROCARE--5-a population-based study. Lancet Oncol. 2014;15(1):23–34. https://doi.org/10.1016/S1470-2045(13)70546-1.
9. Cowppli-Bony A, Uhry Z, Remontet L, Voirin N, Guizard AV, Tretarre B, et al. Survival of solid cancer patients in France, 1989-2013: a population-based study. Eur J Cancer Prev. 2017;26(6):461–8. https://doi.org/10.1097/CEJ.0000000000000372.
10. Cowppli-Bony A, Uhry Z, Remontet L, Guizard AV, Voirin N, Monnereau A, et al. Survie des personnes atteintes de cancer en France métropolitaine 1989-2013. Partie 1 Tumeurs solides. Saint Maurice: Institut de veille sanitaire; 2016.
11. Binder-Foucard F, Bossard N, Delafosse P, Belot A, Woronoff AS, Remontet L, et al. Cancer incidence and mortality in France over the 1980-2012 period: solid tumors. Revue d'epidemiologie et de sante publique. 2014;62(2):95–108. https://doi.org/10.1016/j.respe.2013.11.073.
12. Ferlay J, Soerjomataram I, Ervik M, Dikshit R, Eser S, Mathers C, et al. GLOBOCAN 2012 v1.0. Cancer incidence and mortality worldwide: IARC CancerBase. Lyon: International Agency for Research on Cancer; 2013. (extracted in 2017).
13. Troeung L, Sodhi-Berry N, Martini A, Malacova E, Ee H, O'Leary P, et al. Increasing incidence of colorectal cancer in adolescents and young adults aged 15-39 years in Western

Australia 1982-2007: examination of colonoscopy history. Front Public Health. 2017;5:179. https://doi.org/10.3389/fpubh.2017.00179.
14. Siegel RL, Jemal A, Ward EM. Increase in incidence of colorectal cancer among young men and women in the United States. Cancer Epidemiol Biomarkers Prev. 2009;18(6):1695–8. https://doi.org/10.1158/1055-9965.EPI-09-0186.
15. Brenner DR, Ruan Y, Shaw E, De P, Heitman SJ, Hilsden RJ. Increasing colorectal cancer incidence trends among younger adults in Canada. Prev Med. 2017;105:345–9. https://doi.org/10.1016/j.ypmed.2017.10.007.
16. O'Connell JB, Maggard MA, Liu JH, Etzioni DA, Livingston EH, Ko CY. Rates of colon and rectal cancers are increasing in young adults. Am Surg. 2003;69(10):866–72.
17. Colorectal Cancer Prevention (PDQ(R)): Health Professional Version. PDQ cancer information summaries. Bethesda, MD: National Cancer Institute; 2018.
18. Howlader N, Noone A, Krapcho M, Garshell J, Neyman N, Altekruse S, et al. SEER Cancer statistics review, 1975-2010. [Based on the November 2012 SEER data submission, posted to the SEER web site, April 2013.]. Bethesda, MD: National Cancer Institute; 2013. p. 9.
19. Cong YJ, Gan Y, Sun HL, Deng J, Cao SY, Xu X, et al. Association of sedentary behaviour with colon and rectal cancer: a meta-analysis of observational studies. Br J Cancer. 2014;110(3):817–26. https://doi.org/10.1038/bjc.2013.709.
20. Ma P, Yao Y, Sun W, Dai S, Zhou C. Daily sedentary time and its association with risk for colorectal cancer in adults: a dose-response meta-analysis of prospective cohort studies. Medicine (Baltimore). 2017;96(22):e7049. https://doi.org/10.1097/MD.0000000000007049.
21. Robsahm TE, Aagnes B, Hjartaker A, Langseth H, Bray FI, Larsen IK. Body mass index, physical activity, and colorectal cancer by anatomical subsites: a systematic review and meta-analysis of cohort studies. Eur J Cancer Prev. 2013;22(6):492–505. https://doi.org/10.1097/CEJ.0b013e328360f434.
22. Lippi G, Mattiuzzi C, Cervellin G. Meat consumption and cancer risk: a critical review of published meta-analyses. Crit Rev Oncol Hematol. 2016;97:1–14. https://doi.org/10.1016/j.critrevonc.2015.11.008.
23. Xue K, Li FF, Chen YW, Zhou YH, He J. Body mass index and the risk of cancer in women compared with men: a meta-analysis of prospective cohort studies. Eur J Cancer Prev. 2017;26(1):94–105. https://doi.org/10.1097/CEJ.0000000000000231.
24. Cheng J, Chen Y, Wang X, Wang J, Yan Z, Gong G, et al. Meta-analysis of prospective cohort studies of cigarette smoking and the incidence of colon and rectal cancers. Eur J Cancer Prev. 2015;24(1):6–15. https://doi.org/10.1097/CEJ.0000000000000011.
25. Bagnardi V, Rota M, Botteri E, Tramacere I, Islami F, Fedirko V, et al. Alcohol consumption and site-specific cancer risk: a comprehensive dose-response meta-analysis. Br J Cancer. 2015;112(3):580–93. https://doi.org/10.1038/bjc.2014.579.
26. Zhao Z, Feng Q, Yin Z, Shuang J, Bai B, Yu P, et al. Red and processed meat consumption and colorectal cancer risk: a systematic review and meta-analysis. Oncotarget. 2017;8(47):83306–14. https://doi.org/10.18632/oncotarget.20667.
27. Lowery JT, Ahnen DJ, Schroy PC III, Hampel H, Baxter N, Boland CR, et al. Understanding the contribution of family history to colorectal cancer risk and its clinical implications: a state-of-the-science review. Cancer Am Cancer Soc. 2016;122(17):2633–45. https://doi.org/10.1002/cncr.30080.
28. Adami HO, Bretthauer M, Emilsson L, Hernan MA, Kalager M, Ludvigsson JF, et al. The continuing uncertainty about cancer risk in inflammatory bowel disease. Gut. 2016;65(6):889–93. https://doi.org/10.1136/gutjnl-2015-311003.
29. Lorans M, Dow E, Macrae FA, Winship IM, Buchanan DD. Update on hereditary colorectal cancer: improving the clinical utility of multigene panel testing. Clin Colorectal Cancer. 2018;17:e293. https://doi.org/10.1016/j.clcc.2018.01.001.
30. Win AK, Jenkins MA, Dowty JG, Antoniou AC, Lee A, Giles GG, et al. Prevalence and penetrance of major genes and polygenes for colorectal cancer. Cancer Epidemiol Biomarkers Prev. 2017;26(3):404–12. https://doi.org/10.1158/1055-9965.EPI-16-0693.

31. Jenkins MA, Dowty JG, Ait Ouakrim D, Mathews JD, Hopper JL, Drouet Y, et al. Short-term risk of colorectal cancer in individuals with lynch syndrome: a meta-analysis. J Clin Oncol. 2015;33(4):326–31. https://doi.org/10.1200/JCO.2014.55.8536.
32. Cheynel N, Cortet M, Lepage C, Benoit L, Faivre J, Bouvier AM. Trends in frequency and management of obstructing colorectal cancers in a well-defined population. Dis Colon Rectum. 2007;50(10):1568–75. https://doi.org/10.1007/s10350-007-9007-4.
33. Cheynel N, Cortet M, Lepage C, Ortega-Debalon P, Faivre J, Bouvier AM. Incidence, patterns of failure, and prognosis of perforated colorectal cancers in a well-defined population. Dis Colon Rectum. 2009;52(3):406–11. https://doi.org/10.1007/DCR.0b013e318197e351.
34. Rabeneck L, Paszat LF, Li C. Risk factors for obstruction, perforation, or emergency admission at presentation in patients with colorectal cancer: a population-based study. Am J Gastroenterol. 2006;101(5):1098–103. https://doi.org/10.1111/j.1572-0241.2006.00488.x.
35. Wallace D, Walker K, Kuryba A, Finan P, Scott N, van der Meulen J. Identifying patients at risk of emergency admission for colorectal cancer. Br J Cancer. 2014;111(3):577–80. https://doi.org/10.1038/bjc.2014.300.
36. Murchie P, Smith SM, Yule MS, Adam R, Turner ME, Lee AJ, et al. Does emergency presentation of cancer represent poor performance in primary care? Insights from a novel analysis of linked primary and secondary care data. Br J Cancer. 2017;116(9):1148–58. https://doi.org/10.1038/bjc.2017.71.
37. Sikka V, Ornato JP. Cancer diagnosis and outcomes in Michigan EDs vs other settings. Am J Emerg Med. 2012;30(2):283–92. https://doi.org/10.1016/j.ajem.2010.11.029.
38. Comber H, Sharp L, de Camargo Cancela M, Haase T, Johnson H, Pratschke J. Causes and outcomes of emergency presentation of rectal cancer. Int J Cancer. 2016;139(5):1031–9. https://doi.org/10.1002/ijc.30149.
39. Mitchell ED, Pickwell-Smith B, Macleod U. Risk factors for emergency presentation with lung and colorectal cancers: a systematic review. BMJ Open. 2015;5(4):e006965. https://doi.org/10.1136/bmjopen-2014-006965.
40. Sheringham JR, Georghiou T, Chitnis XA, Bardsley M. Comparing primary and secondary health-care use between diagnostic routes before a colorectal cancer diagnosis: cohort study using linked data. Br J Cancer. 2014;111(8):1490–9. https://doi.org/10.1038/bjc.2014.424.
41. Cleary J, Peters TJ, Sharp D, Hamilton W. Clinical features of colorectal cancer before emergency presentation: a population-based case-control study. Fam Pract. 2007;24(1):3–6. https://doi.org/10.1093/fampra/cml059.
42. Renzi C, Lyratzopoulos G, Card T, Chu TPC, Macleod U, Rachet B. Do colorectal cancer patients diagnosed as an emergency differ from non-emergency patients in their consultation patterns and symptoms? A longitudinal data-linkage study in England. Br J Cancer. 2016;115(7):866–75. https://doi.org/10.1038/bjc.2016.250.

3 Socioeconomic Impact of Emergency Therapies for Colorectal Cancer

Aleix Martínez-Pérez, Carmen Payá-Llorente, and Arturo García-Lozano

3.1 Global Socioeconomic Considerations

Colorectal cancers (CRC) are the third most common malignant tumors worldwide, and they are associated to an increased economic expenditure for healthcare systems due to its high diagnostic, therapeutic, and follow-up costs [1]. Disbursements per patient with CRC over a 5-year period of up to €39,607 (ranging from €33,300 to €49,900) have been estimated using year 2008 values [2], and a rough estimate of the economic burden for colorectal cancer worldwide was to be around USD 14–22 billion [3]. Despite that an elective surgical resection is the gold standard for CRCs curative treatment, up to 30% of CRC patients are presenting as a surgical emergency [4–6]. Emergency surgery for CRC increases postoperative morbidity, mortality, hospital stay, and costs [4, 5, 7]. Curative resection rate is significantly lower, with higher rates of ostomy formation within patients undergoing emergency surgery. Both 5-year overall and cancer-specific survival have been shown impaired for emergency CRC patients compared with those receiving elective procedures [6].

There is substantial heterogeneity in the methodologies and quality of the published economic evaluations of CRC at an elective setting, and only few are specifically focusing the emergency scenario; therefore, the true economic costs of emergent CRC are yet to be fully defined. The main costs of CRC are related to treatment (90%), compared with diagnostic and follow-up costs. Within all the

A. Martínez-Pérez (✉)
Colorectal Surgery Unit, Department of General and Digestive Surgery, Hospital Universitario Doctor Peset, Valencia, Spain

C. Payá-Llorente
Department of General and Digestive Surgery, Hospital Universitario Doctor Peset, Valencia, Spain

A. García-Lozano
Hospital Universitario Doctor Peset, Valencia, Spain

N. de'Angelis et al. (eds.), *Emergency Surgical Management of Colorectal Cancer*, Hot Topics in Acute Care Surgery and Trauma,
https://doi.org/10.1007/978-3-030-06225-5_3

stages, stage I would be the least costly and stage III the most expensive [8]. Those latest patients would present 25% more management-associated costs than those presenting as stage IV. For stage I patients, costs are relatively lower for the treatment (78%) and higher for the follow-up (14.8%) phases [2]. For stages II and III, total costs are mainly influenced by the cost of chemotherapy and biologics, the duration of the treatment with biological agents, and cancer recurrence rates. For stage IV patients, the use of biological agents and chemotherapy presented major impact on costs [2]. Regardless of the stage at diagnosis, primary tumors located at the rectum are most costly than those located at the colon, in all diagnosis, treatment, and follow-up phases of patient's management.

There is a high incidence of emergent presentations (30%) of CRC, which are associated with adverse postoperative and long-term outcomes. Patients receiving surgery after elective admissions had significantly lower adjusted odds of mortality compared with emergent patients, and mean hospital length of stay for elective patients is significantly lower than emergent ones [4, 5]. Thus, increased hospital resources would be required after an important percentage of the total CRC surgeries. Also, the costly treatments needed after the potentially higher recurrences observed for emergency cases could be critical for total expenditures [9]. Finally, increased costs are related to locally advanced and metastatic diseases that, compared to the other stages, are relatively more frequent presented as emergencies than in elective setting [2, 6, 10]. As a result, emergency surgeries for CRC may represent an underestimated cost burden to healthcare systems and society worldwide. Novel strategies for separately evaluate, reduce, and improve the quality of this emergent surgical procedures for CRC should be explored as a global health target.

3.2 Surgical and Long-Term Costs for Healthcare Systems

3.2.1 Types of Costs

Direct costs: Generated by healthcare utilization, they include:

- Hospital and intensive care unit admission periods
- Diagnostic procedures (at presentation and follow-up)
  - Laboratory and radiological investigations
  - Endoscopic exploration and stenting
  - Biopsy and histopathologic evaluation
- Therapeutic procedures
  - Surgical procedure(s) (operating room charges, instrumental)
  - Medication (analgesics, antibiotics, anesthetic drugs, blood transfusion)
  - Chemotherapy, radiotherapy, and biological therapy
  - Other (invasive lines, syringe pumps, physiotherapy, etc.)

- Visits to primary and paramedical healthcare providers after discharge
  - Outpatient visits
  - Wound and stoma care
  - Best supporting care
- Non-medical costs: Generated by expenses for travel to and from healthcare providers

At emergency presentation of CRC, surgery is usually performed immediately following the diagnosis, and as a result, the cost of this and the first required hospitalization would constitute more than 80% of the total direct costs.

Indirect costs: Generated by the impaired ability to work

- Loss of productivity
- Disability allowances
- Out-of-pocket costs to caregivers

Social impairment should also be taken into consideration in those patients and relatives. Quantifying and evaluating the social costs would be mandatory for assessing the real cost-effectiveness of the strategies applied for emergency CRC treatment.

3.2.2 Surgical Costs

Haider et al. identified 162,442 patients undergoing colonic resection for neoplasms, 48,599 at emergency setting, using Nationwide Inpatient Sample (NIS) data between 2001 and 2010 in the USA. The surgical procedure performed as an emergency had a mean cost of USD 22,616.33 per patient, USD 7813.53 more expensive than elective colonic resection in the same population (53% increase) [4]. Shah et al. used a database of CRC patients underwent surgical procedures separating those presenting with a diagnosis requiring emergency surgery (including bowel perforation, peritonitis, or obstruction). Patients receiving emergency surgical procedures spent 51.9% more admission days, produced hospital charges 68.3% higher, and had a nearly four times greater chance of in-hospital death than those who did not [5].

The influence on the total costs produced by the use of laparoscopy has been scarcely evaluated for CRC emergency resections. Koh et al. performed a study over patients who had undergone either emergency laparoscopic or open colectomies for various surgical conditions (i.e., lower gastrointestinal tract bleeding, colonic obstruction, and perforation). Matching was performed for age, gender, surgical diagnosis, and type of surgery. There were no significant differences between the groups for perioperative complications and length of stay. The cost analysis neither demonstrated any significant differences in the total, procedural, and the non-procedural costs between the two groups [11].

3.2.3 Long-Term Costs

Long-term costs for CRC are increasing, mainly associated with the high cost impact of biological agents. For locally advanced tumors, the total costs critically depend on the cost of chemotherapy and biological agents and recurrence rates [2]. Treatment costs for metastatic CRC are substantial, and a new trend for its increasing caused by the rising cost share of biologics has been observed [12]. Disbursements per CRC patient over a 5-year period of up to €39,607 (ranging from €33,300 to €49,900) were estimated using year 2008 values [2]. Moreover, the costs of continuing and advanced care phases would represent between 16.9% and 58.3% of the total long-term costs, depending on CRC stage [8]. In middle-adulthood CRC patients, working patients can expend nearby 3 months out of their employ. A study showed that factors associated with work resumption were, among others, stoma placement, postoperative complications, length of hospital stage, and receiving adjuvant treatments [13]. CRC represented in Spain, during 2011, the loss of 202,784 working days [14].

3.2.4 Reducing the Burden of Emergency Therapies for CRC

Self-expandable metallic stent (SEMS) placement as a bridge to elective surgery for left-sided malignant colonic obstruction appeared as an alternative to the traditional emergency surgical approach. A recent meta-analysis including 8 RCT found a significant lower risk of presenting postoperative complications, and undergoing temporary or permanent stomas, in patients treated with SEMS [15]. Other studies have evaluated the economic impact derived by the use of stenting on emergency setting compared to respective surgery. They showed, together with lesser postoperative morbidity, mortality, and stoma placement rates, decreased costs for patients receiving SEMS preceding elective surgery for the treatment of acute malignant left-sided obstruction [16, 17].

Screening for CRC can avoid an emergency presentation as allows to identify abnormal growths before the cancer development. Consequently, emergency CRC resection is frequently related to a failure of the screening. There is high disparity between countries and continents regarding the recommended screening timing for CRC. Also, several methods are currently available for CRC diagnosis at an asymptomatic phase including stool-based (occult blood, DNA panel), endoscopic, and radiological tests. Although the optimal strategy remains a matter, preventing emergency surgery through the development, promotion, and excellence of CRC screening allows the chance to save and improve lives, and also to save costs [4].

The Guidelines of the American College of Physicians (ACP) recommend [18]:

- To perform individualized assessment of risk for CRC in all adults.
- To screen for CRC in average-risk adults starting at the age of 50 years and in high-risk adults starting at the age of 40 years or 10 years younger than the age at which the youngest affected relative was diagnosed with colorectal cancer.

- To use a stool-based test, flexible sigmoidoscopy, or optical colonoscopy in patients who are at average risk and optical colonoscopy in those who are at high risk. Selection of the test should be based on patient preferences and the benefits and harms and availability of the test.
- To stop screening for colorectal cancer in adults over the age of 75 years or in adults with a life expectancy of less than 10 years.

Other potential solutions for reducing the increased costs associated to emergency presentation of CRC have been proposed, as the creation of dedicated emergency general surgery services. Increased rates of inpatient colonoscopies and definitive surgical procedures on the same admission have been observed after its introduction [19]. Moreover, the development of enhanced recovery pathways and bundles of evidence-based care, such as the proposed for emergency laparotomy, have been shown to improve the postoperative outcomes. The emergency laparotomy pathway quality improvement care (ELPQuiC) consists on the initial assessment with early warning scores, an early antibiotic therapy, less than 6-h time interval between decision and operation, goal-directed fluid resuscitation, and optimal postoperative intensive care [20].

3.3 Quality of Life After Emergency Therapies for CRC

3.3.1 Assessing the Quality of Life After CRC Emergency Surgery

The quality of life of individual patients undergoing both elective and emergency surgical interventions for CRC is crucial when evaluating the full socioeconomic impact of the disease. The World Health Organization define health-related quality of life (HRQOL) as the level of well-being and satisfaction associated with an individual's life and how this level is affected by disease, accidents, and treatments. The predictors of a HRQOL after colorectal surgery involve the impaired physical and social functions, ability to work productively, and the existence of specific symptoms [21]. When managing emergency CRC patients, who usually present with advanced stages, strategies aiming to improve HRQOL are essential. HRQOL evaluation allows to study the impact of disease on survivors and also to elucidate the optimal treatment when two interventions are similar in terms of survival [22].

There have been described multiple instruments for the assessment of HRQOL that could be useful for patients after CRC resection [Table 3.1]. The most frequently used are psychometric questionnaires that could be generic or disease-specific:

- Generic instruments
  - Nottingham Health Profile [23]
  - MOS Short Form 36 (SF-36) [24]
- Cancer-specific instruments
  - Functional Assessment of Cancer Therapy-General (FACT-G) [25]
  - European Organization for the Research and Treatment of Cancer QLQ-C30 (EORTC QLQ-C30) [26]

Table 3.1 Instruments to measure HRQOL in colorectal cancer surgery

Generic	Cancer-specific	CRC-specific	Stoma patients	Functional status
NHP	FACT-G	FACT-C	mCOH-QOL	FIQL
SF-36	EORTC QLQ-C30	EORTC QLQ-CR38	Stoma-QOL	Wexner FIS
SF-6	QoL-CS	EORTC QLQ-CR29	Stoma care QOL index	LARS score
EQ-5D		FCSI		MSKCC BFI
SIP				
6MWT				
QoR-40 and -15				

Nottingham Health Profile (NHP), Short Form 36 (SF-36), 6-Item Short Form Health Survey (SF-6), EuroQol-5 dimension (EQ-5D), Sickness Impact Profile (SIP), 40-item Quality of Recovery Score (QoR-40), 15-item Quality of Recovery Score (QoR-15), 6-minute walk test (6MWT), Functional Assessment of Cancer Therapy-General (FACT-G), European Organization for the Research and Treatment of Cancer QLQ-C30 (EORTC QLQ-C30), Quality of Life–Cancer Survivors (QoL-CS), Functional Assessment of Cancer Therapy–Colorectal Cancer (FACT-C) NCCN/FACT CRC Symptom Index (FCSI), Modificate City of Hope Quality of Life Ostomy Questionnaire (mCOH-QOL), Fecal Incontinence Quality of Life (FIQL), Fecal Incontinence Score (FIS), Memorial Sloan Kettering Cancer Center (MSKCC) Bowel Function Instrument (BFI)

- Colorectal cancer-specific questionnaires
  - Functional Assessment of Cancer Therapy-CRC (FACT-C) [27]
  - QLQ-CR38 [28]
  - QLQ-CR29 [29]

Generic tools allow to compare HRQOL between different diseases, but they are less specific for cancer patients. For CRC patients, an overall, generic instrument comprised of multiple dimensions, supplemented by a disease-specific subscale, has been proposed as the best approach to evaluate HRQOL [22].

3.3.2 Recovery After Colorectal Emergency Surgery

Postoperative recovery not only consists on the restitution of the previous physiological parameters, as social recovery should be also taken into account. Patient's recovery after surgery has then to be considered from a multidimensional perspective. It is divided between early and late periods and comprises psychological and functional recovery, adverse symptomatology, and personal satisfaction [30].

Enhanced recovery after surgery (ERAS) protocols have been developed for colorectal surgery patients aiming to reduce physiological stress and postoperative organ dysfunction through optimization of perioperative care and recovery. They require a multidisciplinary approach in all perioperative phases and appear to reduce times for bowel function recovery and to return to normal activities. ERAS protocols have been applied with safety and effectiveness at emergency colorectal surgery setting, but its use is far to be widespread [31]. Due to the potential benefit for selected patients undergoing emergency operations, development and implementation of specific ERAS protocols after colorectal emergency surgery should be considered.

Late functional complications after CRC emergency surgery have increased together with the improvements on surgical technique and perioperative care that increased the primary anastomosis rates avoiding stoma placements. Those functional problems are more frequent during the first year after surgery. They include fecal incontinence, diarrhea, and constipation, together with frequency, urgency, and difficult evacuations. Those potentially postoperative adverse events should be considered before surgery and thus taken into account at decision-making process during the surgical intervention. Functional problems also depend on the previous patient's status, the surgical procedure performed, and perioperative morbidity. Extensive resections (i.e., subtotal colectomy) may increase bowel dysfunction rates; restricted postoperative social activity is more frequent in ileo-rectal or ileo-sigmoid anastomosis compared with segmental colectomies [32]. Diarrhea has been shown to be more common after right than left hemicolectomy, if less than 16 cm of the sigmoid colon remains, or if more than 10 cm of the terminal ileum is resected [33].

Incontinence are measured usually with the Fecal Incontinence Quality of Life (FIQL) and the Wexner Fecal Incontinence Score (FIS) [34]. The conservative treatment of fecal incontinence would consist on fiber and constipation agents. Surgery is reserved after its failure. The best invasive technique depends on the stage of the disease and patient's anatomy. Sphincteroplasty, sacral nerve stimulation, artificial bowel sphincters, and fecal diversion are the main options. Diarrhea (often associated to incontinence) is usually treated with opioid agonist (e.g., loperamide).

Low anterior rectal resections are lesser performed at emergency setting, but up to 80% of the patients develop bowel dysfunction postoperatively. Despite that the majority of functional impairments improve during the 6–12 first months, symptoms could persist up to 15 years after the surgical resection [35]. The symptoms are included under the term "low anterior resection syndrome" (LARS): fecal urgency, bowel fragmentation, frequent bowel movements, emptying difficulties, incontinence, and increased gas. To assess the severity of LARS, LARS score and the Memorial Sloan Kettering Cancer Center (MSKCC) Bowel Function Instrument (BFI) can be used [36, 37]. The factors associated with the development and severity of LARS are concomitant colonic dysmotility, neorectal pouch dysfunction, and damage to anal sphincter or pelvic nerves [35]. Together with dietary changes and pharmacologic therapies, pelvic floor rehabilitation and sacral nerve stimulation procedures are nowadays in use for the treatment of LARS.

Anastomotic stricture could cause bowel dysfunction in up to 22% of the patients undergoing colorectal resections [38]. Conservative treatments are the first step, including dietary changes and medical therapies. The invasive procedures for the management of postoperative anastomotic strictures include endoscopic balloon dilation, insertion of self-expandable metal stents, endoscopic incisional therapies, and surgery.

3.3.3 Impact of Stoma Formation

Stomas are commonly performed in emergency CRC surgery. Ileostomies or colostomies are widely used for either colonic diversion or decompression. They could be temporary or permanent, also end or loop. Diverting loop ileostomy is used after an emergency low anterior resection with colorectal anastomosis, and in patients with obstructing distal cancer. If feasible, it seems preferable over performing a loop colostomy in such cases, as loop colostomy has more risk of prolapse and sepsis. Ghost ileostomy is a primary anastomosis accompanying pre-staged ileostomy that could be externalized and opened at emergency surgery after a primary anastomotic leak. End colostomies are the most frequent stoma performed in emergency CRC surgery. Its formation could be difficult in obese patients, and they have increased risk for stoma necrosis. Complication rates following stoma formation range between 21% and 70% [39]. They are divided into early (within the first 30 days after surgery) and late complications. Emergency surgery, together with higher body mass index have been observed as a predisposing factors for stoma complications [40].

3.3.3.1 Early Complications

- *Improper stoma site selection* is the most commonly preventable complication of stoma surgery (36). Even in emergency situations, the stoma location should be marked before the interventions, being the surgeon the main responsible (Fig. 3.1a).
- *Dehydration* occur in up to 20% of ileostomy patients, and the risk is higher within the earliest postoperative days [39]. Excessive stoma losses can also lead to other late complications as electrolyte abnormalities, vitamin deficiencies, and malnutrition [41].
- *Stoma retraction* (1–17%) is more common in obese patients and emergency operations [40, 41]. If the stoma retraction develops into complete mucocutaneous separation, it could also lead to peritonitis (Fig. 3.1b).
- *Stoma necrosis* (13%) is also more frequent in obese patients, emergency surgery, and colostomies [42]. Necrosis is secondary to an excessive tension at the mesentery, excessive devascularization, or narrowly spaced sutures. Venous outflow impairment will turn the stoma purple-colored, but the wall is usually viable finally. In contrast, if the arterial inflow is compromised, full-thickness necrosis is presented, and when extension to the fascial layer is noted, surgical revision is mandatory (Fig. 3.1c, d).
- *Peristomal skin irritation* (3–42%) is a common complication more frequent with ileostomies than colostomies. Protruding ileostomies decrease their apparition and severity (Fig. 3.1e).
- *Parastomal infections and abscesses* are uncommon and mostly seen after stoma revision surgery (Fig. 3.1f).

3.3.3.2 Late Complications

- *Parastomal herniation* incidence range between 0% and 48%, being higher for end stomas and for colostomies [40, 41]. The risk factors include obesity, poor nutritional status, site of the wall incision, and emergency surgery. Parastomal

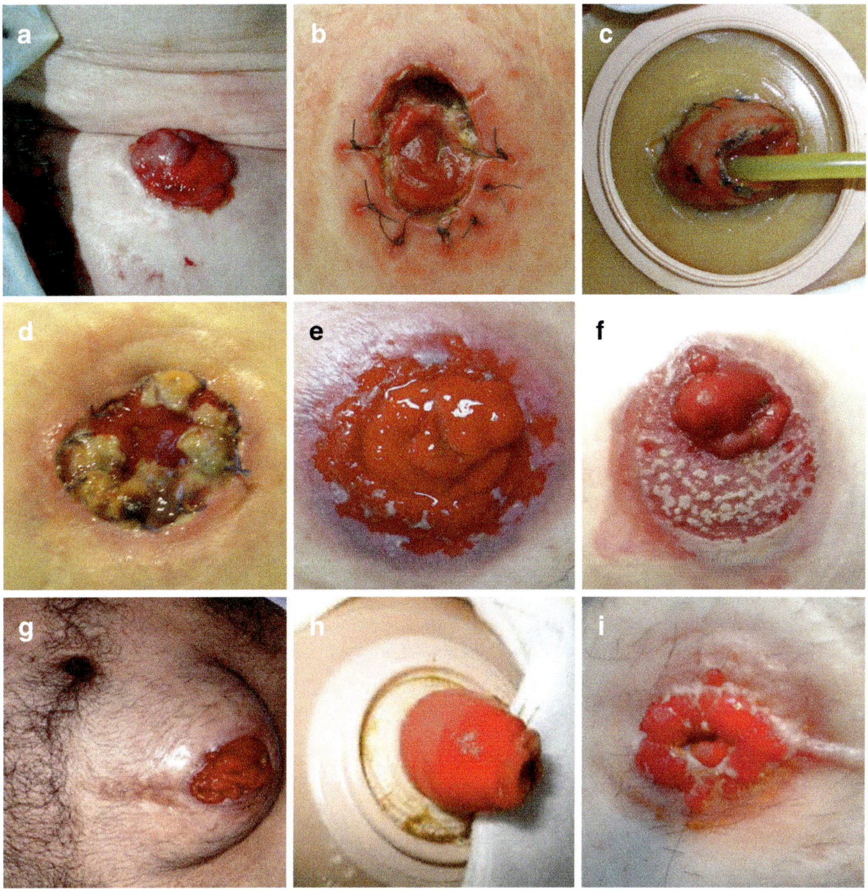

Fig. 3.1 Ostomy complications: (**a**) Improper stoma site selection. (**b**) Colostomy retraction. (**c**) Edema in ileostomy wall with Foley inside the lumen. (**d**) Colostomy wall partial necrosis. (**e**) Ileostomy and skin irritation. (**f**) Skin mycosis surrounding an ileostomy. (**g**) Parastomal hernia. (**h**) Ileostomy prolapse. (**i**) Stoma stenosis

hernias could lead to patient's discomfort, bowel obstruction, and poor appliance fitting. Thus, patients' HRQOL could be critically affected. Symptomatic hernia is an indication of surgical treatment (Fig. 3.1g).

- *Stoma prolapse* (3% of ileostomies, 2% of colostomies) can lead also to pain, poor appliance fitting, obstruction, and incarceration. The highest incidence has been reported for the loop transverse colostomy [42] (Fig. 3.1h).
- *Stoma stenosis* (2–15%) earliest symptom could be a noisy stoma when flatus passing [39] (Fig. 3.1i).

3.3.3.3 Quality of Life in Ostomy Patients

Patients undergoing a stoma placement refer lower overall quality of life, body image, and poorer social activity when compared with CRC patients who had no stoma. Changes in lifestyle, dietary restrictions, and social isolation are frequent within them. Eighteen percent to 26% of the patients with colostomies experience negative psychological symptoms within the first 3 months of surgery; and these symptoms are commonly anxiety and depression [43]. Moreover, also ostomy caregivers present a relatively higher depression and anxiety than other caregivers [44].

There have been described different instruments for measuring the HRQOL at ostomy patients. The City of Hope Quality of Life Ostomy Questionnaire (COH-QOL) is the most used. This questionnaire was described in 1983 and was further revised and validated for stoma patients [45]. Improved preoperative assessment and counseling with longer follow-up by the stoma specialist would be helpful in the management of these patients. However, the most effective method of preventing a stoma complication remains to be avoiding their formation.

References

1. Ferlay J, Soerjomataram I, Dikshit R, Eser S, Mathers C, Rebelo M, et al. Cancer incidence and mortality worldwide: sources, methods and major patterns in GLOBOCAN 2012. Int J Cancer. 2015;136(5):E359–86. https://doi.org/10.1002/ijc.29210.
2. Tilson L, Sharp L, Usher C, Walsh C, Whyte S, O'Ceilleachair A, et al. Cost of care for colorectal cancer in Ireland: a health care payer perspective. Eur J Health Econ. 2012;13(4):511–24. https://doi.org/10.1007/s10198-011-0325-z.
3. Redaelli A, Cranor CW, Okano GJ, Reese PR. Screening, prevention and socioeconomic costs associated with the treatment of colorectal cancer. Pharmacoeconomics. 2003;21(17):1213–38.
4. Haider AH, Obirieze A, Velopulos CG, Richard P, Latif A, Scott VK, et al. Incremental cost of emergency versus elective surgery. Ann Surg. 2015;262(2):260–6. https://doi.org/10.1097/SLA.0000000000001080.
5. Shah NA, Halverson J, Madhavan S. Burden of emergency and non-emergency colorectal cancer surgeries in West Virginia and the USA. J Gastrointest Cancer. 2013;44(1):46–53. https://doi.org/10.1007/s12029-012-9455-5.
6. McArdle CS, Hole DJ. Emergency presentation of colorectal cancer is associated with poor 5-year survival. Br J Surg. 2004;91(5):605–9. https://doi.org/10.1002/bjs.4456.
7. Kelly M, Sharp L, Dwane F, Kelleher T, Comber H. Factors predicting hospital length-of-stay and readmission after colorectal resection: a population-based study of elective and emergency admissions. BMC Health Serv Res. 2012;12:77. https://doi.org/10.1186/1472-6963-12-77.
8. Corral J, Castells X, Molins E, Chiarello P, Borras JM, Cots F. Long-term costs of colorectal cancer treatment in Spain. BMC Health Serv Res. 2016;16:56. https://doi.org/10.1186/s12913-016-1297-6.
9. Chen TM, Huang YT, Wang GC. Outcome of colon cancer initially presenting as colon perforation and obstruction. World J Surg Oncol. 2017;15(1):164. https://doi.org/10.1186/s12957-017-1228-y.
10. Ghazi S, Berg E, Lindblom A, Lindforss U, Low-Risk Colorectal Cancer Study G. Clinicopathological analysis of colorectal cancer: a comparison between emergency and elective surgical cases. World J Surg Oncol. 2013;11:133. https://doi.org/10.1186/1477-7819-11-133.
11. Koh FH, Tan KK, Tsang CB, Koh DC. Laparoscopic versus an open colectomy in an emergency setting: a case-controlled study. Ann Coloproctol. 2013;29(1):12–6. https://doi.org/10.3393/ac.2013.29.1.12.
12. Song X, Zhao Z, Barber B, Gregory C, Cao Z, Gao S. Cost of illness in patients with metastatic colorectal cancer. J Med Econ. 2011;14(1):1–9. https://doi.org/10.3111/13696998.2010.536870.
13. Gordon LG, Beesley VL, Lynch BM, Mihala G, McGrath C, Graves N, et al. The return to work experiences of middle-aged Australian workers diagnosed with colorectal cancer: a matched cohort study. BMC Public Health. 2014;14:963. https://doi.org/10.1186/1471-2458-14-963.

14. Vicente-Herrero MT, Terradillos-Garcia MJ, Ramirez-Iniguez-de la Torre MV, Capdevila-Garcia LM, Lopez-Gonzalez AA. [Colorectal cancer in Spain: temporary disability and preventive occupational strategies]. Rev Gastroenterol Mex 2013;78(2):75–81. doi:https://doi.org/10.1016/j.rgmx.2013.01.005.
15. Arezzo A, Passera R, Lo Secco G, Verra M, Bonino MA, Targarona E, et al. Stent as bridge to surgery for left-sided malignant colonic obstruction reduces adverse events and stoma rate compared with emergency surgery: results of a systematic review and meta-analysis of randomized controlled trials. Gastrointest Endosc. 2017;86(3):416–26. https://doi.org/10.1016/j.gie.2017.03.1542.
16. Flor-Lorente B, Baguena G, Frasson M, Garcia-Granero A, Cervantes A, Sanchiz V, et al. Self-expanding metallic stent as a bridge to surgery in the treatment of left colon cancer obstruction: cost-benefit analysis and oncologic results. Cir Esp. 2017;95(3):143–51. https://doi.org/10.1016/j.ciresp.2016.12.014.
17. Singh H, Latosinsky S, Spiegel BM, Targownik LE. The cost-effectiveness of colonic stenting as a bridge to curative surgery in patients with acute left-sided malignant colonic obstruction: a Canadian perspective. Can J Gastroenterol. 2006;20(12):779–85.
18. Qaseem A, Denberg TD, Hopkins RH Jr, Humphrey LL, Levine J, Sweet DE, et al. Screening for colorectal cancer: a guidance statement from the American College of Physicians. Ann Intern Med. 2012;156(5):378–86. https://doi.org/10.7326/0003-4819-156-5-201203060-00010.
19. Anantha RV, Brackstone M, Parry N, Leslie K. An acute care surgery service expedites the treatment of emergency colorectal cancer: a retrospective case-control study. World J Emerg Surg. 2014;9(1):19. https://doi.org/10.1186/1749-7922-9-19.
20. Huddart S, Peden CJ, Swart M, McCormick B, Dickinson M, Mohammed MA, et al. Use of a pathway quality improvement care bundle to reduce mortality after emergency laparotomy. Br J Surg. 2015;102(1):57–66. https://doi.org/10.1002/bjs.9658.
21. Cohen RD. The quality of life in patients with Crohn's disease. Aliment Pharmacol Ther. 2002;16(9):1603–9.
22. Dunn J, Lynch B, Aitken J, Leggett B, Pakenham K, Newman B. Quality of life and colorectal cancer: a review. Aust N Z J Public Health. 2003;27(1):41–53.
23. Hunt SM, McKenna SP, McEwen J, Williams J, Papp E. The Nottingham Health Profile: subjective health status and medical consultations. Soc Sci Med A. 1981;15(3 Pt 1):221–9.
24. Ware JE Jr, Sherbourne CD. The MOS 36-item short-form health survey (SF-36). I. Conceptual framework and item selection. Med Care. 1992;30(6):473–83.
25. Cella DF, Tulsky DS, Gray G, Sarafian B, Linn E, Bonomi A, et al. The Functional Assessment of Cancer Therapy scale: development and validation of the general measure. J Clin Oncol. 1993;11(3):570–9. https://doi.org/10.1200/JCO.1993.11.3.570.
26. Sprangers MA, Cull A, Bjordal K, Groenvold M, Aaronson NK. The European Organization for Research and Treatment of Cancer. Approach to quality of life assessment: guidelines for developing questionnaire modules. EORTC Study Group on Quality of Life. Qual Life Res. 1993;2(4):287–95.
27. Ward WL, Hahn EA, Mo F, Hernandez L, Tulsky DS, Cella D. Reliability and validity of the Functional Assessment of Cancer Therapy-Colorectal (FACT-C) quality of life instrument. Qual Life Res. 1999;8(3):181–95.
28. Sprangers MA, te Velde A, Aaronson NK. The construction and testing of the EORTC colorectal cancer-specific quality of life questionnaire module (QLQ-CR38). European Organization for Research and Treatment of Cancer Study Group on Quality of Life. Eur J Cancer. 1999;35(2):238–47.
29. Whistance RN, Conroy T, Chie W, Costantini A, Sezer O, Koller M, et al. Clinical and psychometric validation of the EORTC QLQ-CR29 questionnaire module to assess health-related quality of life in patients with colorectal cancer. Eur J Cancer. 2009;45(17):3017–26. https://doi.org/10.1016/j.ejca.2009.08.014.
30. Bowyer A, Jakobsson J, Ljungqvist O, Royse C. A review of the scope and measurement of postoperative quality of recovery. Anaesthesia. 2014;69(11):1266–78. https://doi.org/10.1111/anae.12730.

31. Lohsiriwat V. Enhanced recovery after surgery vs conventional care in emergency colorectal surgery. World J Gastroenterol. 2014;20(38):13950–5. https://doi.org/10.3748/wjg.v20.i38.13950.
32. You YN, Chua HK, Nelson H, Hassan I, Barnes SA, Harrington J. Segmental vs. extended colectomy: measurable differences in morbidity, function, and quality of life. Dis Colon Rectum. 2008;51(7):1036–43. https://doi.org/10.1007/s10350-008-9325-1.
33. Yde J, Larsen HM, Laurberg S, Krogh K, Moeller HB. Chronic diarrhoea following surgery for colon cancer-frequency, causes and treatment options. Int J Colorectal Dis. 2018;33:683. https://doi.org/10.1007/s00384-018-2993-y.
34. Jorge JM, Wexner SD. Etiology and management of fecal incontinence. Dis Colon Rectum. 1993;36(1):77–97.
35. Martellucci J. Low anterior resection syndrome: a treatment algorithm. Dis Colon Rectum. 2016;59(1):79–82. https://doi.org/10.1097/DCR.0000000000000495.
36. Emmertsen KJ, Laurberg S. Low anterior resection syndrome score: development and validation of a symptom-based scoring system for bowel dysfunction after low anterior resection for rectal cancer. Ann Surg. 2012;255(5):922–8. https://doi.org/10.1097/SLA.0b013e31824f1c21.
37. Temple LK, Bacik J, Savatta SG, Gottesman L, Paty PB, Weiser MR, et al. The development of a validated instrument to evaluate bowel function after sphincter-preserving surgery for rectal cancer. Dis Colon Rectum. 2005;48(7):1353–65. https://doi.org/10.1007/s10350-004-0942-z.
38. Ridtitid W, Siripun A, Rerknimitr R. Stricture at colorectal anastomosis: to dilate or to incise. Endosc Int Open. 2018;6(3):E340–E1. https://doi.org/10.1055/s-0043-122495.
39. Shabbir J, Britton DC. Stoma complications: a literature overview. Colorectal Dis. 2010;12(10):958–64. https://doi.org/10.1111/j.1463-1318.2009.02006.x.
40. Kann BR. Early stomal complications. Clin Colon Rectal Surg. 2008;21(1):23–30. https://doi.org/10.1055/s-2008-1055318.
41. Bafford AC, Irani JL. Management and complications of stomas. Surg Clin North Am. 2013;93(1):145–66. https://doi.org/10.1016/j.suc.2012.09.015.
42. Krishnamurty DM, Blatnik J, Mutch M. Stoma complications. Clin Colon Rectal Surg. 2017;30(3):193–200. https://doi.org/10.1055/s-0037-1598160.
43. Wade BE. Colostomy patients: psychological adjustment at 10 weeks and 1 year after surgery in districts which employed stoma-care nurses and districts which did not. J Adv Nurs. 1990;15(11):1297–304.
44. Cotrim H, Pereira G. Impact of colorectal cancer on patient and family: implications for care. Eur J Oncol Nurs. 2008;12(3):217–26. https://doi.org/10.1016/j.ejon.2007.11.005.
45. Grant M, Ferrell B, Dean G, Uman G, Chu D, Krouse R. Revision and psychometric testing of the City of Hope Quality of Life-Ostomy Questionnaire. Qual Life Res. 2004;13(8):1445–57. https://doi.org/10.1023/B:QURE.0000040784.65830.9f.

4 Acute Care and Surgical Risk Assessment

Arezo Kanani, Hartwig Kørner, and Kjetil Soreide

4.1 Introduction

Colorectal cancer presents as an emergency in about 15–20% of the patients with colon cancer and about 5% of those with rectal cancer [1–4] with regional variations and some reporting emergency presentations as high as 33% [5]. An oncologic emergency is defined as an "acute, potentially life-threatening condition in a cancer patient that has developed as a result of malignant disease or its treatment" [6].

It is important to meet the acutely ill patient with colorectal cancer with optimal knowledge due to associated high perioperative mortality of up to 20% and morbidity of 40–50% [1–3]. Colorectal cancer usually presents in an emergent setting through one of either three ways, *obstruction*, *perforation*, or *hemorrhage*, with prevalence from high to low in mentioned order [2]. Acute obstruction occurs in 8–29% [2, 5, 6] and stands for 77–85% of emergency colorectal cancer operations [2, 5]. Emergency presentation may also occur during either neoadjuvant or palliative treatment, with some drugs such as bevacizumab (an anti-angiogenesis inhibitor) reported to predispose to perforations. For the sake of clarity, this chapter will discuss the patient with colorectal cancer that presents as an emergency.

Conflict of interest: None declared.

A. Kanani
Department of Gastrointestinal Surgery, Stavanger University Hospital, Stavanger, Norway

H. Kørner
Department of Gastrointestinal Surgery, Stavanger University Hospital, Stavanger, Norway

Clinical Medicine, University of Bergen, Bergen, Norway

K. Soreide (✉)
Department of Gastrointestinal Surgery, Stavanger University Hospital, Stavanger, Norway

Clinical Medicine, University of Bergen, Bergen, Norway

Clinical Surgery, University of Edinburgh and Royal Infirmary of Edinburgh, Edinburgh, UK

N. de'Angelis et al. (eds.), *Emergency Surgical Management of Colorectal Cancer*, Hot Topics in Acute Care Surgery and Trauma,
https://doi.org/10.1007/978-3-030-06225-5_4

Once it has been established the patient's symptoms is caused by an acute colorectal condition, acute care should be initiated. The clinician has to decide together with the patient what will be the next steps of treatment adjusted to risk and perceived benefit. In this chapter, we will highlight important aspects of the acute care and surgical risk assessment to better manage this patient group presenting as an emergency.

4.2 Acute Care and Emergency Assessment

Colorectal cancer presenting as an emergency imposes multiple challenges. As 60% of these patients are ≥70 years [7], they usually have comorbidities, which both aggravate their serious condition and may challenge the effect of treatment. The patients may often present with a locally advanced or disseminated disease associated with deranged physiology and will hence tolerate surgery less well [3, 4, 6, 8–10]. Typically, patients often present late at evening or night, when more junior surgeons are on call and less experienced staff available.

A structured approach (Fig. 4.1) to this complicated patient group is advised for better management. In some cases, despite the fact that patients experience symptoms early, they have a delay in contact with the healthcare system. These patients are usually older with dementia, come from low socioeconomic background, or

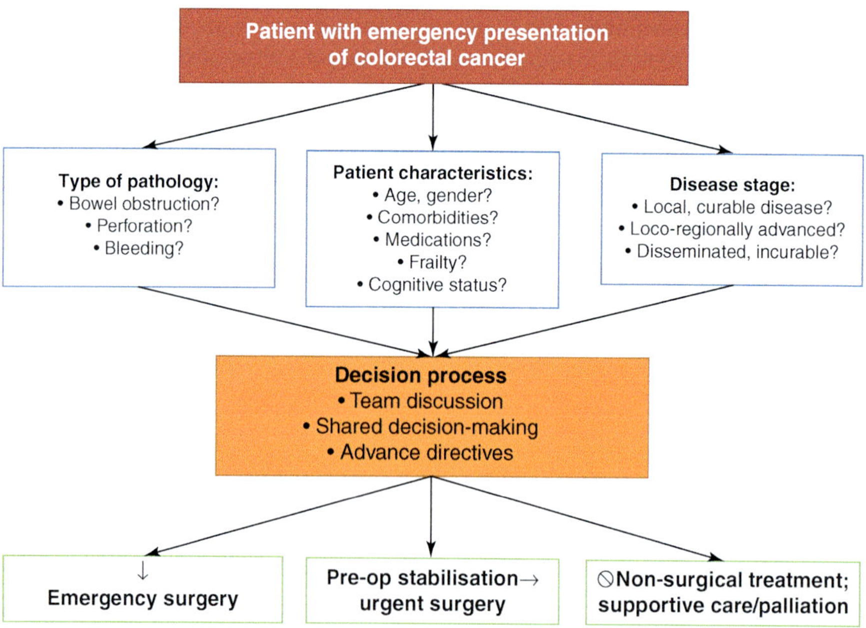

Fig. 4.1 Structured approach to the patient with acute presentation of colorectal cancer

have non-Caucasian background [1]. A few patients also have an extreme hospital anxiety and thus postpone contact with health care.

Acute care assessment includes to diagnose the **pathology causing the acute condition**, i.e., obstruction, perforation or hemorrhage, the *patient's characteristics* in terms of acute changes of physiology (sepsis, electrolyte and fluid derangements, anemia) and preexisting comorbidities, use of medications and cognitive function, and *stage of cancer disease*, i.e., locoregional or systemic disease. Moreover, as patients may present at various stations of their disease trajectory, and with differing perspectives for their remaining life time, the doctor in charge should try to identify the patient's preferences with regard to goals and intensity of further treatment. Thus, aims for cure or palliation should be set out early: limitations to use of resources and organ support and, if any, limitations to resuscitation or advanced organ support if required during the course of management (Fig. 4.2).

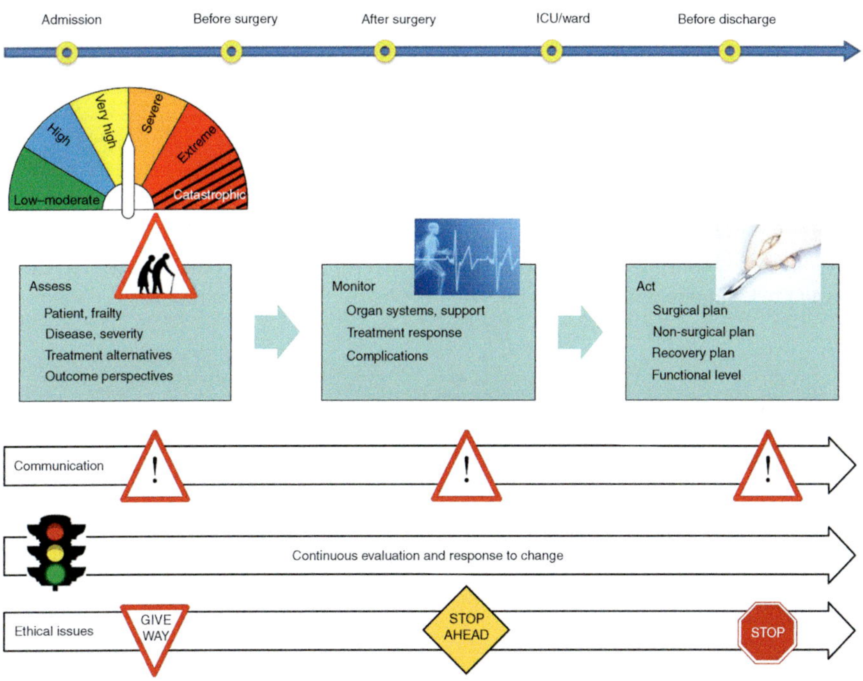

Fig. 4.2 Creating a road map in the pathway of care during emergency surgery. Caring for all, but particular the geriatric patient with a surgical emergency is complex and needs to be tailored to the individual based on associated comorbidity and frailty, disease severity, treatment alternatives, and the wishes of the patient. Continued assessment of interventions and effect, timely and repeated communication, and cautious reflection on aspects of care should be incorporated into decision-making. ICU, intensive care unit. Reproduced with permission from John Wiley [15] Desserud KF, Veen T, Søreide K. Emergency general surgery in the geriatric patient. Br J Surg 2016;103(2):e52–61

4.2.1 Clinical Assessment

One of the first challenges is to determine the condition's degree of emergency. The first priority is to assess if the patient needs immediate surgery or if time allows for optimizing the patient for surgery within the next 24–72 h. The findings of generalized peritonitis combined with signs of systemic inflammatory response (sepsis) indicate the need for urgent surgery, while patients with signs of bowel obstruction usually profit from appropriate fluid and electrolyte replacement and diagnostic imaging. Most patients with hemorrhage from a colorectal cancer can be stabilized with blood transfusions and correction of coagulation disorders and prepared for endoscopic diagnosis and treatment.

In order to achieve a rapid and comprehensive assessment of the emergency presentation of a colorectal cancer, a proper clinical evaluation based on symptoms and physical examination has to be supplemented with biochemical blood analyses, blood typing, and radiological imaging. A full contrast-enhanced computerized tomography imaging of the abdomen and chest should be obtained whenever possible, as this will provide fast and highly reliable information on the pathological condition of the acute illness, as well as the stage of cancer disease. This information is essential to determine a treatment plan.

4.2.2 Type of Acute Presentation

Obstruction is the most frequent acute presentation [2, 5, 6, 11]. In contrast to small bowel obstruction, large bowel obstruction develops over longer time and therefore rarely presents like a fulminant small bowel obstruction with caliber leap. Therefore, the need of immediate surgery is far less frequent, and focus should be on stabilizing the patient and plan the next step of treatment [11]. Surgical treatment depends on the localization of the cancer and the stage of disease and is described in other chapters in this book.

Perforation is the less common but a far more serious acute presentation of colorectal cancer [11]. The cecum is the most frequent site of perforation due to a distal bowel obstruction: increased intraluminal pressure and tension lead to compromised microcirculation of the cecum (according to La Place's law) and thus result in necrosis of the bowel wall [2, 5, 6]. Tenderness and pain in the right lower quadrant, palpation of a dilated cecum, and a diameter of 10 cm or above on imaging should increase the suspicion of imminent bowel perforation. In some cases, a CT scan will reveal intramural gas in the cecal wall as a sign of ischemia and necrosis. In this case, urgent surgery should be considered. However, when the ileocecal valve is insufficient, the small intestines will absorb the increased pressure and fluid contents of the colon, and dilated small bowel segments are seen on imaging studies. In some cases, the perforation can be contained with limited contamination or abscess formation. These patients can initially be treated with antibiotics and drainage before final surgical treatment [2, 5, 11].

Acute hemorrhage is the least common acute presentation. In contrast to chronic occult blood loss due to colorectal cancer, patients with macroscopic hemorrhage from the colon usually present with dark red bloody discharge and seldom with melena as seen in upper gastrointestinal bleeding. Most patients with acute bright-red bloody discharge are diagnosed with rectal cancer. However, bleeding from colorectal cancer rarely induces hemorrhagic shock as seen in bleeding from the upper gastrointestinal tract.

4.2.3 Staging

Consideration of the stage of the cancer is essential for planning. Colorectal cancer emergencies may be due to either localized disease (e.g., a small local, effectively obstructing tumor localized in the large bowel), locally advanced disease that affects other organs, or in the setting of disseminated, and often incurable disease if metastases at multiple sites. Accurate knowledge of stage is an important backstage of treatment decisions, as stage of disease is the most important prognostic factor for long-term outcome for the patient. If liver-alone metastases are present, the potential for a curative goal of surgery should always be entertained. Information of stage is vital to assess where the patient is in the trajectory of cancer disease course, i.e., curable or a non-curable state, or advanced disease with short life expectance or with likely controllable (but not curable) disease with longer life expectancy. Together with other important factors such as the patient's own perspectives and wishes for remaining lifetime, the planned course of action needs to be discussed with patients' preferences incorporated, whenever possible. In this context, empathetic and clear communication with the patient as well as the patient's surrogates will be crucial for a satisfactory course of diagnosis, treatment, and outcome of acutely ill patients with colorectal cancer.

4.2.4 Patient-Related Factors

Aging is caused by accumulation of damaged genetic material by extrinsic (radiation, diet) and intrinsic (free radicals) factors [12]. Such changes over time determine the physiological reserves of the patient in terms of frailty, sarcopenia, anemia, poor nutritional status, and reduced immune system [12]. The degree of biological aging varies between patients and determines physiological reserve, response to insult, and ability to recover from stress. Age as a pure numeric parameter is therefore not an absolute factor as such for surgical or other treatment, but should be seen in the context of biological age [5, 7, 8]. The patient may present with various degrees of the cancer cachexia syndrome, i.e., the loss of protein mass due to metabolic changes induced by often advanced cancer disease [13, 14]. Thus, age and body weight may serve as proxy surrogate markers for patient risk and other comorbidities.

4.2.5 Comorbidity

Comorbidities are strong predictors of mortality [15]. In patients over 70 years with multiple comorbidities, mortality can be higher than 50% and over 90% in patients above 90 years [15]. Multiple studies have shown that high age, emergency surgery, sepsis, frailty, and high ASA score are associated with increased mortality [15].

Cardiovascular and respiratory diseases are important to consider. Patients with congestive heart failure or previous heart attack are more prone to adverse effects of hypovolemia and anemia due to limited cardiac output and are at the same time exposed for the risk of resuscitation fluid overload. The NYHA classification of daily function, e.g., class III or IV, can quickly give an idea of the heart condition and may be supplied by echocardiography.

Assessment of hydration status is particularly important before anesthesia and should be done in close cooperation with the anesthesiologist [3]. When the patient is given general anesthesia and muscle relaxation, the body is in a state of systemic vasodilation. Changes of the intraperitoneal pressure, either decrease in open or increase in laparoscopic surgery, decrease venous return to the heart and consequently reduce cardiac output. In worst case this can lead to serious hypovolemia and cardiac arrest before the surgery has started [16]. Therefore, it is important to rehydrate and replenish circulating volume or blood losses before surgery whenever possible with crystalloid fluids or blood transfusion. If the patient has electrolyte imbalances, one can choose fluid resuscitation with 0.9% saline with/without added electrolytes. If this is not sufficient, adding vasopressors, such as dopamine and norepinephrine, is indicated [15, 17]. It is important to remember that a geriatric patient might be in shock even with a systolic blood pressure of 110 mmHg due to their reduced functional capacity [15]. In contrast, over resuscitation with colloids increases blood loss by diluting clotting factors and disturbs hemostasis [16, 18].

Underlying *pulmonary diseases* and reduced compliance of the chest wall and the lungs contribute to worsen hypoxia in the already critically ill patient [15]. Cellular hypoxia causes cellular dysfunction which can lead to systemic inflammatory response syndrome and organ dysfunction. However, it is important to keep in mind that hypoxia is not always caused by respiratory or circulatory failure, but may be caused by a distended abdomen due to bowel obstruction or peritonitis that presses the diaphragm upwards and reduces the volume of the thoracic cavity. Increased abdominal pressure can also impair the venous return to the heart. In this case, a nasogastric tube is indicated to decompress the gastrointestinal tract as an effective measure to restore physiology [16].

Acute *renal injury* is a potentially life-threatening condition in the critically ill patient [19]. Sepsis and nephrotoxic drugs stand for 50% and 25% of causes of acute kidney failure in intensive care units. Major surgery, hypovolemia, and nephrotoxic radiological contrast agents are common causes in the acute colorectal patient. Renal function is measured by serum creatinine levels and urinary output [19]. Acute renal failure inhibits secretion of acidosis and bicarbonate production (i.e., metabolic acidosis), which affects cardiac contractility and electrical conduction, reduces venous vasoconstriction, increases total peripheral vascular resistance, and further impairs oxygen delivery [19]. This has serious consequences in the acute colorectal patient and challenges anesthesia. Early resuscitation and treating sepsis is therefore crucial to prevent or reverse acute renal failure [19].

Electrolyte disturbances are common and often related to renal failure. In example, severe hypo- or hyperpotassemia can cause cardiac abnormalities and in worst case give arrhythmias that lead to cardiac arrest [19]. Potassium abnormalities also interfere with neuromuscular transmission. Suxamethonium (Curacit) is a muscle relaxant given under introduction of anesthesia and can worsen hyperpotassemia. It is therefore important to correct electrolyte imbalances preoperatively. Insulin-glucose infusion induces shift of the extracellular potassium into the intracellular space, and thus decreases the adverse effect of hyperpotassemia on the heart and muscular system [19]. Alternatively, sodium bicarbonate infusion causes alkalosis, which leads to release of intracellular hydrogen molecules into the blood in exchange with extracellular potassium [19].

Anemia combined with iron deficiency is common and is associated with increased mortality, thus it is a poor prognostic factor [20]. Particularly elderly patients with coronary artery disease are at risk. However, correcting anemia by blood transfusion should be restricted to patients with severe anemia (i.e., hemoglobin <8 mg/L) or clear symptoms of anemia, as multiple studies have shown that blood transfusion is associated with reduced survival of cancer, increased recurrence rate and postoperative infections [3, 16, 20]. Other adverse side effects of blood transfusion include transmission of blood-borne pathogens and transfusion-related acute lung injury (TRALI), a syndrome which causes acute hypoxemia and noncardiogenic pulmonary edema [20].

Hematological disorders are important to consider preoperatively. If the patient suffers from von Willebrand factor (vWF) disease, hemophilia types A or B, or idiopathic thrombocytopenic purpura (ITP), a hematologist should be consulted. Desmopressin is administered to increase vWF; FVIII or factor IX is administered in cases of hemophilia. For patients with ITP, high-dose corticosteroids and intravenous immunoglobulins are recommended [20, 21]. Surgery causes a thrombogenic stress response. Adequate anticoagulation, currently given as low fragment heparin, is important to prevent thromboembolic complications such as deep venous thrombosis or lung emboli.

Frailty is a consequence of age-related decrease in physiological reserve and resistance to stress and a common condition in the acute care setting. It is estimated that 6–15% of the elderly patient group are frail [8]. It is characterized by a distinct phenotype consisting of minimum three of the five following traits: unintentional weight loss, self-reported fatigue, diminished physical activity, impairment of grip strength, and reduced gait speed [4, 8, 15]. Frailty increases the patient's individual risk of disease-related mortality, falls, institutionalization, and hospitalization [8, 15]. A comprehensive geriatric assessment that is often used in research and in elective patients is too comprehensive for use in the acute care [7, 15, 22]. While frailty is strongly associated with poor outcome, there is currently no universal agreed definition for its assessment in the emergency setting.

Malnutrition due to reduced caloric and protein intake is common in elderly patients over 70 years of age and is considered as a marker of frailty because many malnourished patients also present with altered cognition, impaired mobility, and deranged quality of life [8]. A malnourished patient with emergent colorectal disease is more prone to adverse complications after surgery, such as anastomotic leak, wound infection, respiratory infection, and longer hospitalization due to delayed recovery [8, 23]. In contrary to the cancer cachexia syndrome, the effects of malnutrition can be reversed by nutritional support, which is obviously irrelevant in the acute setting. On the other hand, obesity also imposes challenges by increased risk of atelectasis and respiratory failure, thus increasing complication rate [24].

4.2.6 Medications

A complete list of all medications is of great importance for assessment of the acute colorectal cancer patient, as most drugs may cause both known and unknown adverse effects and interactions.

Anticoagulant and antiplatelet medications can cause bleeding that may be difficult to manage. Knowledge of these types of medications are important before performing surgery to know how to counteract their effects (Table 4.1). The traditionally most used drugs, acetylsalic acid and warfarine, are increasingly replaced by novel types of anticoagulants.

Using corticosteroids for more than 30 days prior to surgery and in doses higher than 20 mg/day induces immune suppression and reduced collagen formation and increases the risk of impaired wound healing, anastomosis leakage, and postoperative infections [23].

Angiotensin-converting enzyme inhibitors can during anesthesia mask hypovolemia and contribute to acute kidney injury.

Nonsteroidal anti-inflammatory drugs have adverse effects on the heart, kidneys, and lungs. They can also cause perforation of bowel.

In patients with vascular and heart disorders, beta-blockers should not be discontinued during surgery [17].

Table 4.1 Antiplatelet and anticoagulant medications with description of their effect and available antidote

Medication	Effect	Antidote
Acetylsalicylic acid	Inhibits platelet aggreagation	None, platelet transfusion can be tried
Clopidogrel	Inhibits platelet activation	None, platelet transfusion can be tried
Heparin	Creates complex with antithrombin III, inhibits clotting factors IXa, Xa, Xia, XIIa	Protamine sulfate
Fondaparinux (Arixtra)	Indirect factor Xa inhibitor	None
Rivaroxaban (Xarelto), Apixaban (Eliquis)	Direct factor Xa inhibitor	None
Dabigatran (Pradaxa)	Direct thrombin inhibitor	Praxbind

4.2.7 Cognitive Function

The cognitive function of the patient is an important factor in several aspects. First, it is the base for meaningful communication and shared decision-making. Secondly, preexisting dementia is often related to reduced life expectancy and may have severe impact on decisions regarding the intensity of treatment to be chosen. Thirdly, normal premorbid cognitive function may be compromised by the acute illness. When cognitive function is impaired, it is prudent to involve the patient's family caregivers or surrogates [15]. In this context, it is also highly important to formulate advanced directives and to discuss the patient's preferences with regard to actions to be taken when adverse events occur [15]. In this context, complete staging of the cancer disease is indispensable prognostic knowledge. The presence of widely disseminated disease should initiate contact with the palliative multidisciplinary team whenever possible to preserve best possible quality of life during the remaining lifetime of the patient and for coping of the family with the loss of their beloved one.

4.2.8 Preoperative Stabilization

Most patients who do not require immediate surgery will profit from stabilization on an intensive or high-dependency care unit (described in the respective chapters). Here we briefly mention challenges in the intensive care unit, since many of the patients are in demand of advanced resuscitation. This part of the disease trajectory has to be done with close cooperation between the surgeon and the intensivists (Fig. 4.2). It is important to remember that the aim is not complete resuscitation, but to improve the patient's physiology to better cope with the emergent state and planned surgery. In the emergency setting, studies show that complete resuscitation in favor of delaying surgery does not improve perioperative mortality nor 5-year survival [3].

4.3 Surgical Risk Assessment

At emergent presentation, the perioperative mortality of colorectal cancer is reported up to 20% and morbidity of 40–50% [1–3, 10], as compared to approximately 3% in elective and 18% in elderly patients [7, 9, 25]. Perioperative mortality consists of surgical complications and those associated to the condition of the critically ill patient.

Surgical risk assessment depends on a combination of knowledge of clinical information of the individual patient, supplied by surgeons' sound knowledge of relevant studies in the literature and personal experience. Inevitably, this results in a subjective assessment of the patient. Therefore, sound discussions based on good collegial relationship are encouraged as they will contribute to more favorable patient outcomes.

Table 4.2 ASA risk score

ASA classification	Definition
ASA I	A normal healthy patient
ASA II	A patient with mild systemic disease
ASA III	A patient with severe systemic disease
ASA IV	A patient with severe systemic disease that is a constant threat to life
ASA V	A moribund patient who is not expected to survive without the operation
ASA VI	A declared brain-dead patient whose organs are being removed for donor purposes

ASA denotes the American Society of Anesthesiologists

In order to achieve a more objective assessment with better prognostic information, several risk scores have been developed. The most used score is the ASA (American Society of Anesthesiologists, Table 4.2) grading showing a statistically significant association between mortality and morbidity [2]. ASA takes both the patient's current state and comorbid conditions into account. The patient is graded from 1 to 5, where 1 is previously healthy and where 5 is a patient with critically ill/life-threatening condition [26, 27].

The Acute Physiological and Chronic Health Evaluation (APACHE II) score is mostly used in the ICU, but can also be used in the emergency patient to assess the physiological consequence of the acute illness while taking into account the patient's previous status and age [9, 16, 25, 28]. However, most scores work best on a group level for comparison and are less good in individual outcome prediction.

The Physiological and Operative Severity Score (POSSUM) uses 12 physiological variables and 6 operative variables to predict mortality and morbidity within 30 days after performed surgery [25, 29]. It has also been used to compare individual performance between surgeons and surgical institutions. Because POSSUM consistently over-predicted mortality, it was further developed to different specialty-specific models, two of them being CR-POSSUM, colorectal POSSUM, and P-POSSUM, Portsmouth POSSUM. They predict mortality more accurately compared to POSSUM; however, they do not predict morbidity [25]. It should also be noted that both POSSUM and P-POSSUM are found to underestimate morbidity and mortality in patients who were admitted acutely and in patients of older age and therefore should be used with caution in these settings [9, 25, 28]. These scores are best for comparison of outcomes and risk between groups rather than decision-making for the individual patient.

Taken together, assessing the emergency patient with colorectal cancer includes stage, type of acute presentation, comorbidities, medications, patient's cognitive state, and preferences for further treatment. For the patient to make a well-informed decision, the risks of surgery in addition to the underlying disease must be declared. The diagnosis of disseminated incurable disease or severe comorbidity should initiate a sound reflection on possible treatments and involvement of the palliative team [30].

References

1. Wallace D, Walker K, Kuryba A, Finan P, Scott N, van Der Meulen J. Identifying patients at risk of emergency admission for colorectal cancer. Br J Cancer. 2014;111(3):577.
2. Schwenter F, Morel P, Gervaz P. Management of obstructive and perforated colorectal cancer. Expert Rev Anticancer Ther. 2010;10(10):1613–9.
3. Cuffy M, Abir F, Audisio RA, Longo WE. Colorectal cancer presenting as surgical emergencies. Surg Oncol. 2004;13(2):149–57.
4. Torrance ADW, Powell SL, Griffiths EA. Emergency surgery in the elderly: challenges and solutions. Open Access Emerg Med. 2015;7:55.
5. Baer C, Menon R, Bastawrous S, Bastawrous A. Emergency presentations of colorectal cancer. Surg Clin. 2017;97(3):529–45.
6. Bosscher M, Van Leeuwen B, Hoekstra H. Surgical emergencies in oncology. Cancer Treat Rev. 2014;40(8):1028–36.
7. Kristjansson SR, Nesbakken A, Jordhøy MS, Skovlund E, Audisio RA, Johannessen H-O, et al. Comprehensive geriatric assessment can predict complications in elderly patients after elective surgery for colorectal cancer: a prospective observational cohort study. Crit Rev Oncol Hematol. 2010;76(3):208–17.
8. Kristjansson SR, Farinella E, Gaskell S, Audisio RA. Surgical risk and post-operative complications in older unfit cancer patients. Cancer Treat Rev. 2009;35(6):499–502.
9. Tekkis P, Kessaris N, Kocher H, Poloniecki J, Lyttle J, Windsor A. Evaluation of POSSUM and P-POSSUM scoring systems in patients undergoing colorectal surgery. Br J Surg. 2003;90(3):340–5.
10. McArdle C, Hole D. Emergency presentation of colorectal cancer is associated with poor 5-year survival. Br J Surg. 2004;91(5):605–9.
11. Helsedirektoratet. Nasjonalt handlingsprogram med retningslinjer for diagnostikk, behandling og oppfølging av kreft i tykktarm og endetarm. Oslo: Helsedirektoratet; 2017.
12. Aunan J, Watson M, Hagland H, Søreide K. Molecular and biological hallmarks of ageing. Br J Surg. 2016;103(2):e29.
13. Lieffers JR, Mourtzakis M, Hall KD, McCargar LJ, Prado CM, Baracos VE. A viscerally driven cachexia syndrome in patients with advanced colorectal cancer: contributions of organ and tumor mass to whole-body energy demands. Am J Clin Nutr. 2009;89(4):1173–9.
14. Porporato P. Understanding cachexia as a cancer metabolism syndrome. Oncogenesis. 2016;5(2):e200.
15. Desserud K, Veen T, Søreide K. Emergency general surgery in the geriatric patient. Br J Surg. 2016;103(2):e52.
16. Stahel PF. Schein's common sense emergency abdominal surgery. 4th ed. London: BioMed Central; 2015.
17. McConnell KW, Coopersmith CM. Organ failure avoidance and mitigation strategies in surgery. Surg Clin. 2012;92(2):307–19.
18. American College of Surgeons Committee on T. Advanced trauma life support: ATLS: student course manual. 9th ed. Chicago, IL: American College of Surgeons; 2012.
19. Maxwell RA, Bell CM. Acute kidney injury in the critically ill. Surg Clin. 2017;97(6):1399–418.
20. Douglas WG, Uffort E, Denning D. Transfusion and management of surgical patients with hematologic disorders. Surg Clin. 2015;95(2):367–77.
21. Van PY, Schreiber MA. Hematologic issues in the geriatric surgical patient. Surg Clin. 2015;95(1):129–38.
22. Biffl WL, Biffl SE. Rehabilitation of the geriatric surgical patient: predicting needs and optimizing outcomes. Surg Clin. 2015;95(1):173–90.
23. Hübner M, Hahnloser D. Perioperative management. Coloproctology. New York, NY: Springer; 2017. p. 409–19.
24. Pelosi P, Gregoretti C. Perioperative management of obese patients. Best Pract Res Clin Anaesthesiol. 2010;24(2):211–25.

25. Richards CH, Leitch FE, Horgan PG, McMillan DC. A systematic review of POSSUM and its related models as predictors of post-operative mortality and morbidity in patients undergoing surgery for colorectal cancer. J Gastrointest Surg. 2010;14(10):1511–20.
26. American Society of Anesthesiologists. ASA physical status classification system. Washington, DC: American Society of Anesthesiologists; 2014. Available from: https://www.asahq.org/resources/clinical-information/asa-physical-status-classification-system.
27. Daabiss M. American Society of Anaesthesiologists physical status classification. Indian J Anaesth. 2011;55(2):111.
28. Oliver C, Walker E, Giannaris S, Grocott M, Moonesinghe S. Risk assessment tools validated for patients undergoing emergency laparotomy: a systematic review. Br J Anaesth. 2015;115(6):849–60.
29. Al-Homoud S, Purkayastha S, Aziz O, Smith JJ, Thompson MD, Darzi AW, et al. Evaluating operative risk in colorectal cancer surgery: ASA and POSSUM-based predictive models. Surg Oncol. 2004;13(2-3):83–92.
30. Søreide K, Desserud KF. Emergency surgery in the elderly: the balance between function, frailty, fatality and futility. Scand J Trauma Resusc Emerg Med. 2015;23(1):10.

Complicated Colorectal Cancer: Role of Imaging

5

Athena Galletto, Laurence Baranes, Sebastien Mulé, Edouard Herin, Melanie Chiaradia, Marjane Djabbari, Rym Kharrat, Benhalima Zegai, Frederic Pigneur, and Alain Luciani

5.1 Introduction

Colorectal cancer is the third most common cancer and the fourth most common cancer cause of death globally, accounting for roughly 1.2 million new cases and 600,000 deaths per year [1]. Incidence is low at ages younger than 50 years, but strongly increases with age. Median age at diagnosis is about 70 years in developed countries [2]. Colorectal cancer develops mostly without any symptoms in the early stages. In 15–30% of cases, however, CRC patients present with symptoms of acute abdomen such as bowel perforation, obstruction, or gastrointestinal bleeding [3]. Those complications mostly occur in elderly patients and are associated with poor prognosis [4]. These poor outcomes start at their initial hospital admission and also impacts long-term survival [3]. Elderly patients with CRC may be specifically at risk for emergent presentation because of medical comorbid conditions, insufficient screening, unrecognized symptoms, and inadequate overall access to the health-care

A. Galletto · L. Baranes · M. Chiaradia · M. Djabbari · R. Kharrat · B. Zegai · F. Pigneur
Service d'Imagerie Médicale, Assistance Publique Hôpitaux de Paris,
Hôpitaux Universitaires Henri Mondor, Créteil Cedex, France

S. Mulé · A. Luciani (✉)
Service d'Imagerie Médicale, Assistance Publique Hôpitaux de Paris,
Hôpitaux Universitaires Henri Mondor, Créteil Cedex, France

Faculté de Médecine de Créteil, UPEC, Créteil, France

INSERM IMRB U955 Equipe 18, Créteil, France
e-mail: alain.luciani@aphp.fr

E. Herin
Service d'Imagerie Médicale, Assistance Publique Hôpitaux de Paris,
Hôpitaux Universitaires Henri Mondor, Créteil Cedex, France

Faculté de Médecine de Créteil, UPEC, Créteil, France

N. de'Angelis et al. (eds.), *Emergency Surgical Management of Colorectal Cancer*,
Hot Topics in Acute Care Surgery and Trauma,
https://doi.org/10.1007/978-3-030-06225-5_5

system [4]. Imaging hence plays a key role in this setting. Its first objective is to provide the earliest diagnosis of any complication. Its second objective is increasingly dealing with interventional therapy of some complications associated with colorectal cancer treatment. This chapter will go through the role of imaging in the four major complications occurring in colorectal cancer setting, with a special focus on the pre-therapeutic imaging strategy in complicated or advanced CRC.

5.2 Obstruction

Bowel obstruction is the most frequent complication associated with colon cancer. The reported frequency of patients with obstructive colon cancer ranges from 8% to 59% [5]. Bowel obstruction is more frequent in tumors of the descending colon because of a smaller diameter of the left colon. Currently, CT with multiplanar reconstruction is the best imaging technique to investigate a patient with suspected bowel obstruction: it allows the positive diagnosis of the obstruction but also ensures the precise location of the transition point—precise zone between dilated bowel loops and normal bowel loops—usually ensuring an appropriate identification of the cause of the obstruction [6]. During a large bowel obstruction, CT typically shows a distension of the large bowel, possibly associated with small bowel distension when the tumor is located close to the ileocecal valve or when the ileocecal valve is not continent. In CRC-related bowel obstruction, the transition point appears as an irregular circumferential thickening of the colon wall [7] (Fig. 5.1).

Long-lasting large bowel obstruction may be complicated with ischemia and perforation of the proximal colon due to the increased pressure above the tumor [5]. Diastatic perforation of the caecum can occur when the ileocecal valve is continent, due to a closed loop obstruction, in which two points of the bowel are occluded. A cecal distension of more than 9 cm has been shown to be associated with this perforation ($p = 0.002$) [8]. Ischemic lesions of the obstructed colon may precede perforation. CT findings of this pre-perforative ischemia include the absence of enhancement of the colonic wall, parietal pneumatosis, and possible presence of air in the mesenteric and portal vein (aeroportia) (Fig. 5.1). The presence of peritoneal fluid may be reactive to the obstruction, but should raise suspicion for bowel perforation or peritoneal carcinomatosis.

Obstructive CRC and related complications usually require urgent surgical management, although about 35% occur in patients with advanced, metastatic, or non-operable disease [9]. As a result, morbidity and mortality rates in cases of emergency surgery in these situations are very high: in a study, Wong et al. [3] demonstrated that emergency patients were less likely to have a curative resection (60.2%) than elective patients (78%; $p < 0.0001$) and they were more likely to die within 30 days of the operation (9.1% vs. 2.1%); moreover, the 5-year survival rate for all operated CRCs was 39.2% (95% CI, 32.4–46.1) for all emergency patients and 64.7% (95% CI, 61.9–67.5) for all elective patients; whether the all-cause

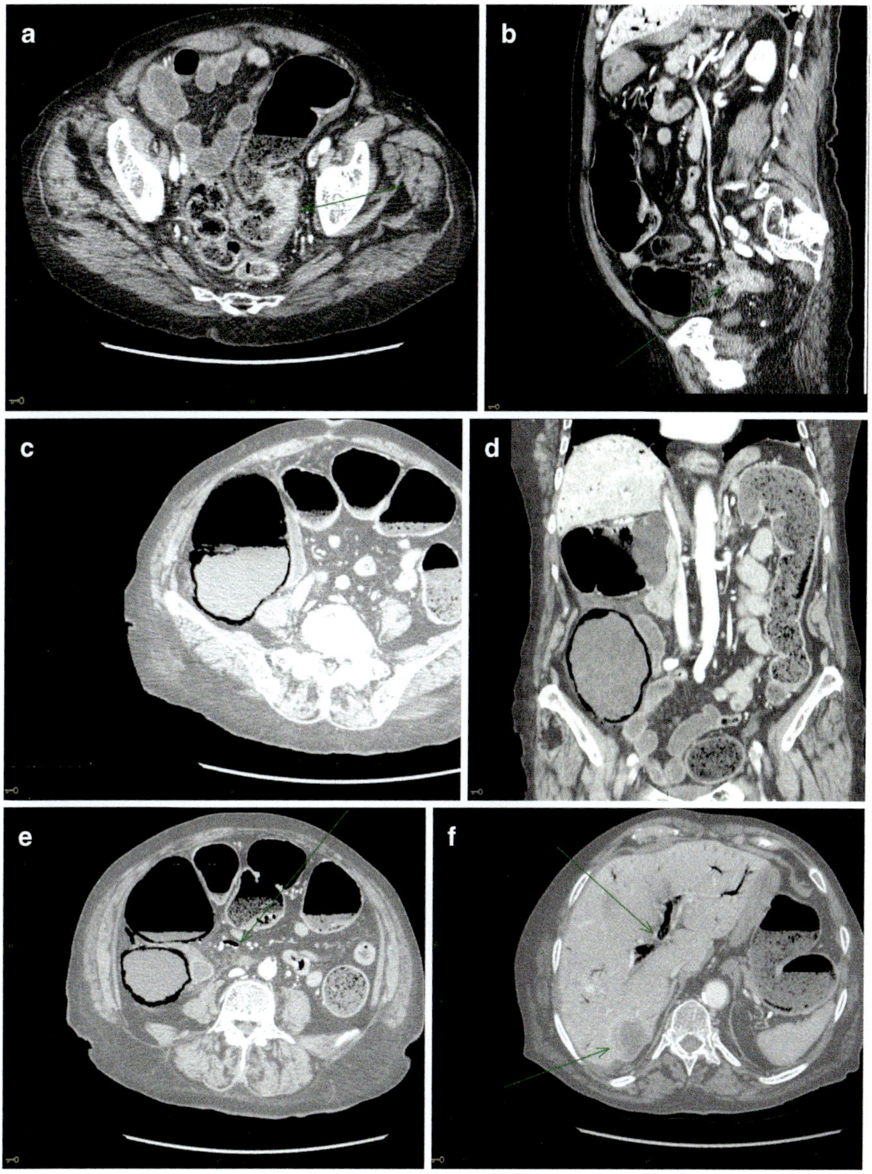

Fig. 5.1 An 89-year-old patient admitted for abdominal pain. (**a**) Contrast-enhanced abdominal CT scan displays an important colonic distension over a sigmoid parietal thickening (arrow on axial view). (**b**) Sagittal view of the contrast-enhanced, portal venous phase CT scan shows the sigmoid parietal tumor (arrow). (**c**) The entire colon is distended with fecal stasis predominating in the cecum. (**d**) Parietal pneumatosis within the cecal wall is also visible. (**e**) Gas is also present within the mesenteric vein. (**f**) Presence of gas in the portal vein (arrow). The CT shows a hepatic metastasis (arrow)

mortality for all curatively resected colon cancers was 51.6% (95% CI, 41.4–61.8) for all emergency curatively resected colon patients and 75.6% (95% CI, 71.8–79.4%) for all elective curatively resected colon patients ($p < 0.0001$). Therefore, alternatives to surgery such as colonic stenting have been developed to treat obstructive CRC, either in the setting of advanced and metastatic disease or as a bridge to surgery. The colonic stents, initially placed under fluoroscopic control alone, are currently almost always placed under endoscopic and fluoroscopic control. Zhang et al. showed that the use of a stent as a bridge to surgery for obstructive left-sided colorectal cancer could increase the chance of primary anastomosis and reduce the need for stoma creation (RR, 0.70; 95% CI, 0.50–0.99; $p = 0.04$) and postprocedural complications (RR, 0.42; 95% CI, 0.24–0.71; $p = 0.001$). Stent insertion before subsequent surgery has no effect on perioperative mortality and long-term survival [10].

5.3 Perforation

Intestinal perforation may occur in two settings: at the tumor site itself, secondary to tumor necrosis or adjacent inflammation, or cranially, as a result of increased intraluminal pressure caused by bowel obstruction or mucin-producing neoplasms. Spontaneous bowel perforation occurs through ischemia and necrosis of the intestinal wall [11]. Neoplastic cells infiltrate the colonic wall and subsequently undergo necrosis during rapid tumor growth or under ischemic conditions, both of which result in vulnerability to perforation. In addition, vascular occlusion by neoplastic infiltration, direct tumor emboli, and increased intraluminal pressure secondary to bowel obstruction may induce or accelerate bowel ischemia. Perforation is also more common in patients after radiotherapy or during chemotherapy [4, 11].

The incidence of bowel perforation in patients with CRC ranges from 1.2% to 10.0% [12–14]. Perforation occurs most commonly in the sigmoid colon and cecum and less frequently in the ascending and descending colon [11, 15] (Fig. 5.2).

Perforated CRCs present a life-threatening emergency and require immediate surgery. Several studies have shown a high postoperative mortality rate in perforated CRCs (considered alone or along with other emergency presentations), ranging from 11% to 40%. Cheynel et al. demonstrated that the 5-year overall cumulative recurrence rate was higher for perforated than for uncomplicated CRC (45.2% vs. 29.7%; $p = 0.003$) and that perforation was an independent risk factor for local recurrence or peritoneal carcinomatosis ($p = 0.004$), but not for distant metastasis (excluding peritoneal carcinomatosis; ($p = 0.55$)). Moreover, they showed that perforated CRC was associated with a higher postoperative mortality rate than the uncomplicated type (20.2% vs. 6.6%; $p < 0.001$). They found out that the overall 5-year relative survival rate, including postoperative mortality, was 37% for patients with a perforation and 49.2% for patients who chose elective surgery ($p = 0.006$). After exclusion of immediate postoperative mortality, these percentages reached 47.3% and 53%, respectively ($p = 0.014$) [16].

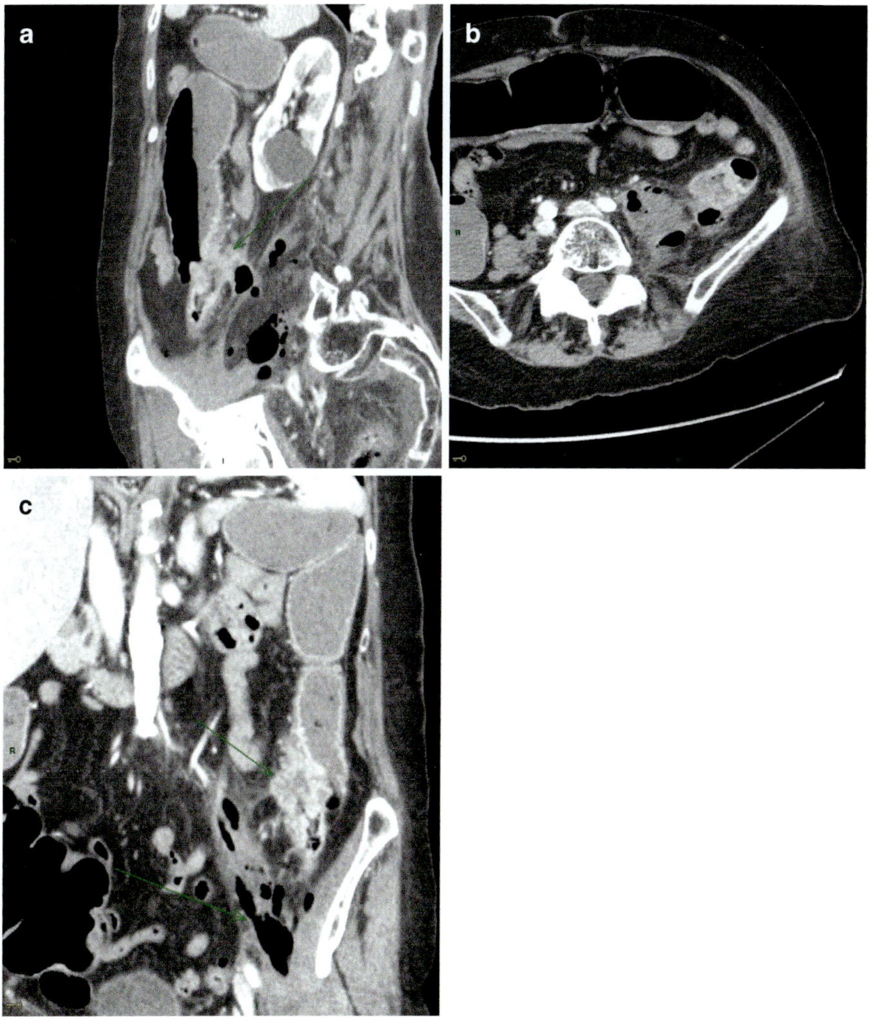

Fig. 5.2 (**a**–**c**) An 86-year-old woman; CT performed for abdominal pain. The CT showed colonic perforation over an exophytic mass of the left side colon (arrows) perforated in the retroperitoneal space adjacent to a collection within the iliopsoas lodge extending towards the inguinal region

Interestingly, the presence of a perforated T4 CRC results in higher 30-day mortality, but does not impact long-term oncological outcomes compared to patients with non-perforated T4 CRC [12].

CT is the cornerstone of the initial workup and follow-up of CRC in this precise setting, as the clinical presentation is usually that of an acute abdomen. CT can actually show pneumoperitoneum, pericolonic inflammatory changes and abscesses, as well as a colorectal mass [17] (Figs. 5.2 and 5.3). CT is extremely sensitive for the detection of free air in the abdomen [6]: Udayasankar et al. demonstrated that the

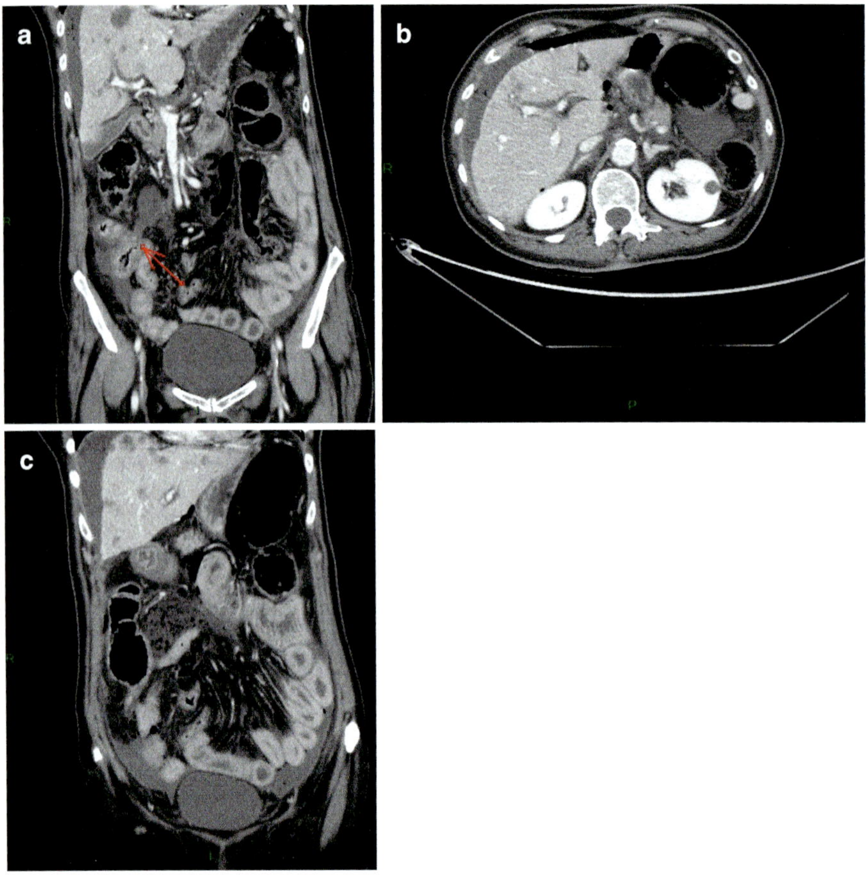

Fig. 5.3 (**a**–**c**) A 70-year-old woman admitted for abdominal pain having a history of cecal mass treated by chemotherapy for 3 months. CT shows a colonic perforation in the region of the colonic neoplastic mass (Arrow, coronal view of CT scan, **a**). Perforation is visible within the peritoneal cavity: free air in the prehepatic space is visible (**b**), as well as a fecal intra-abdominal collection (**c**). The perforation site is visible as a thin interruption of the abdominal wall. The CT shows hepatic metastases (**a**–**c**)

sensitivity, specificity, and positive predictive value of ultralow-dose CT for the detection of free air could reach 100%, 98.5%, and 91.7%, respectively [18].

Although a large amount of free air is typically observed in perforated CRC, more commonly, the perforation can be suspected when the CT scan displays small amount of small air bubbles with peritoneal fluid and mesenteric stranding in the pericolic fat [6]. Of note, the administration of a rectal contrast material can help to find the site of perforation. As with all other causes of colonic perforation (diverticulitis, trauma, ischemic colitis, severe colitis, and volvulus), perforated colon cancer can also present as a localized perforation with formation of an

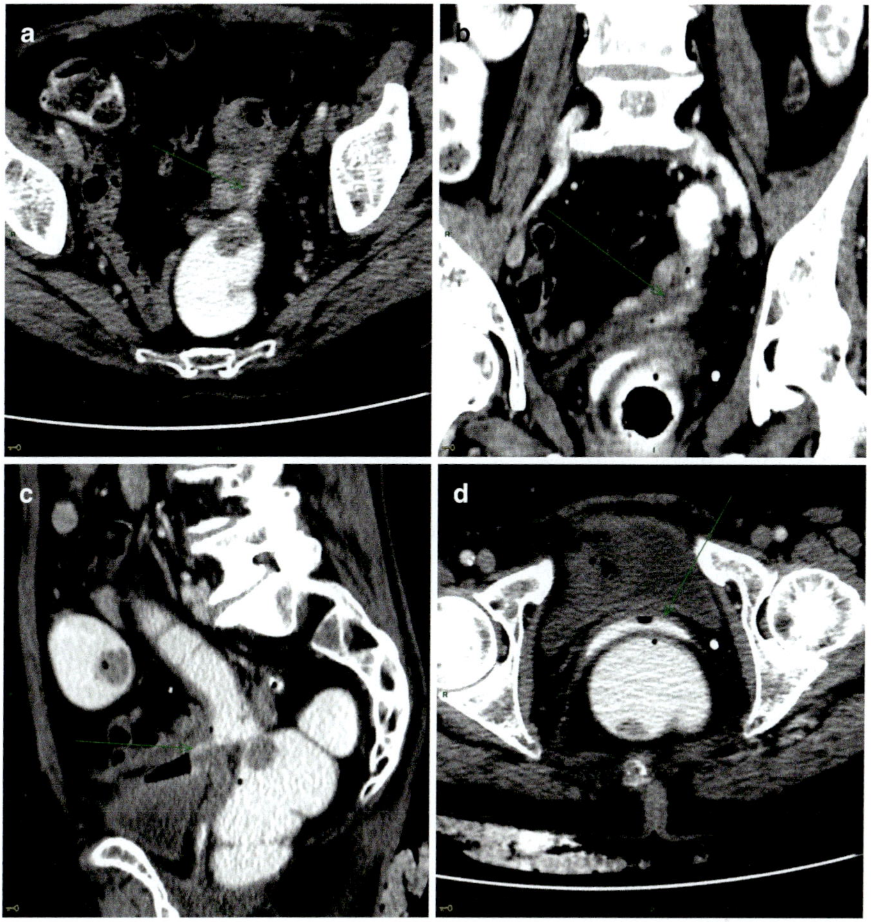

Fig. 5.4 A 78-year-old woman with sigmoid adenocarcinoma and dirty vaginal discharge. CT scan with rectal opacification and intravenous contrast agent administration was performed. (**a**–**c**) Axial, coronal, and sagittal planes showing sigmoid cancer stenosis and fistulous tract from the sigmoid to vagina. (**d**) Presence of contrast and air into the vagina

abscess or a fistula toward the bladder, the female genital tract, or the small bowel (Fig. 5.4).

In order to differentiate colonic perforation that is caused by cancer from that caused by various benign conditions, it is mandatory to identify the irregular wall thickening of the colon wall. However, the analysis of the colonic wall can be challenging in the absence of bowel preparation and, with severe pericolonic inflammation, presence of a large abscess or peritoneal fluid. Radiologists and clinicians should hence be cautious when dealing with acute abdominal presentations associated with bowel distension and free air and should study carefully the entire bowel lumen and wall for subtle signs associated with CRC association.

5.4 Infection

Perforation and infiltration of adjacent organs, with abscess formation, are an uncommon initial presentation of CRC, occurring in 0.3–0.4% of cases [17, 19].

The most frequent location of abscesses is the peritoneal cavity, including the paracolic spaces and the pelvic cavity; fistula formation or inflammation spreading along intra-abdominal planes may lead to abscesses formation in unusual locations such as the retroperitoneum, abdominal wall, perirectal space, psoas muscle, and thigh or subcutaneously on the trunk [19]. Furthermore, abscess-forming CRC that occur in the right lower quadrant or the pelvic cavity can be mistaken for inflammatory conditions (diverticulitis, appendicitis with perforation, and pelvic inflammatory or infectious diseases). Differentiating between diverticulitis and sigmoid CRC is a frequent clinical challenge with a considerable overlap in CT features [20] (Fig. 5.5). A major pericolic fat stranding adjacent to a poorly thickened colonic wall is generally the most significant CT finding in favor of an inflammatory or infectious condition. This severe pericolonic fat stranding leads to an engorgement of the vasa recta that feeds the colon, a finding known as the centipede sign [21, 22]. The preservation of the colonic layering inside a thickened bowel wall is another important feature in favor of the diagnosis of benign inflammatory or infectious conditions, while a marked, asymmetric wall thickening, with loss of a stratified enhancement that involves a short segment of the colon, supports the diagnosis of a CRC. Third, a sudden transition from a normal to an abnormal bowel wall is in favor of malignancy, whereas a smooth and gradual transition is usually present in benign conditions.

Goh et al. have reported the presence of a localized mass (present in 85% of patients with cancer vs. 10% of patients with diverticulitis) and a pericolonic abscess (seen in one 5% of 20 patients with cancer vs. 50% of patients with diverticulitis) to be reliable discriminators between patients with cancer and those with diverticulitis [20]. Moreover, the presence of pericolonic lymphadenopathy is more common in CRC than in benign conditions: pericolonic lymph nodes have 71% sensitivity and 85% specificity for cancer [23]. Other parameters found to have both high sensitivity and specificity for the diagnosis of diverticulitis rather than colon cancer are the presence of non-inflamed diverticula, inflamed diverticula, and minimal degree of enhancement [24]. Finally, the presence of intralesional calcifications and the absence of pericolic fat stranding can be in favor of the diagnosis of a mucinous carcinoma vs. an abscess [17].

Despite all these features, there is no sure imaging sign allowing for a definitive radiological diagnosis of abscessed colorectal cancer, and patients above 50 with sigmoid diverticulitis, and abscess or mass formation, should undergo medical therapy, drainage when indicated, and later colonoscopy to rule out CRC [25]. However, radiologists again should be cautious before draining a pericolonic abscess and should attempt to rule out CRC in these specific situations.

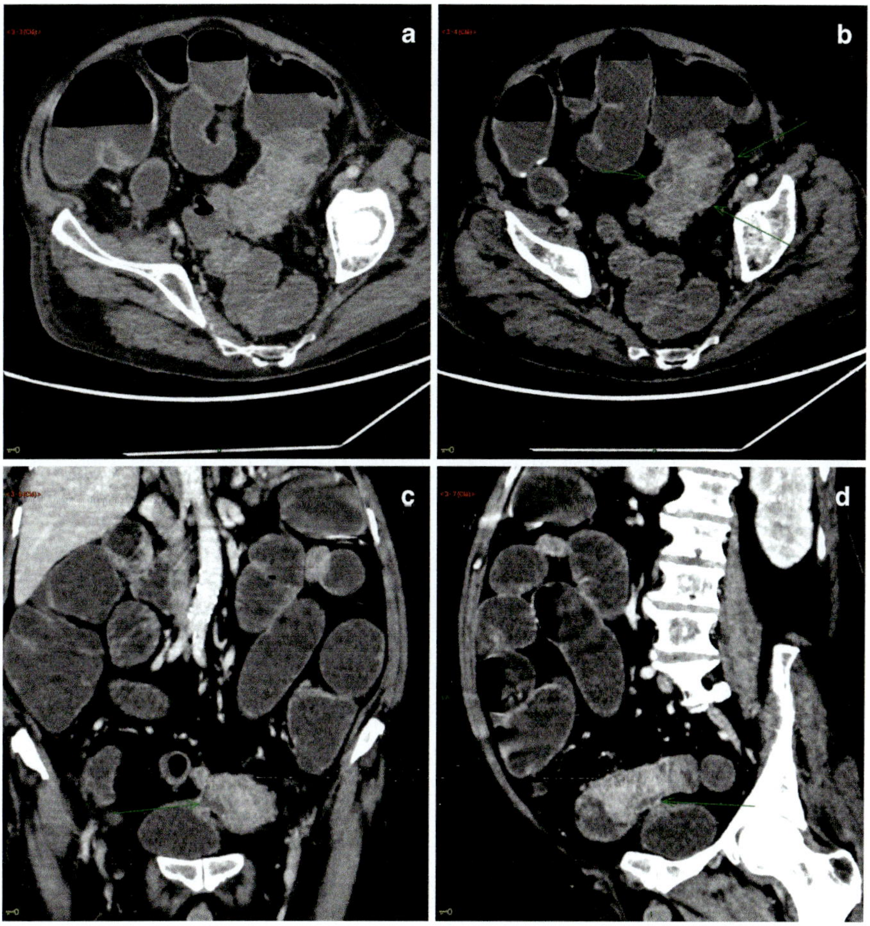

Fig. 5.5 A 58-year-old man, CT performed for abdominal pain and diarrhea since 1 month associated with inflammatory biologic syndrome. (**a**) Irregular sigmoid parietal thickening with bowel obstruction. (**b**) Intraparietal abscesses (arrows). (**c**, **d**) Communication between the bladder and abscess. Rectosigmoidoscopy showed diverticula, parietal edema, and no stenosis. Biopsy showed chronic inflammatory lesions without malignancy sign

5.5 Hemorrhage

CRC accounts for 2–11% of all lower gastrointestinal bleedings [26]. The first-line modality to investigate lower gastrointestinal bleeding is colonoscopy. Digital subtraction angiography (DSA) may be indicated for patients with active colonic bleeding who cannot be hemodynamically stabilized or undergo bowel preparation for emergent colonoscopy or after a failed endoscopic hemostasis attempt [27]. In order to plan the DSA with embolization, a multi detector CT angiography must be performed to localize the bleeding site and to analyze arterial anatomy [28, 29]. In the setting of acute lower gastrointestinal bleeding, its sensitivity has been reported to reach 91–92% [30].

Protocol of CT angiography includes an unenhanced phase, an arterial phase, and a portal venous phase [31]. The contrast medium needs to have a high iodine concentration and should be injected at rate no smaller than 4 mL/s. Arterial phase is obtained by using a bolus tracking with a region of interest positioned in the abdominal aorta [28]. On multidetector CT angiography, the extravasation of contrast medium may appear linear, jet-like, swirled, ellipsoid, or pooled. The venous phase is considered useful for the evaluation of progressive contrast extravasation [32, 33]. CT angiography provides a validated road map for further endovascular hemostatic intervention in patients with positive blush. In a swine model, colonic bleeding rates of 0.4 mL/min are detectable [34]. Dobritz et al. showed that rates of bleeding above 0.25 mL/min could be detected by MDCT on an experimental model with a sensitivity of 97% and specificity of 100% using arterial and portal venous phase images [35]. Therefore, a negative CT angiography predicts a low-flow bleeding process and is a good predictor of spontaneous improvement of a lower gastrointestinal bleeding without further intervention [35]. Chan et al. studied 115 CTAs performed for lower GI hemorrhage (37 positive for active bleeding, 78 negative): 77.4% of patients with lower GI bleed who had an initial negative CTA did not rebleed without the need for radiological or surgical intervention [36] (Fig. 5.6).

The goal of endovascular therapy is to provide a super-selective embolization to the bleeding vessel while allowing mucosal viability via collateral circulation and hence minimizing the risk of bowel infarction [37]. The treatment of the bleeding episode by arterial embolization reduces the potential mortality of an immediate surgery that can reach 8.2% [38]. Arteriography successively studies the superior and the inferior mesenteric artery and the anterior division of the internal iliac artery. Embolization is performed as selectively and distally as possible using microcoils (2–3 mm). Besides treatment failure and bleeding recurrence, the main risk of the procedure is bowel ischemia. In an analysis including 338 patients (1992–2006) with lower gastrointestinal bleeding of multiple causes treated by arterial embolization, the technical success was 96%, and the recurrence (within 30 days) was 22%. Minor complications were seen in 26%, and major complications were seen in 17%. The most common major complication was bowel infarction [26].

5.6 Preoperative Workup of Complicated Colorectal Cancer

In cases where rescue surgery is not required, the pretreatment workup of patients with complicated CRC has some specificities. Abdominal CT is already available and may have already detected liver or lymph node metastases or peritoneal carcinosis. Taking into account the higher risk of metastatic disease in these patients, an extensive workup including liver MRI, thoracic CT, and PET CT which increases

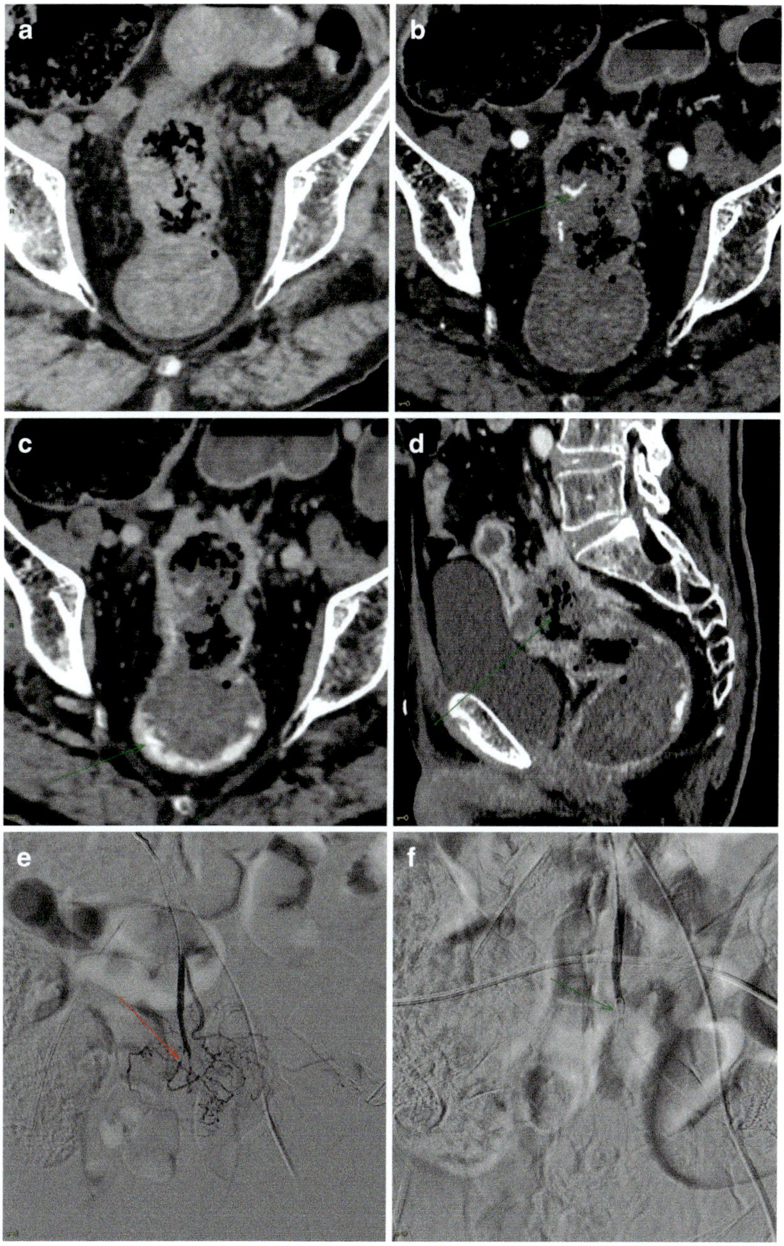

Fig. 5.6 An 80-year-old patient, with rectal bleeding, and CT performed for hemorrhagic shock. (**a**) Unenhanced CT scan showing rectal hematic content and irregular wall. (**b**) Active arterial bleeding of the sigmoid wall: linear extravasation of contrast (arrow). (**c**) Increase of the contrast extravasation on the venous phase (arrow). (**d**) Sagittal view showing irregular thickening of the colic wall (arrow). (**e**) Selective arteriography of inferior mesenteric artery showing irregular sigmoid artery (arrow). (**f**) Control after embolization with microcoils showing a good result (arrow)

the sensitivity of the detection of distant metastases is recommended [39]. MRI is more sensitive than CT to detect hepatic metastasis with respective reported figures of 81% versus 75%. MRI shows a better sensitivity than CT in per-patient ($p = 0.05$) and in per-lesion analysis ($p < 0.000$) [40].

In one study, PET/CT showed a higher specificity than CT in detecting suspected hepatic and extrahepatic metastases of gastrointestinal cancers and has an impact of nearly 40% on changement in patient management strategies [41]. In another one, the sensitivity of PET was equivalent to CT one's for hepatic sites (both 79%), but was superior for extrahepatic abdominal sites (63% and 25%, respectively). PET provided additional information in five patients, mainly by revealing abdominal extrahepatic metastases, but falsely upstaged three patients [42].

In the particular case of rectal cancer, a rectal MRI must be performed to analyze the locoregional staging before treatment [39].

CT colonoscopy or virtual colonoscopy (CTC) has proven to be a valid tool in identifying both primary and synchronous colonic lesions. CTC is beneficial after incomplete optical colonoscopy to assess the proximal colon [17]. It has a sensitivity of 93% and a specificity of 97% for detecting polyps >1 cm. Sensitivity and specificity fall to 86% and 86%, respectively, for polyps measuring <1 cm [43]. It can be particularly useful in obstructive colorectal cancer when colonoscopy cannot cross the primary tumor. Flor et al. verified that an obstructing colorectal cancer does not affect colon distension, this allowing visualization with CT colonography [44].

Overall, CT remains the cornerstone of imaging management of complicated CRC. It ensures the early diagnosis of occlusion, perforation, and hemorrhage and helps an accurate planning of DSA when needed in cases of active bleeding. However, it is important to recon the role of complete imaging workup when dealing with patients suspected of CRC facing acute complications, as long-term outcomes are driven by the detection of distant metastases.

Last interventional therapy can be required, especially for abscess drainage and endovascular embolization in cases of active persistent bleeding.

References

1. Ferlay J, Soerjomataram I, Dikshit R, Eser S, Mathers C, Rebelo M, et al. Cancer incidence and mortality worldwide: sources, methods and major patterns in GLOBOCAN 2012. Int J Cancer. 2015;136(5):E359–86.
2. Siegel R, DeSantis C, Virgo K, Stein K, Mariotto A, Smith T, et al. Cancer treatment and survivorship statistics, 2012. CA Cancer J Clin. 2012;62(4):220–41.
3. Wong SKC, Jalaludin BB, Morgan MJ, Berthelsen AS, Morgan A, Gatenby AH, et al. Tumor pathology and long-term survival in emergency colorectal cancer. Dis Colon Rectum. 2008;51(2):223–30.
4. McGillicuddy EA, Schuster KM, Davis KA, Longo WE. Factors predicting morbidity and mortality in emergency colorectal procedures in elderly patients. Arch Surg. 2009;144(12):1157–62.
5. Biondo S, Kreisler E, Millan M, Fraccalvieri D, Golda T, Martí Ragué J, et al. Differences in patient postoperative and long-term outcomes between obstructive and perforated colonic cancer. Am J Surg. 2008;195(4):427–32.

6. Horton KM, Abrams RA, Fishman EK. Spiral CT of colon cancer: imaging features and role in management. Radiographics. 2000;20(2):419–30.
7. Taourel P, Kessler N, Lesnik A, Pujol J, Morcos L, Bruel JM. Helical CT of large bowel obstruction. Abdom Imaging. 2003;28(2):267–75.
8. Sabbagh C, Siembida N, Yzet T, Robert B, Chivot C, Browet F, et al. What are the predictive factors of caecal perforation in patients with obstructing distal colon cancer? Colorectal Dis. 2018;20:688.
9. Carraro PG, Segala M, Cesana BM, Tiberio G. Obstructing colonic cancer: failure and survival patterns over a ten-year follow-up after one-stage curative surgery. Dis Colon Rectum. 2001;44(2):243–50.
10. Zhang Y, Shi J, Shi B, Song C-Y, Xie W-F, Chen Y-X. Self-expanding metallic stent as a bridge to surgery versus emergency surgery for obstructive colorectal cancer: a meta-analysis. Surg Endosc. 2012;26(1):110–9.
11. Kim SW, Kim HC, Yang DM. Perforated tumours in the gastrointestinal tract: CT findings and clinical implications. Br J Radiol. 2012;85(1017):1307–13.
12. Abdelrazeq AS, Scott N, Thorn C, Verbeke CS, Ambrose NS, Botterill ID, et al. The impact of spontaneous tumour perforation on outcome following colon cancer surgery. Colorectal Dis. 2008;10(8):775–80.
13. Badía JM, Sitges-Serra A, Pla J, Ragué JM, Roqueta F, Sitges-Creus A. Perforation of colonic neoplasms. A review of 36 cases. Int J Colorectal Dis. 1987;2(4):187–9.
14. Biondo S, Martí-Ragué J, Kreisler E, Parés D, Martín A, Navarro M, et al. A prospective study of outcomes of emergency and elective surgeries for complicated colonic cancer. Am J Surg. 2005;189(4):377–83.
15. Catalano O. [Perforated carcinoma of the colorectum. Computerized tomography findings]. Radiol Med 1997;93(1–2):83–86.
16. Cheynel N, Cortet M, Lepage C, Ortega-Debalon P, Faivre J, Bouvier A-M. Incidence, patterns of failure, and prognosis of perforated colorectal cancers in a well-defined population. Dis Colon Rectum. 2009;52(3):406–11.
17. Kim SW, Shin HC, Kim IY, Kim YT, Kim C-J. CT findings of colonic complications associated with colon cancer. Korean J Radiol. 2010;11(2):211–21.
18. Udayasankar UK, Li J, Baumgarten DA, Small WC, Kalra MK. Acute abdominal pain: value of non-contrast enhanced ultra-low-dose multi-detector row CT as a substitute for abdominal radiographs. Emerg Radiol. 2009;16(1):61–70.
19. Tsai H-L, Hsieh J-S, Yu F-J, Wu D-C, Chen F-M, Huang C-J, et al. Perforated colonic cancer presenting as intra-abdominal abscess. Int J Colorectal Dis. 2007;22(1):15–9.
20. Goh V, Halligan S, Taylor SA, Burling D, Bassett P, Bartram CI. Differentiation between diverticulitis and colorectal cancer: quantitative CT perfusion measurements versus morphologic criteria--initial experience. Radiology. 2007;242(2):456–62.
21. Pereira JM, Sirlin CB, Pinto PS, Jeffrey RB, Stella DL, Casola G. Disproportionate fat stranding: a helpful CT sign in patients with acute abdominal pain. Radiographics. 2004;24(3):703–15.
22. Fernandes T, Oliveira MI, Castro R, Araújo B, Viamonte B, Cunha R. Bowel wall thickening at CT: simplifying the diagnosis. Insights Imaging. 2014;5(2):195–208.
23. Chintapalli KN, Esola CC, Chopra S, Ghiatas AA, Dodd GD. Pericolic mesenteric lymph nodes: an aid in distinguishing diverticulitis from cancer of the colon. AJR Am J Roentgenol. 1997;169(5):1253–5.
24. Shen S-H, Chen J-D, Tiu C-M, Chou Y-H, Chiang J-H, Chang C-Y, et al. Differentiating colonic diverticulitis from colon cancer: the value of computed tomography in the emergency setting. J Chin Med Assoc. 2005;68(9):411–8.
25. Lecleire S, Nahon S, Alatawi A, Antonietti M, Chaput U, Di-Fiore A, et al. Diagnostic impact of routine colonoscopy following acute diverticulitis: a multicenter study in 808 patients and controls. United Eur Gastroenterol J. 2014;2(4):301–6.
26. Strate LL, Naumann CR. The role of colonoscopy and radiological procedures in the management of acute lower intestinal bleeding. Clin Gastroenterol Hepatol. 2010;8(4):333–43. quiz e44.

27. ASGE Standards of Practice Committee, Pasha SF, Shergill A, Acosta RD, Chandrasekhara V, Chathadi KV, et al. The role of endoscopy in the patient with lower GI bleeding. Gastrointest Endosc. 2014;79(6):875–85.
28. Geffroy Y, Rodallec MH, Boulay-Coletta I, Jullès M-C, Fullès M-C, Ridereau-Zins C, et al. Multidetector CT angiography in acute gastrointestinal bleeding: why, when, and how. Radiographics. 2011;31(3):E35–46.
29. Valek V, Husty J. Quality improvement guidelines for transcatheter embolization for acute gastrointestinal nonvariceal hemorrhage. Cardiovasc Intervent Radiol. 2013;36(3):608–12.
30. Jaeckle T, Stuber G, Hoffmann MHK, Jeltsch M, Schmitz BL, Aschoff AJ. Detection and localization of acute upper and lower gastrointestinal (GI) bleeding with arterial phase multi-detector row helical CT. Eur Radiol. 2008;18(7):1406–13.
31. Ernst O, Bulois P, Saint-Drenant S, Leroy C, Paris J-C, Sergent G. Helical CT in acute lower gastrointestinal bleeding. Eur Radiol. 2003;13(1):114–7.
32. Zahid A, Young CJ. Making decisions using radiology in lower GI hemorrhage. Int J Surg. 2016;31:100–3.
33. Tew K, Davies RP, Jadun CK, Kew J. MDCT of acute lower gastrointestinal bleeding. AJR Am J Roentgenol. 2004;182(2):427–30.
34. Kuhle WG, Sheiman RG. Detection of active colonic hemorrhage with use of helical CT: findings in a swine model. Radiology. 2003;228(3):743–52.
35. Dobritz M, Engels H-P, Schneider A, Wieder H, Feussner H, Rummeny EJ, et al. Evaluation of dual-phase multi-detector-row CT for detection of intestinal bleeding using an experimental bowel model. Eur Radiol. 2009;19(4):875–81.
36. Chan V, Tse D, Dixon S, Shrivastava V, Bratby M, Anthony S, et al. Outcome following a negative CT Angiogram for gastrointestinal hemorrhage. Cardiovasc Intervent Radiol. 2015;38(2):329–35.
37. Evangelista PT, Hallisey MJ. Transcatheter embolization for acute lower gastrointestinal hemorrhage. J Vasc Interv Radiol. 2000;11(5):601–6.
38. McArdle CS, Hole DJ. Emergency presentation of colorectal cancer is associated with poor 5-year survival. Br J Surg. 2004;91(5):605–9.
39. Expert Panel on Gastrointestinal Imaging, Fowler KJ, Kaur H, Cash BD, Feig BW, Gage KL, et al. ACR Appropriateness Criteria® pretreatment staging of colorectal cancer. J Am Coll Radiol. 2017;14(5S):S234–44.
40. Floriani I, Torri V, Rulli E, Garavaglia D, Compagnoni A, Salvolini L, et al. Performance of imaging modalities in diagnosis of liver metastases from colorectal cancer: a systematic review and meta-analysis. J Magn Reson Imaging. 2010;31(1):19–31.
41. Polat E, Bostanci EB, Aksoy E, Karaman K, Poyraz NY, Duman U, et al. The impact of PET/CT on the management of hepatic and extra hepatic metastases from gastrointestinal cancers. Eur J Radiol. 2015;84(6):1165–70.
42. Truant S, Huglo D, Hebbar M, Ernst O, Steinling M, Pruvot F-R. Prospective evaluation of the impact of [18F]fluoro-2-deoxy-D-glucose positron emission tomography of resectable colorectal liver metastases. Br J Surg. 2005;92(3):362–9.
43. Halligan S, Altman DG, Taylor SA, Mallett S, Deeks JJ, Bartram CI, et al. CT colonography in the detection of colorectal polyps and cancer: systematic review, meta-analysis, and proposed minimum data set for study level reporting. Radiology. 2005;237(3):893–904.
44. Flor N, Ceretti AP, Mezzanzanica M, Rigamonti P, Peri M, Tresoldi S, et al. Impact of contrast-enhanced computed tomography colonography on laparoscopic surgical planning of colorectal cancer. Abdom Imaging. 2013;38(5):1024–32.

Principles of Colonoscopy for Colorectal Cancer Emergency

6

Federica Gaiani, Franca Patrizi, Iradj Sobhani, and Gian Luigi de'Angelis

Endoscopy plays a fundamental role in the management of colorectal cancer (CRC).

Colonoscopy has been demonstrated to be the most cost-effective method for colorectal cancer screening and diagnosis.

However, despite the number of procedures performed worldwide is increasing and the introduction of screening programs is spreading, approximately 15–30% of CRC patients present as a surgical emergency, the most common causes being obstruction, perforation, or bleeding [1].

In the acute management of CRC, colonoscopy can be helpful in providing a histological diagnosis as well as a therapeutic approach in case of bleeding or obstruction.

6.1 Bleeding Colorectal Cancer

Acute lower gastrointestinal bleeding (LGIB) accounts for about 20% of all gastrointestinal (GI) bleeding [2] and is usually defined as overt bleeding from the GI tract distal to the ligament of Treitz.

F. Gaiani (✉) · G. L. de'Angelis
Gastroenterology and Endoscopy Unit, University Hospital of Parma, University of Parma, Parma, Italy
e-mail: gianluigi.deangelis@unipr.it

F. Patrizi
Gastroenterology and Interventional Endoscopy Unit, AUSL Bologna, Bologna, Italy
e-mail: franca.patrizi@ausl.bologna.it

I. Sobhani
Gastroenterology Department, Henri Mondor Hospital, University Paris-Est CRETEIL (UPEC), Creteil, France
e-mail: iradj.sobhani@aphp.fr

N. de'Angelis et al. (eds.), *Emergency Surgical Management of Colorectal Cancer*, Hot Topics in Acute Care Surgery and Trauma,
https://doi.org/10.1007/978-3-030-06225-5_6

The estimated annual incidence of hospitalization for LGIB is 20/100,000 adults, even though between the third and ninth decades, this rate increased 200-fold [3].

Although most patients with acute LGIB have favorable outcomes, morbidity and mortality are increased in older patients and in those with comorbidities [2].

The usual manifestation of LGIB is hematochezia (maroon or red blood passed per rectum). In rare cases, if the bleeding source is located in the cecum/right colon, the patient can present with melena (black, tarry stools) [2]. Notably, approximately 15% of patients with presumed LGIB are ultimately found to have an upper GI bleeding [4].

Little data are available on the association between CRC and bleeding-related symptoms. Colorectal cancer accounts for up to 17% of all etiologies in patients with LGIB [5–7].

Moreover, a nationwide, population-based, retrospective study showed that 74% of CRC patients presented with bleeding-related symptoms [8].

Although CRC presents more commonly with an occult bleeding [7], overt bleeding has been reported to be common, ranging from 37% to 58% in different studies [8].

The probability of bleeding depends both from characteristics of the neoplasia (vascularization of the neoplastic tissue, proportion of necrotized tissue) and the clinical context, particularly concerning to ongoing treatments.

In 2014, Hreinsson et al. showed that overt and occult bleeders had almost half the odds of non-bleeders to have metastases at diagnosis as bleeding-related symptoms can lead to early diagnostic tests. Overt bleeders were significantly less likely than non-bleeders to have obstructive symptoms, while occult bleeders had a significantly higher frequency of proximal cancer compared with non-bleeders [8].

6.1.1 Clinical Management

The initial assessment of the patient presenting with acute LGIB should include an accurate evaluation of vital signs and physical examination (with rectal examination), a focused medical history, and laboratory testing, in order to establish the entity of bleeding, perform a risk stratification strategy, and define the best timing for diagnostic exams [2].

Medical history should lead through differential diagnosis by the evaluation of bleeding episodes (nature, duration, etc.) and the presence of any associated symptom (abdominal pain, alteration of bowel habits, and weight loss).

Past relevant medical elements include prior abdominal and/or vascular surgery, prior episodes, or known GI bleeding-associated conditions (peptic ulcer disease, diverticular disease, inflammatory bowel disease, or pelvic radiation therapy) [2].

The evaluation of comorbidities is also important to obtain a risk assessment and stratification, which can help in defining the likelihood of an adverse outcome, the level of care, and the timing of colonoscopy.

Particular attention should be paid to pharmacological history, looking for recent or usual administration of drugs which may influence bleeding risk (nonsteroidal anti-inflammatory drugs (NSAIDs), antiplatelet agents, and anticoagulants) [7].

Table 6.1 Risk factors of poor outcome for patients with LGIB

Medical history	Cardiopulmonary, renal, hepatic disease [2, 40, 41]
	Age >60 years [42]
	Smoking [42]
	Aspirin use [40, 41]
	History of diverticulosis or angioectasia [2]
Characteristics of bleeding	Ongoing bleeding (gross blood on initial digital rectal examination and recurrent hematochezia) [2]
	Gross blood on initial rectal exam [43]
	Bright red rectal bleeding [42]
	Bleeding in first 4 h of hospitalization [40, 41]
	Rebleeding [42]
Vital signs and clinical evaluation	Hemodynamic instability at presentation (tachycardia, hypotension, and syncope) [2, 40, 41]
	Systolic blood pressure <100 mmHg [40, 41, 44]
	Altered mental status [44]
	Heart rate >100 b.p.m. [40, 41]
	Abnormal vital signs after 1 h [43]
	Non-tender abdomen [40, 41]
Laboratory tests	Elevated creatinine >150 μM [42]
	Anemia (initial hematocrit ≤35%) [42, 43]
	Prothrombin time >1.2 control [44]

Risk factors of poor outcome include hemodynamic instability at presentation, ongoing bleeding, comorbidities, age >60 years, a history of diverticulosis or angioectasia, an elevated creatinine, and anemia (Table 6.1). Intensive care monitoring should be assured for patients with high-risk features.

At initial evaluation, in the presence of hypovolemia and hemodynamic instability, a prompt resuscitation with intravenous liquids should be ensured.

Laboratory testing should include a complete blood count, serum electrolytes, urea nitrogen and creatinine, coagulation tests, blood type, and cross match.

Some patients will require blood transfusion, depending of entity of bleeding and comorbidities.

There might be the necessity of platelet and fresh frozen plasma transfusions, depending, respectively, on platelet count (might be superior to 50×10^9 /L) and quantity of packed RBCs transfused, according to the trauma literature [9, 10].

LGIB in patients on anticoagulation or antiplatelet agents requires an individualized approach [2].

Overall, a multidisciplinary approach involving prescribing specialist (cardiologist/neurologist), hematologist, and endoscopist is necessary when managing patients on antithrombotic medications.

In case of an acute LGIB and concomitant therapy with vitamin K antagonists (VKA), the decision of performing an acute reversal should be based on the entity and the persistence of bleeding, on the thromboembolic risk, on hemodynamic instability, and on the presence of comorbidities.

Studies on the management of upper GI bleeding recommend that endoscopy should not be postponed to correct coagulopathy in patients with a INR ≤ 2.5 and serious GI bleeding [11]. Moreover, a modest elevation in INR (1.5–2.7) does not seem to increase the risk of rebleeding after endoscopic hemostasis [12, 13].

Regarding the acute reversal of anticoagulation, treatment options depend on clinical setting.

All patients with major bleeding and INR > 5 should have vitamin K administered and VKA stopped. In critical actively bleeding patients with persistent or intermittent hemodynamic instability, coagulation factors should be administered even in case of therapeutic INR ranges. The 4-factor prothrombin complex concentrate (PCC) (or the 3-factor PCC if the 4F is not available) rather than fresh frozen plasma (FFP) should be used. Infusion of vitamin K (5–10 mg iv infusion over 30 min) is recommended [11].

On the other hand, in case of minor GI bleeding not causing anemia, there is no need for urgent anticoagulation reversal [14] and oral or low-dose intravenous vitamin K administration.

Direct oral anticoagulants (DOACs), including dabigatran, rivaroxaban, edoxaban, and apixaban, have to be carefully managed in case of active bleeding. It is important to determine the time of last DOAC intake and measure the value of creatinine clearance to predict the half-life time of the drug, together with complete count and clotting screen. In the absence of renal or hepatic failure, DOAC's clearance and subsequent loss of efficacy are rapid and predictable, occurring gradually over 12–24 h. For this reason, in the presence of a significant bleeding without hemodynamic compromise, temporary drug withdrawal may be the only therapeutic measure associated to fluid replacement to maintain diuresis. In this situation, endoscopy may be differed for 12–24 h. In case of severe bleeding, DOACs should be stopped, and general resuscitation interventions should be promptly started. Hemodialysis for clearing dabigatran, gastric lavage in case of recent overdose of DOACs, or off-label use of PCC might be considered in overt GI bleeding with shock. In this last case, emergency endoscopy may be appropriate. A reversal agent is available for dabigatran (idarucizumab), and further molecules for the other DOACs are under evaluation for FDA approval [14].

For patients on antiplatelet agents with life-threating or serious GI bleeding, options include stopping these agents and/or administration of platelets. It is recommended to consult a cardiologist before stopping antiplatelet agents in case of significant bleeding in patients with recent (within 90 days) acute coronary syndrome or with recently placed intracoronary stent (within 1 year for drug-eluting intracoronary stent or within 30 days for a bare metal stent placement) [10].

6.1.2 Aim and Timing of Colonoscopy

The role of colonoscopy in the management of acute LGIB is crucial not only for a diagnostic purpose (with histological evaluation) but also for localizing the source of bleeding and attempting hemostasis. Identifying the source of bleeding in overt LGIB poses a diagnostic challenge [7].

During endoscopic evaluation, a differential diagnosis between CRC and other common causes of acute severe LGIB (diverticulosis, ischemic colitis, inflammatory bowel disease, vascular ectasia, polyps or post-polypectomy bleeding, hemorrhoids) is mandatory [2].

Every effort should be made during colonoscopy to accurately inspect the colonic mucosa, with terminal ileum intubation and use of water-jet irrigation device to facilitate the removal of residual material.

The diagnostic yield of colonoscopy in these patients ranges from 48% to 90% [15, 16].

In high-risk patients with signs and symptoms on ongoing bleeding, after resuscitation, it is recommended to perform an urgent (within 12–24 h of admission) colonoscopy. This approach is safe and may facilitate the identification and treatment of bleeding lesions [17].

Bowel preparation for urgent colonoscopy is recommended (4–6 L of polyethylene glycol solution in 3–4 h) to facilitate the cecal intubation rate [17]. Urgent colonoscopy should be performed within 1–2 h of preparation completion.

For patients remaining unstable after resuscitation and those intolerant to colonoscopy preparation (even via nasogastric tube), computed tomographic angiography as a diagnostic test should be considered (with subsequent radiographic intervention if necessary).

A surgical consultation should be requested, as surgery for acute LGIB can be considered as a "rescue" option after failure of endoscopic and radiological treatments: in any case, every effort should be attempted to localize the source of bleeding before surgical resection.

In hemodynamically stable patients at presentation with low-risk clinical features and no serious comorbidities or in those with high-risk clinical features without signs or symptoms of ongoing bleeding, nonurgent (next available) colonoscopy should be performed after adequate colonic purge [2, 18].

It is important to underline that endoscopic hemostasis in CRC is rarely required because bleeding is usually limited and slow, resulting from erosion of the mucosal surface [7]; moreover, hemorrhage is generally diffuse from the neoplastic mass, and hemostasis is not durable.

For these reasons, patients are usually treated with supportive medical and surgical care. Nevertheless, in some rare cases, bleeding in CRC may result in a brisk hemorrhage, and endoscopic treatment may be attempted [3].

The therapeutic role of endoscopy is to buy time for the surgeon and oncologist to decide on further management.

Different endoscopic hemostatic techniques have been demonstrated to be safe and effective in the setting of GI bleeding, evaluated by several randomized controlled studies and meta-analyses addressed to focus on hemostatic treatment for the upper GI tract. So far, for acute LGIB, endoscopic treatments have only been investigated in non-randomized or retrospective cohort studies or described in case reports. Generally speaking, the possible options of treatment include injection therapy, contact thermal therapies (bipolar/multipolar electrocoagulation, heat probe), noncontact thermal therapy (argon plasma coagulation APC), band ligation, mechanical therapy with metallic clips, and spraying of topical hemostatic agents [2].

The endoscopist has to select the best modality of hemostasis depending on the characteristics and localization of the source of bleeding and on his experience with the different endoscopic devices.

Contact thermal therapy and endoscopic clip placement are the preferred hemostatic techniques in case of well-localized bleeding from a visible vessel, a rare manifestation in CRC [7, 19].

APC has been described as a preferred therapy in bleeding CRC as this technique allows a uniform cauterization of limited depth (approximately 3 mm) in a relatively large area [20].

An emerging endoscopic treatment includes hemostatic sprays/powders, which are applied through the working channel of the endoscope and may control actively bleeding lesions by creating a mechanical barrier layer upon bleeding mucosa [21].

Theoretically, hemostatic powders are a good alternative to APC as they are able to cover the whole surface area of the tumor. A few cases have been described in the literature, with very good success rate and no adverse event reported [22].

6.2 Obstructive Colorectal Cancer

Colorectal cancer may present with colonic obstruction in up to 15–20% of cases [23]. In this emergency setting, endoscopy may be required with several aims.

Firstly, colonoscopy may be necessary to determine the etiology of obstruction and, eventually, to provide tissue for diagnosis. Secondly, through endoscopy, it is possible to direct surgical resection by tattooing the pathological colonic segment.

Last, but not least, endoscopic treatment may be applied in specific clinical situations.

In case of colonic obstruction, it is necessary to take into account all the possible underlying causes.

Among malignant causes, colorectal cancer is responsible for as much as three-fourths of all malignant colonic obstruction. With regard to the location, the majority of colonic obstructing adenocarcinomas arise in the left colon, most commonly in the sigmoid colon [2].

Other malignant causes are metastatic cancer and locally advanced pelvic tumors.

Benign causes include volvulus, stenotic Crohn's disease, diverticulitis, anastomotic strictures, radiation injury, ischemia, foreign bodies, and intussusception.

6.2.1 Clinical Management

From a clinical point of view, patients with colonic obstruction present with abdominal pain of variable intensity and localization, associated to abdominal distension. Nausea or vomiting may be present.

When peritoneal signs with fever and guarding/rebound tenderness are present, surgical consultation should not be delayed [24] for suspected complete colonic obstruction or gangrenous bowel. In these cases, endoscopy is contraindicated due to the high risk of perforation.

After clinical examination and blood tests to detect an eventual septic status, an upright or decubitus plain abdominal radiograph is usually performed. If the site of occlusion is located in the large bowel, the colonic diameter is dilated with air-fluid levels proximal to the obstructing site.

In this clinical setting, it is recommended absolute bowel rest, intravenous hydration, electrolyte correction, placement of a nasogastric tube for proximal gut decompression, and intravenous broad-spectrum antibiotics in septic patients.

After X-ray confirmation of large bowel obstruction, computed tomography (CT) images should be performed to provide information about site and etiology of obstructing disease.

Accordingly, with ESGE guidelines, a contrast-enhanced CT scan is recommended as the primary diagnostic tool when malignant colonic obstruction is suspected, with sensitivity and specificity, respectively, of 96% and 93%. Moreover, CT scan provides adequate information about etiology in about 81% of cases [25, 26].

Once the diagnosis of colonic obstruction is confirmed by clinical and radiological examinations, in the absence of specific contraindications, endoscopy may be performed for a diagnostic and therapeutic purpose.

Endoscopic exploration of the left colon in an emergency setting is usually feasible, as it requires only cleansing enemas for preparation, whereas a complete colonoscopy may be more challenging because it requires a colonoscopy bowel preparation in patients with high risk of perforation [24].

6.2.2 Endoscopic Treatment of Colonic Obstruction

Usually, malignant colonic obstruction is treated by conventional emergency surgery which includes resection or diversion procedures [24]. Nevertheless, these interventions are associated with considerable mortality and morbidity rates, respectively, of 15–20% and 40–50% [27]. Moreover, the quality of life of these patients can be permanently impacted because a considerable proportion of ostomies created in urgency cannot be reversed [28].

In this context, endoscopy has to be considered an alternative solution in selected cases for a less invasive, either definitive or temporary treatment of the obstruction.

At present, the placement of self-expanding metallic stents (SEMS) is the endoscopic technique of choice for the treatment of malignant obstruction, both as bridge to surgery and for palliation.

Tumor debulking applying endoscopic laser therapy, APC and snare tissue resection with or without APC have been used in selected patients unwilling and/or unfit for surgery. However, these techniques are not standardized, and their effectiveness has been reported for a limited time and in small case series [24, 29].

Abdominal gas decompression with endoscopic placement of a transanal tube can improve the clinical condition of obstruction. Nevertheless, this technique is not routinely used because of several limitations, including the frequent tube dysfunction and obstruction and the inability to use the device indefinitely for palliation [24].

6.2.3 Self-Expanding Metallic Stents (SEMS)

Colonic stent placement is indicated only in the presence of obstructive symptoms due to left-sided (distal to splenic flexure) colonic cancer diagnosed at endoscopy or CT scan [25].

Stenting is not recommended in the absence of symptoms because of the increasing complication rate without appreciable benefits [3].

Evidence of perforation is the only absolute contraindication for colonic stenting. It is also reported a lower success rate of colonic stenting in the presence of peritoneal carcinomatosis and rectal tumor located at less than 5–10 cm from the anal verge [30], as frequently complicates with pain, tenesmus, incontinence, and stent migration.

The main complications of SEMS placement are perforation (0–12.8%), stent failure (0–11.7%), stent migration (0–4.9%), re-obstruction, pain, and bleeding.

Regarding proximal colonic obstruction, emergency resection is considered to be the treatment of choice [26], even though SEMS may be the treatment of choice when an extracolonic malignant obstruction is present. In this situation, although there is a lower success rate of stenting compared to primary colonic obstructing malignancies, it is accepted a less invasive palliative procedure to avoid surgery in patients who usually have a short survival [31].

A multidisciplinary evaluation (surgeon, endoscopist, and oncologist) is advocated before SEMS placement to define the best approach for each different clinical setting.

Colonic stenting should be performed in selected high-volume centers by experienced endoscopists who are skilled in the use of fluoroscopy, since usually stents are inserted through the endoscope with a combined technique (endoscopy and fluoroscopy) (Fig. 6.1).

Considering clinical indications, it is well established that colonic stenting is the emergency procedure of choice as a bridge to elective surgery in patients with an increased risk of postoperative mortality (age ≥70 years and/or ASA status ≥3) [25] and symptomatic left-sided colonic obstruction.

Some studies demonstrated that SEMS placement results in increased primary anastomosis rate, reduced stoma creation rate, and decreased complication rate compared to emergency surgery [32, 33].

Anyway, several points are still debated about outcomes of SEMS placement. In particular, oncological safety, long-term outcomes, and indications for young patients and fit for surgery have to be considered [25, 34].

Although SEMS allow colonic decompression without the morbidity and mortality of emergency surgery, this has to be balanced with the oncological outcomes in patients with a curable colonic cancer.

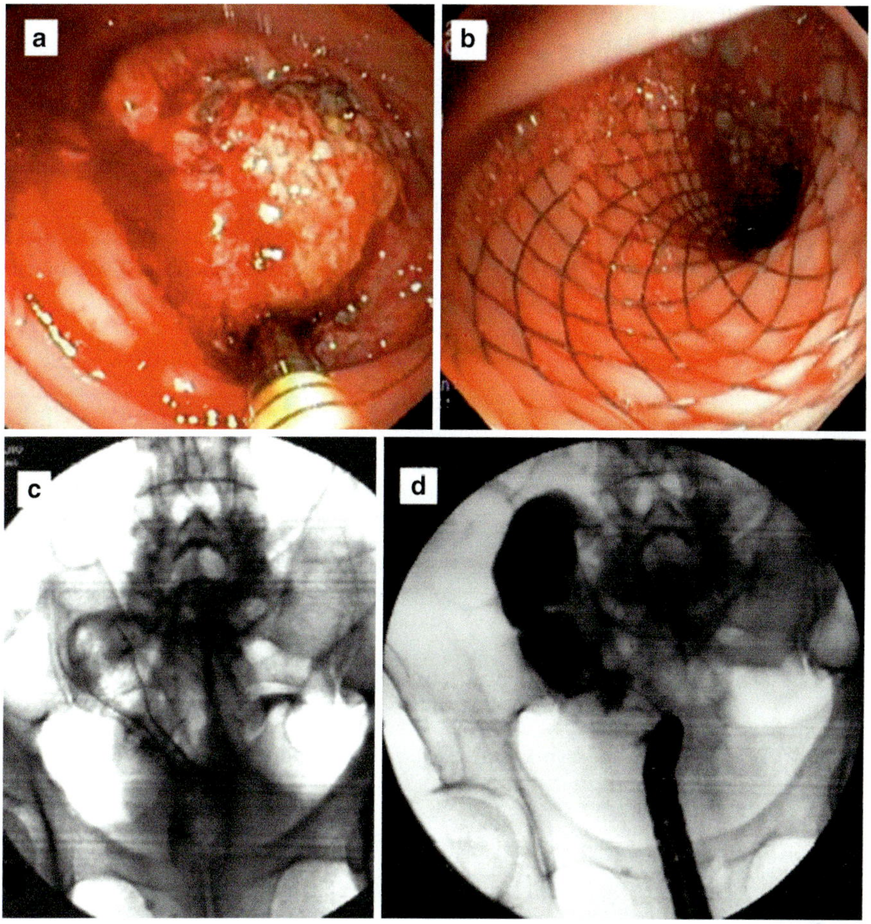

Fig. 6.1 (**a**) Obstructing cancer of the sigmoid colon; insertion of a through-the-scope SEMS. (**b**) SEMS placement, endoscopic view. (**c**) SEMS placement, fluoroscopic view. (**d**) Fluoroscopic control with contrast injection after SEMS placement

SEMS placement as a bridge to elective surgery does not seem to have effect on perioperative mortality and long-term survival compared to emergency surgery. On the other hand, there is evidence [35] of a higher disease recurrence rate in SEMS as bridge-to-surgery patients, together with a lower 5-year overall survival and increased cancer-related mortality. These poor outcomes are worsened by SEMS-related perforation.

Overall, SEMS placement as a bridge-to-surgery is not recommended as a standard treatment for fit-for-surgery potentially curable patients with left-sided malignant colonic obstruction [3, 10].

In high surgical risk patients, elective surgery should be performed within 10 days after stenting as bridge-to-surgery. Moreover, preoperative CT colonography or colonoscopy through the stent are appropriate tools to examine the colon proximal to the obstructing malignancy in order to exclude synchronous tumors.

With regard to the palliative setting, SEMS placement is recommended as the technique of choice, allowing a significant reduction of the hospital stay, complication rate, and need of colostomy [32, 36]. The technical success of stent placement has demonstrated to range between 88% and 100% [37]. Moreover, SEMS placement guarantees an earlier start of chemotherapy compared to surgery with no significant difference in the overall morbidity rate [38].

SEMS placement is not recommended in patients who are being treated or considered for further treatment with antiangiogenic drugs (e.g., bevacizumab), as these treatments have been reported to increase the risk of perforation after SEMS placement. On the other hand, chemotherapeutics different from antiangiogenic agents can be safely used in patients after palliative stenting [39].

References

1. Anantha RV, Brackstone M, Parry N, Leslie K. An acute care surgery service expedites the treatment of emergency colorectal cancer: a retrospective case-control study. World J Emerg Surg. 2014;9(1):19.
2. Strate LL, Gralnek IM. ACG clinical guideline: management of patients with acute lower gastrointestinal bleeding. Am J Gastroenterol. 2016;111(5):755.
3. Barnett A, Cedar A, Siddiqui F, Herzig D, Fowlkes E, Thomas CR Jr. Colorectal cancer emergencies. J Gastrointest Cancer. 2013;44(2):132–42.
4. Laine L, Shah A. Randomized trial of urgent vs. elective colonoscopy in patients hospitalized with lower GI bleeding. Am J Gastroenterol. 2010;105(12):2636–41. quiz 42.
5. Hreinsson JP, Gumundsson S, Kalaitzakis E, Bjornsson ES. Lower gastrointestinal bleeding: incidence, etiology, and outcomes in a population-based setting. Eur J Gastroenterol Hepatol. 2013;25(1):37–43.
6. Committee ASoP, Gurudu SR, Bruining DH, Acosta RD, Eloubeidi MA, Faulx AL, et al. The role of endoscopy in the management of suspected small-bowel bleeding. Gastrointest Endosc. 2017;85(1):22–31.
7. Committee ASoP, Pasha SF, Shergill A, Acosta RD, Chandrasekhara V, Chathadi KV, et al. The role of endoscopy in the patient with lower GI bleeding. Gastrointest Endosc. 2014;79(6):875–85.
8. Hreinsson JP, Jonasson JG, Bjornsson ES. Bleeding-related symptoms in colorectal cancer: a 4-year nationwide population-based study. Aliment Pharmacol Ther. 2014;39(1):77–84.
9. Shaz BH, Dente CJ, Nicholas J, MacLeod JB, Young AN, Easley K, et al. Increased number of coagulation products in relationship to red blood cell products transfused improves mortality in trauma patients. Transfusion. 2010;50(2):493–500.
10. Dzik WH, Blajchman MA, Fergusson D, Hameed M, Henry B, Kirkpatrick AW, et al. Clinical review: Canadian National Advisory Committee on Blood and Blood Products--Massive transfusion consensus conference 2011: report of the panel. Crit Care. 2011;15(6):242.
11. Barkun AN, Bardou M, Kuipers EJ, Sung J, Hunt RH, Martel M, et al. International consensus recommendations on the management of patients with nonvariceal upper gastrointestinal bleeding. Ann Intern Med. 2010;152(2):101–13.
12. Shingina A, Barkun AN, Razzaghi A, Martel M, Bardou M, Gralnek I, et al. Systematic review: the presenting international normalised ratio (INR) as a predictor of outcome in patients with upper nonvariceal gastrointestinal bleeding. Aliment Pharmacol Ther. 2011;33(9):1010–8.
13. Rubin TA, Murdoch M, Nelson DB. Acute GI bleeding in the setting of supratherapeutic international normalized ratio in patients taking warfarin: endoscopic diagnosis, clinical management, and outcomes. Gastrointest Endosc. 2003;58(3):369–73.

14. Radaelli F, Dentali F, Repici A, Amato A, Paggi S, Rondonotti E, et al. Management of anticoagulation in patients with acute gastrointestinal bleeding. Dig Liver Dis. 2015;47(8):621–7.
15. Strate LL, Syngal S. Timing of colonoscopy: impact on length of hospital stay in patients with acute lower intestinal bleeding. Am J Gastroenterol. 2003;98(2):317–22.
16. Davila RE, Rajan E, Adler DG, Egan J, Hirota WK, Leighton JA, et al. ASGE Guideline: the role of endoscopy in the patient with lower-GI bleeding. Gastrointest Endosc. 2005;62(5):656–60.
17. Hassan C, Bretthauer M, Kaminski MF, Polkowski M, Rembacken B, Saunders B, et al. Bowel preparation for colonoscopy: European Society of Gastrointestinal Endoscopy (ESGE) guideline. Endoscopy. 2013;45(2):142–50.
18. Romano C, Oliva S, Martellossi S, Miele E, Arrigo S, Graziani MG, et al. Pediatric gastrointestinal bleeding: perspectives from the Italian Society of Pediatric Gastroenterology. World J Gastroenterol. 2017;23(8):1328–37.
19. Kaltenbach T, Watson R, Shah J, Friedland S, Sato T, Shergill A, et al. Colonoscopy with clipping is useful in the diagnosis and treatment of diverticular bleeding. Clin Gastroenterol Hepatol. 2012;10(2):131–7.
20. Nozoe Y, Araki Y, Fukushima H, Shirouzu K. A case of argon plasma coagulation therapy for hemorrhagic rectal tumor in a highly aged patient. Kurume Med J. 2004;51(2):159–61.
21. Martin S, Armstrong A. An unusual haemorrhagic complication of an anastomotic leak and a novel method of controlling the haemorrhage. Ann R Coll Surg Engl. 2017;99(3):e116–e9.
22. Mourad FH, Leong RW. Role of hemostatic powders in the management of lower gastrointestinal bleeding: a review. J Gastroenterol Hepatol. 2018;33:1445.
23. Billingsley KG, Morris AM, Dominitz JA, Matthews B, Dobie S, Barlow W, et al. Surgeon and hospital characteristics as predictors of major adverse outcomes following colon cancer surgery: understanding the volume-outcome relationship. Arch Surg. 2007;142(1):23–31. discussion 2.
24. Committee ASoP, Harrison ME, Anderson MA, Appalaneni V, Banerjee S, Ben-Menachem T, et al. The role of endoscopy in the management of patients with known and suspected colonic obstruction and pseudo-obstruction. Gastrointest Endosc. 2010;71(4):669–79.
25. van Hooft JE, van Halsema EE, Vanbiervliet G, Beets-Tan RG, DeWitt JM, Donnellan F, et al. Self-expandable metal stents for obstructing colonic and extracolonic cancer: European Society of Gastrointestinal Endoscopy (ESGE) Clinical Guideline. Gastrointest Endosc. 2014;80(5):747–61.e1–75.
26. Frago R, Ramirez E, Millan M, Kreisler E, del Valle E, Biondo S. Current management of acute malignant large bowel obstruction: a systematic review. Am J Surg. 2014;207(1):127–38.
27. Tekkis PP, Kinsman R, Thompson MR, Stamatakis JD. Association of Coloproctology of Great Britain I. The Association of Coloproctology of Great Britain and Ireland study of large bowel obstruction caused by colorectal cancer. Ann Surg. 2004;240(1):76–81.
28. Martinez-Santos C, Lobato RF, Fradejas JM, Pinto I, Ortega-Deballon P, Moreno-Azcoita M. Self-expandable stent before elective surgery vs. emergency surgery for the treatment of malignant colorectal obstructions: comparison of primary anastomosis and morbidity rates. Dis Colon Rectum. 2002;45(3):401–6.
29. Solecki R, Zajac A, Richter P, Szura M. Bifocal esophageal and rectal cancer palliatively treated with argon plasma coagulation. Surg Endosc. 2004;18(2):346.
30. Yoon JY, Jung YS, Hong SP, Kim TI, Kim WH, Cheon JH. Clinical outcomes and risk factors for technical and clinical failures of self-expandable metal stent insertion for malignant colorectal obstruction. Gastrointest Endosc. 2011;74(4):858–68.
31. Trompetas V, Saunders M, Gossage J, Anderson H. Shortcomings in colonic stenting to palliate large bowel obstruction from extracolonic malignancies. Int J Colorectal Dis. 2010;25(7):851–4.
32. Zhang Y, Shi J, Shi B, Song CY, Xie WF, Chen YX. Self-expanding metallic stent as a bridge to surgery versus emergency surgery for obstructive colorectal cancer: a meta-analysis. Surg Endosc. 2012;26(1):110–9.

33. Lee JH, Yoon JY, Park SJ, Hong SP, Kim TI, Kim WH, et al. The learning curve for colorectal stent insertion for the treatment of malignant colorectal obstruction. Gut Liver. 2012;6(3):328–33.
34. Di Saverio S, Birindelli A, Segalini E, Novello M, Larocca A, Ferrara F, et al. "To stent or not to stent?": immediate emergency surgery with laparoscopic radical colectomy with CME and primary anastomosis is feasible for obstructing left colon carcinoma. Surg Endosc. 2018;32(4):2151–5.
35. Sabbagh C, Browet F, Diouf M, Cosse C, Brehant O, Bartoli E, et al. Is stenting as "a bridge to surgery" an oncologically safe strategy for the management of acute, left-sided, malignant, colonic obstruction? A comparative study with a propensity score analysis. Ann Surg. 2013;258(1):107–15.
36. Tilney HS, Lovegrove RE, Purkayastha S, Sains PS, Weston-Petrides GK, Darzi AW, et al. Comparison of colonic stenting and open surgery for malignant large bowel obstruction. Surg Endosc. 2007;21(2):225–33.
37. Fiori E, Lamazza A, De Cesare A, Bononi M, Volpino P, Schillaci A, et al. Palliative management of malignant rectosigmoidal obstruction. Colostomy vs. endoscopic stenting. A randomized prospective trial. Anticancer Res. 2004;24(1):265–8.
38. Zhao XD, Cai BB, Cao RS, Shi RH. Palliative treatment for incurable malignant colorectal obstructions: a meta-analysis. World J Gastroenterol. 2013;19(33):5565–74.
39. van Halsema EE, van Hooft JE, Small AJ, Baron TH, Garcia-Cano J, Cheon JH, et al. Perforation in colorectal stenting: a meta-analysis and a search for risk factors. Gastrointest Endosc. 2014;79(6):970–82.e7. quiz 83.e2, 83.e5.
40. Strate LL, Orav EJ, Syngal S. Early predictors of severity in acute lower intestinal tract bleeding. Arch Intern Med. 2003;163(7):838–43.
41. Strate LL, Saltzman JR, Ookubo R, Mutinga ML, Syngal S. Validation of a clinical prediction rule for severe acute lower intestinal bleeding. Am J Gastroenterol. 2005;100(8):1821–7.
42. Newman J, Fitzgerald JE, Gupta S, von Roon AC, Sigurdsson HH, Allen-Mersh TG. Outcome predictors in acute surgical admissions for lower gastrointestinal bleeding. Colorectal Dis. 2012;14(8):1020–6.
43. Velayos FS, Williamson A, Sousa KH, Lung E, Bostrom A, Weber EJ, et al. Early predictors of severe lower gastrointestinal bleeding and adverse outcomes: a prospective study. Clin Gastroenterol Hepatol. 2004;2(6):485–90.
44. Kollef MH, O'Brien JD, Zuckerman GR, Shannon W. BLEED: a classification tool to predict outcomes in patients with acute upper and lower gastrointestinal hemorrhage. Crit Care Med. 1997;25(7):1125–32.

Management of Colonoscopy Complications

7

Osvaldo Chiara, Stefania Cimbanassi, and Arianna Birindelli

7.1 Introduction

Colonoscopy is widely performed for diagnosis and treatment of large bowel diseases and for colorectal cancer screening in developed countries.

Colonoscopy is generally safe and well tolerated, and major complications are uncommon. A systematic review including 57,742 screening colonoscopies from 12 studies showed 162 (0.28%) serious adverse events [1]. Bleeding and perforation more commonly occur following interventional colonoscopy, with a sevenfold increased risk after polypectomy [2].

Complications after colonoscopy range from asymptomatic and self-limiting to severe conditions which require prompt diagnosis and treatment, to avoid serious and life-threatening consequences. In this chapter, medical and surgical complications after colonoscopy were reviewed, with a focus on diagnostic pathway and therapeutic approach.

O. Chiara (✉)
Surgery, University of Milano, Milano, Italy

General Surgery and Trauma Team Division, ASST Niguarda Hospital Milano, Milano, Italy
e-mail: osvaldo.chiara@ospedaleniguarda.it, osvaldo.chiara@unimi.it

S. Cimbanassi
General Surgery and Trauma Team Division, ASST Niguarda Hospital Milano, Milano, Italy
e-mail: stefania.cimbanassi@ospedaleniguarda.it

A. Birindelli
Department of Surgery, University of Bologna, Bologna, Italy

N. de'Angelis et al. (eds.), *Emergency Surgical Management of Colorectal Cancer*,
Hot Topics in Acute Care Surgery and Trauma,
https://doi.org/10.1007/978-3-030-06225-5_7

7.2 Miscellaneous of Cardiopulmonary Adverse Events After Colonoscopy

Dehydration due to bowel preparation or pathologic conditions (e.g., bowel obstruction) is a risk factor for hypotension and cardiovascular adverse events during and after sedation [3].

A painful endoscopy may cause patient anxiety inducing cardiovascular events such as tachycardia, bradycardia, hypotension, or hypertension.

In predisposed patients, large bowel insufflation can trigger vasovagal reactions with fluctuations in systemic blood pressure and heart rate. In addition, patients affected by pulmonary chronic diseases, obesity, hypertension, coronary artery disease, and advanced age show an increased risk of cardiovascular adverse events, such as arrhythmias, hyper-hypotension, and myocardial ischemia during colonoscopy, with an incidence between 0.2% and 0.5% [4].

As far as the respiratory complications are concerned, excessive sedation may cause prolonged hypoxia, hypercapnia, hypotension, and aspiration. It was demonstrated that the association between midazolam and opioids increases the risk of hypoxia, as compared to the use of midazolam alone [5]. Therefore, in patients with risk factors, this association should be avoided as much as possible, preferring gaseous analgesia (nitrous oxide) [3] or minimum effective dose of opioids.

All patients receiving sedation should be monitored with at least pulse oximetry and noninvasive blood pressure. Prolonged endoscopic procedures cause patient discomfort and deep sedation with support of anesthesiologist is advisable.

In case of cardiovascular or respiratory complications, the procedure should be immediately discontinued and appropriate treatment given.

7.3 Perforation

7.3.1 Mechanism

Iatrogenic colonic perforation (ICP) is the most worrying complication after colonoscopy. It can occur either in diagnostic or therapeutic procedures. During diagnostic or screening procedures, it may be caused by an excessive pneumatic distension (barotrauma) or by the direct mechanical damage to the colonic wall caused by the tip or the side of the endoscope as it is pushed forward. In these cases, perforation occurs generally during the procedure itself, and it is usually larger than 2 cm. Rarely, a muscular tear may evolve in a full-thickness perforation in the following days. In interventional endoscopies (e.g., polypectomies), the mechanism of perforation can be the same described for diagnostic procedures, or due to thermal/electrical injury of the colonic wall. In the latter case, perforation and symptoms are commonly 24–72 h delayed [6]. If the colonic wall damage is full-thickness, usually it leads to a diffuse peritonitis, while if it is partial-thickness, the perforation can be concealed and confined by surrounding tissues with the development of a pericolic abscess.

7.3.2 Incidence

A recent study [7] including 56,882 colonoscopies reported an incidence of full-thickness large bowel perforation of 0.07% (40 cases). A Spanish study reported an incidence of ICP of 0.09% (15 out of 16,285) [8], while a Dutch review [9] of 30,366 endoscopic procedures of the colon reported ICP in 35 patients (0.12%). In an overview of studies published from 2001 to 2009 analyzing 969,913 colonoscopies [10], incidence of ICP ranged from 0.032 to 0.14.

Higher risk of ICP has been associated with low-volume practice, female sex (greater colonic length, more mobile transverse colon), age over 75 years old (four-to sixfold rise, reduced wall strength), diverticular disease, previous abdominal surgery (especially pelvic), colonic obstruction (risk of over-insufflation), colonoscopy when compared to sigmoidoscopy (2–4 times greater), and multiple comorbidities (diabetes mellitus, chronic pulmonary disease, congestive heart failure, myocardial infarction, cerebrovascular disease, peripheral vascular disease, renal insufficiency, liver disease, and dementia). According to Anderson et al., trainees have a nonsignificant higher incidence of ICP compared with experienced endoscopist [11].

Therapeutic colonoscopies are generally at higher risk for ICP, with an incidence of 0.17% [7]. In particular, polypectomy for polyps larger than 10 mm in the right colon or 20 mm in the left, multiple polypectomies, the use of argon plasma coagulation, endoscopic mucosal resection (EMR), and endoscopic submucosal dissection (ESD) for colorectal neoplasia have been found to have an increased risk of ICP [12]. In fact, according to a meta-analysis of four Japanese studies, procedure-related complications occurred in 5.8% of EMR and 8.4% of ESD [13]. In a recent meta-analysis, stenting of either benign or neoplastic strictures has been associated with 7.4% of ICPs: type of stent, benign etiology and Crohn disease, bevacizumab therapy, and re-dilation have been identified as risk factors [14]. Balloon dilatation of rectal anastomotic strictures has demonstrated an ICP rate of 1.1% [15].

7.3.3 Diagnosis

The diagnosis of ICP can be immediate or delayed, also in relation to the mechanism of perforation. In a retrospective evaluation of ICPs in a single institution [11], 68% were identified on the day of endoscopy, 23% on day 1 or 2 after endoscopy, and 9% after 2 weeks from the procedure. The results of a survey of 30,336 colonoscopies showed an average of 0.36 days delay in diagnostic endoscopies, as compared with 1.5 days delay after therapeutic procedures [9].

The diagnosis of ICP is based on clinical, laboratory, and radiologic findings. Sometimes, diagnosis of ICP derives from the direct visualization of the colonic defect or intraperitoneal structures during endoscopy [16], while other ICP patients develop symptoms hours after the endoscopy. In two large clinical series, the most consistent symptoms were abdominal pain (from 74% to 95%), guarding/rebound tenderness with localized or diffuse peritonitis (82.5%), tachycardia (62.5%), leukocytosis (40%), fever (38%), rectal bleeding (15%), and abdominal distension only (6.6%). A small number of patients with ICP (5%) remained asymptomatic. An unusual clinical sign is delayed subcutaneous emphysema and ongoing necrotizing infection of the abdominal wall [7, 8].

Perforations of intraperitoneal segments of the colon (cecum, transverse colon, sigmoid colon) more often lead to free intraperitoneal fluid and air (large amount in the case of barotrauma from over-insufflation), whereas perforations of the ascending, descending colon and rectum or wall injuries contained in supplying mesentery result in retroperitoneal air. Mixed situations are possible if perforation is in between an intra- and extraperitoneal area [17]. When an ICP is clinically suspected, imaging investigations can greatly contribute to the diagnosis. Upright plain abdominal radiographs can detect free peritoneal air, but they are insensitive to the presence of free fluid. CT scan, instead, is much more effective in the diagnosis of extra-luminal air [16]. It can detect even small amounts of both free intraperitoneal air and fluid, pointing out foci of gas congregating near the perforation site. In retroperitoneal perforations, CT scan shows air tracking along mesenteric and retroperitoneal fascial planes, sometimes up to the mediastinum, the neck, and the abdominal or chest wall. In some cases, pneumatosis of the colonic wall or of the mesenteric and portal venous system can be identified. Double contrast CT (intravenous and rectal) may be useful to detect concealed or sealed-off perforations which are eligible for nonoperative management [18].

7.3.4 Treatment

According to the timing of diagnosis and the extent of peritonitis, the management of ICP includes endoscopic repair, nonoperative management, or emergency surgery, as defined in recent WSES guidelines [19]. All patients with ICP should obtain a surgical consultation and should be admitted to a surgical ward with a 24/7 emergency theater availability, since an initial success of endoscopic or nonoperative treatment does not rule out the need for delayed surgery [20].

Endoscopic repair is possible in patients with adequate preparation, when the recognition occurs intra-procedurally or within 4 h and in the presence of adequate endoscopic skills and equipment. Nowadays, many endoscopic devices are available for closure of parietal defects. Through-the-scope (TTS) clips or over-the-scope (OTSC) clips are both effective to close small defects (<1 cm for TTS and <2 cm for OTSC) [21, 22]. A recent and promising option for larger defects is the overstitch endoscopic suturing device (Apollo Endosurgery, Austin, TX, USA) [23]. Finally, partially or fully covered stents could potentially close a colonic perforation, but data about this option are not available. In general, the most important issue about endoscopic repair of ICP is the difficulty to evaluate the completeness of the closure. A persistent leak may lead to intra-abdominal abscesses or fecal peritonitis [24]. A standard radiologic or CT scan control with contrast enema after endoscopic closure is performed in some institutions, but a negative test cannot exclude a delayed leak.

Nonoperative management (NOM) of ICP is appropriate in selected patients with adequate bowel preparation, free air without free fluid, localized pain without fever, and hemodynamic stability. NOM is usually feasible in small, sealed-off perforations after a therapeutic colonoscopy, when the clinical conditions are fair and CT scan confirms the absence of a diffuse peritonitis [25]. The so-called post-polypectomy electrocoagulation syndrome is a clinical condition characterized by fever, laboratory inflammatory signs, and localized pain, it is due to a full-thickness burn of colon wall by electrocoagulation, and it can be usually managed conservatively. Every time a NOM strategy has been chosen, a regular clinical and laboratory (WBC, CRP, PCT) follow-up is required, with 2–6 days bowel rest and wide-spectrum antibiotic therapy. In cases of clinical or laboratory worsening, a CT scan is recommended. If this confirms the progression of the peritonitis, with increase of free air and fluid, surgery becomes mandatory. Of note, a delayed surgery after a period of NOM usually requires more extensive and challenging procedures and is associated with a less favorable outcome [16].

Emergency surgical management of ICP is indicated when the patient presents clinical or radiological signs of diffuse peritonitis, with severe systemic inflammation or sepsis or in case of a failed endoscopic treatment or NOM.

The choice of the surgical technique, laparoscopy or laparotomy, is left to the surgeon discretion, according to individual skills and intraoperative findings. Surgical options range from direct suture, wedge resection, colonic resection with or without primary anastomosis or stoma, and colostomy by exteriorization of the perforation. In ICP in patients with colonic carcinoma, surgery must follow the principles of oncologic surgery. Extent of injury, perfusion conditions on its edges, grade of contamination, and hemodynamic stability of the patient are the most important factors for the choice of the most appropriate surgical technique [19, 26]. Nowadays, laparoscopy may be considered the first-line approach for the surgical management of ICP [19]. Depending on the surgeon's skill, the definitive surgical procedure (simple suture, wedge resection, segmental resection with anastomosis or stoma, exteriorization of the perforation) may be all performed laparoscopically. In general, laparoscopic treatment of ICP is associated with shorter hospital length of stay and fewer postoperative complications [27–29]. Open surgery is mandatory in hemodynamically unstable patients and advisable when extensive adhesions for multiple previous surgery are anticipated, in case of very large defects of the colonic wall, and when surgery is delayed with diffuse fecal peritonitis. A damage control approach, with bowel resection, open abdomen, and delayed bowel anastomosis or stoma formation, is an option to be considered in very sick patients, as suggested by current guidelines (Fig. 7.1) [30, 31].

7.4 Bleeding

7.4.1 Mechanism and Incidence

Bleeding is a complication occurring after operative colonoscopies (polypectomy, biopsy) with an incidence from 0.1% to 1% [32]. Cutting or mixed current device is most commonly associated with immediate hemorrhage, while coagulation current is

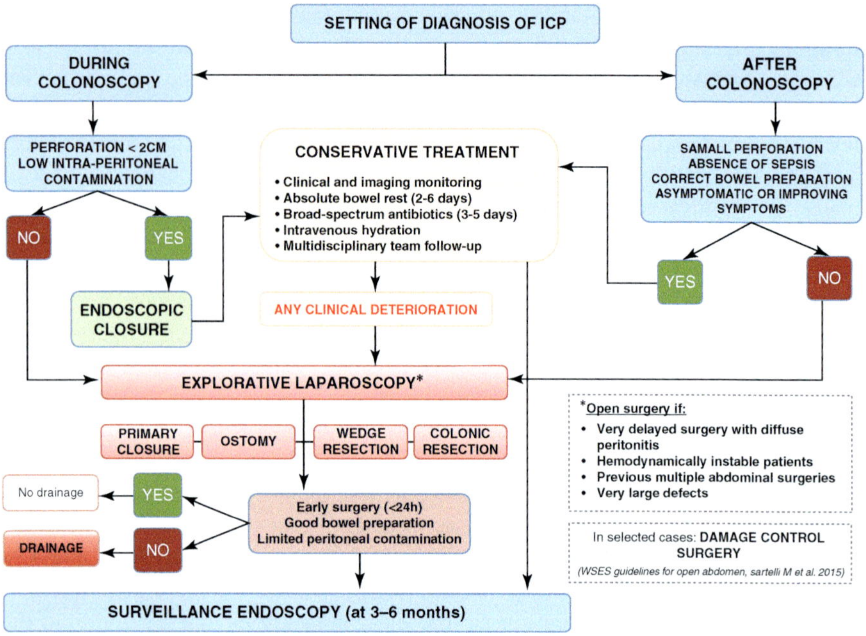

Fig. 7.1 Algorithm for the management of ICP [30]

associated with delayed bleeding (5–7 days, rarely up to 4 weeks) [33]. Higher rate of hemorrhagic complications was reported in resection of polyps larger than 2 cm or multiple polypectomies, polyps located in the right colon, and sessile polyps with villous or tubule-villous histotype [34]. Anticoagulant or dual antiplatelet therapy and coagulation disorders are risk factors for post-procedural bleeding as well. Recommendations to decrease the risk of post-polypectomy bleeding include the injection of saline (with adrenaline) in the submucosal layer, the grip of polypoid tissue into the diathermic snare not exceeding 2 cm, the adjunct of clips to clamp visible vessels, and the use for small polyps of mini-snare without electrocautery [35].

7.4.2 Treatment

Endoscopic hemostasis should be the first-line treatment of post-polypectomy hemorrhage. If the source of bleeding can be identified and is small, it can be controlled using submucosal injection of adrenaline, or a TTS clip [36]. For larger vessels, the use of OTSC is associated with a high rate of success [37]. Hemostasis with electrocautery should be used with caution, particularly in the right colon where it may cause transmural burn, post-polypectomy electrocoagulation syndrome, and delayed perforation. When endoscopic approach fails to control hemorrhage, angio-embolization of the bleeding vessel may be an option. An endoscopic and/or CT scan follow-up is necessary to verify the viability of bowel after endovascular treatment [38]. Surgery is the last chance to stop hemorrhage when endoscopy has been unsuccessful and angio-embolization is ineffective or not available. Laparotomy is usually the first-line surgical approach because of hemodynamic instability. The surgical treatment is commonly a colonic resection of the bleeding bowel segment with or without anastomosis according to the patient's general conditions.

7.5 Unusual Complications

An unusual complication of colonoscopy is the injury to the spleen, caused by traction on the spleno-colic ligament during insufflation or direct mechanical trauma, while the endoscope is pushed forward [39]. In these cases, treatment ranges from nonoperative management in hemodynamically stable patients to splenectomy.

Another surgical complication is the strangulation of hernias due to the increase of abdominal pressure during insufflation [40]. If the attempt of hernia reduction fails, emergency hernia repair is indicated.

Large bowel intraluminal gas explosion during colonoscopy has been reported [41], caused by a high concentration of methane in the presence of oxygen when electrocautery energy is used for an operative procedure. An inadequate cleaning of the bowel and the use of nonabsorbable sugars (mannitol, lactulose, sorbitol) may be additional contributing factors. The use of CO_2 instead of air has been proposed as a preventive measure [42].

7.6 Conclusions

Thousands of colonoscopies are performed every day worldwide with a fundamental role in the prevention, diagnosis, and treatment of tumors and benign diseases of the rectum and colon. Complications are rare, but they are associated with unpleasant prolonged hospital stay, unexpected operation, stoma formation, abdominal sepsis, and even death. In ICPs, the 30-day morbidity and mortality rates have been reported as high as 21–53% and 0–26%, respectively [43]. The endoscopist should be aware of risk factors, and special precaution should be taken, particularly in patients with advanced age and several comorbidities. In diagnostic endoscopy, endoscope progression should be gently performed and loop formation avoided. Alternative maneuvers (compression, decubitus changes) should be used in the case of pain, and when persistent difficulty in progression is observed, it is better to abandon the procedure. Air should be insufflated judiciously to avoid barotrauma, especially if bowel obstruction is suspected. CO_2 should be used to further minimize bowel distension, abdominal discomfort, and risk of perforation and explosion. In endoscopic polypectomies, the amount of tissue included in the loop should be a maximum of 2 cm, and pre-polypectomy submucosal injection of saline solution is recommended to reduce the risk of electrocoagulative damage of muscularis propria. Mixed current mode limits the depth of tissue damage, and cold techniques are more advisable to excise polyps smaller than 5 mm.

The awareness of possible complications, risk factors, and preventive and treatment measures should be in the armamentarium of the endoscopist, in order to select the appropriate approach in each clinical condition, reduce the rate of endoscopic complications, and diagnose and treat them as promptly as possible.

References

1. Whitlock EP, Lin JS, Liles E, Beil TL, Fu R. Screening for colorectal cancer: a targeted updated systematic review for the US preventive services task force. Ann Intern Med. 2008;149: 638–58.
2. Rabeneck L, Paszt LF, Hilsden RJ, et al. Bleeding and perforation after outpatient colonoscopy and their risk factors in usual clinical practice. Gastroenerology. 2008;135:1899–906.
3. https://www.cochrane.org/CD008506/COLOCA_the-use-of-nitrous-oxide-gas-during-colonoscopy-procedures.
4. Cotton PB, Eisen GM, Aabakken L, et al. A lexicon for endoscopic adverse events: report of an ASGE workshop. Gastrointest Endosc. 2010;71:446–54.
5. Triantafillidis JK, Merikas E, Nikolakis D, Papalois AE. Sedation in gastrointestinal endoscopy: current issues. World J Gastroenterol. 2013;19:463–81.
6. Manta R, Tremolaterra F, Arezzo A, Verra M, et al. Complications during colonoscopy: prevention, diagnosis and management. Tech Coloproctol. 2015;19:505–13.
7. Samalavicius NE, Kazanavicius D, Lunevicius TP, et al. Incidence, risk, management and outcomes of iatrogenic full-thickness large bowel injury associated with 56882 colonoscopies in 14 Lithuanian hospitals. Surg Endosc. 2013;27:1628–163.
8. Martinez MTG, Poblador AR, Raposo LG, Fernandez AMG, Nunez JRC. Perforation after colonoscopy: our 16 year experience. Rev Esp Enferm Dig. 2007;99:588–92.
9. Luning TH, Keemer-Gels ME, Barendregt WB, Tan ACITL, Rosman C. Colonoscopic perforations: a review of 30,366 patients. Surg Endosc. 2007;21:994–7.
10. Lohsiriwat V. Colonoscopy perforation: incidence, risk factors, management and outcome. World J Gatroenterol. 2010;16:425–30.
11. Anderson ML, Pasha TM, Leighton JA. Endoscopic perforation of the colon: lesson from a 10-year study. Am J Gastroenterol. 2000;95:3418–22.
12. Heldwein W, Dollhopf M, Rosch T, et al. The Munich Polypectomy Study (MUPS): prospective analysis of complications and risk factors in 4000 colonic snare polypectomies. Endoscopy. 2005;37:1116–22.
13. Wang J, Zhang XH, Ge J, Yang CM, Liu JY, Zhao SL. Endoscopic submucosal dissection vs endoscopic mucosal resection for colorectal tumors: a meta-analysis. World J Gastroenterol. 2014;20:8282–7.
14. Van Halsema EE, Van Hooft JE, Small AJ, et al. Perforations in colorectal stenting: a meta-analysis and a search for risk factors. Gastrointest Endosc. 2014;79:970–82.
15. Ragg J, Garimella V, Cast J, Hunter IA, Hartley JE. Balloon dilatation of benign rectal anastomotic strictures: a review. Dig Surg. 2012;29:287–91.
16. Iqbal CW, Culliname DC, Schuller HJ, Sawyer MD, Zietlow SP, Farley DR. Surgical management and outcomes of 165 colonoscopic perforations from a single institution. Arch Surg. 2008;14:6722–5.
17. Kim DH, Pickhard PJ, Taylor AJ, Menias CO. Imaging evaluation of complications at optical colonoscopy. Curr Probl Diagn Radiol. 2008;4:165–77.
18. Shanmuganathan K, Mirvis SE, Chiu WC, Killeen KL, Scalea TM. Triple contrast helical T in penetrating torso trauma: a prospective study to determine peritoneal violation and the need for laparotomy. Am J Roentgenol. 2001;177:1247–56.
19. De Angelis N, Di Saverio S, Chiara O, Sartelli M, Martinez-Perez A, Patrizi F, et al. 2017 WSES guidelines for the management of iatrogenic colonoscopy perforation. World J Emerg Surg. 2018;13:5–25.

20. Committee ASoP, Fisher DA, Maple JT, Ben-Menachem T, Cash BD, Decker GA, et al. Complications of colonoscopy. Gastrointest Endosc. 2011;74:745–52.
21. Byeon JS. Colonic perforation: can we manage it endoscopically? Clin Endosc. 2013;46:495–9.
22. Weiland T, Fehlker M, Gottwald T, Schurr MO. Performance of the OTSC system in the endoscopic closure of iatrogenic gastrointestinal perforations: a systematic review. Surg Endosc. 2013;27:2258–74.
23. Stavropoulos SN, Modayil R, Friedel D. Current applications of endoscopic suturing. World J Gastrointest Endosc. 2015;7:777–89.
24. Cho SB, Lee WS, Joo YE, Kim HR, Park CH, Kim HS, Choi SK, Rew JS. Therapeutic options for iatrogenic colon perforation: feasibility of endoscopic clip closure and predictors of the need for early surgery. Surg Endosc. 2012;6:473–9.
25. Lohsiriwat V, Sujarittanakarn S, Akaraviputh T, Lertakyamanee N, Lohsiriwt D, Kachinthorn U. What are the risk factors of colonoscopic perforations? BMC Gastroenterol. 2009;9:71–8.
26. Shin DK, Shin SY, Park CY, Jin SM, Cho YH, Kim WH, et al. Optimal methods for the management of iatrogenic colonoscopic perforation. Clin Endosc. 2016;49:282–8.
27. Di Saverio S, Patrizi F, Bassi M, Birindelli A, Nigro F, Cennamo V. Minimally invasive laparoscopic management of colonoscopic perforation avoiding laparotomy and colostomy: when and how to perform primary repair - a video vignette. Colorectal Dis. 2016;18:817–8.
28. Agresta F, Michelet I, Mainente P, Bedin N. Laparoscopic management of colonoscopic perforations. Surg Endosc. 2000;14:592–3.
29. Coimbra C, Bouffluoux L, Kohnen L, Deroover A, Dresse D, Denoel A, Honore P, Detry O. Laparoscopic repair of colonoscopic perforation: a new standard? World J Surg. 2010;34:1949–53.
30. De'Angelis N, Di Saverio S, Chiara O, et al. 2017 WSES guidelines for the management of iatrogenic colonoscopy perforation. World J Emerg Surg. 2018;13:5.
31. Chiara O, Cimbanassi S, Biffl W, Leppaniemi A, Henry S, Scalea T, et al. International consensus conference on open abdomen in trauma. J Trauma Acute Care Surg. 2016;80:173–83.
32. Warren JL, Klabunde CN, Mariotto AB, et al. Adverse events after outpatients colonoscopy in the Medicare population. Ann Intern Med. 2009;150:849–57.
33. Parra-Blanco A, Kaminaga N, Kojima T, Endo Y, Tajiri A, Fujita R. Colonoscopic polypectomy with cutting current: is it safe? Gastrointest Endosc. 2000;51:676–81.
34. Saito Y, Uraoka T, Yamaguchi Y, et al. A prospective multicenter study of 1111 colorectal submucosal dissections. Gastrointest Endosc. 2010;72:1217–25.
35. Parikh ND, Zanocco K, Keswani RN, Gawron AJ. A cost efficacy decision analysis of prophylactic clip placement after endoscopic removal of large polyps. Clin Gastroenterol Hepatol. 2013;11:1319–24.
36. Luigiano C, Ferrara F, Ghersi S, et al. Endoclip assisted resection of large peduncolated colorectal polyps: technical aspects and outcome. Dig Dis Sci. 2010;55:1726–31.
37. Jacques J, Legros R, Chaussade S, Sautereau D. Endoscopic hemostasis: an overview of procedures and clinical scenarios. Dig Liver Dis. 2014;46:766–76.
38. Manta R, Galloro G, Mangiavillano B, et al. Over-the-scope clip (OTSC) represents an effective endoscopic treatment for acute GI bleeding after failure of conventional techniques. Surg Endosc. 2013;27:3162–4.
39. Soh B, Chan S. The use of superselective mesenteric embolization as a first line management of acute lower gastrointestinal bleeding. Ann Med Surg. 2017;17:27–32.
40. Rao KV, Beri GD, Sterling MJ, Salen G. Splenic injury as a complication of colonoscopy: a case series. Am J Gastroenterol. 2009;104:1604–5.
41. Chae HS, Kim SS, Han SW, et al. Herniation of the large bowel through a post-traumatic diaphragmatic defect during colonoscopy: report of a case. Dis Colon Rectum. 2002;45:1261–2.
42. Ladas SD, Karamanolis G, Ben-Soussan E. Colonic gas explosion during therapeutic colonoscopy with electrocautery. World J Gastroenterol. 2007;13:5295–8.
43. Riss S, Akan B, Mikola B, et al. CO2 insufflation during colonoscopy decreases post-interventional pain in deeply sedated patients: a randomized controlled trial. Wien Klin Wochenschr. 2009;121:464–8.

Emergencies Related to Primary Colon Cancer: Multidisciplinary Management of Colon Obstruction, Perforation and Bleeding Due to Colon Cancer in the Absence of Metastatic Disease

8

Erika Picariello, Claudia Zaghi, Paola Fugazzola, Matteo Tomasoni, Enrico Cicuttin, Luca Ansaloni, and Federico Coccolini

Abbreviations

CRC	Colorectal cancer
CT scan	Computed tomography
DC	Damage control
HP	Hartmann procedure
LBO	Large bowel obstruction
LCO	Left colon obstruction
OLCC	Obstructed left colon cancer
ORCC	Obstructed right colon cancer
RC	Right colectomy
RPA	Resection and primary anastomosis
SEMS	Self-expanding metallic stents
TD	Tube decompression

E. Picariello (✉) · C. Zaghi · P. Fugazzola · M. Tomasoni · E. Cicuttin · L. Ansaloni
F. Coccolini
General, Emergency and Trauma Surgery Department, Bufalini Hospital, Cesena, FC, Italy

N. de'Angelis et al. (eds.), *Emergency Surgical Management of Colorectal Cancer*,
Hot Topics in Acute Care Surgery and Trauma,
https://doi.org/10.1007/978-3-030-06225-5_8

8.1 Introduction

Interest in colorectal cancer (CRC) is still high because of the relevance of the disease. In the last 50 years, there have been large improvements about survival, due to screening programs, accurate and preoperative staging, and a multidisciplinary treatments [1, 2].

However, when the first appearance occurs in emergency clinical scenario like occlusion, perforation, or bleeding, diagnosis, life-saving strategies, obstruction release, and oncological issues are a challenging matter. Physician and surgeon must be skilled in identifying the right balance between saving-life procedures and oncological issues.

Emergency settings related to colorectal cancer are not so rare:

- Large bowel complications are the 47% of gastrointestinal emergencies [3]; large bowel obstruction (LBO) represents almost the 80%, while perforation ranges the 20% of the emergency [4–7].
- Bleeding has been thought to occur about 6–10% of patients with advanced cancer [8].
- CRC presents as urgencies or emergencies in a wide range from 7% to 40% [3].
- In the 75% of cases, CRC obstruction is located distal to the splenic flexure, and the most common location is the sigmoid colon [9].
- In almost 70% of cases, perforation occurs at the tumor site; in almost 30% of cases proximal to the tumor site [3, 10, 11].

8.2 Clinical Presentation

8.2.1 Occlusion

When LBO presents acutely, the most common symptoms are crampy abdominal pain, abdominal bloating, and absence of bowel movement and flatus; vomiting is less frequent. When LBO presents subacutely, there are a gradual development of symptoms, changes in bowel movement, and recurrent left lower quadrant abdominal pain.

Abdominal examination shows abdominal distension, tenderness, and hyperactive or absence of bowel sounds. A rectal cancer may be directly palpable at the rectal exploration [12–14].

Laboratory test evaluates electrolyte imbalances, elevated urea nitrogen, and metabolic alkalosis as consequences of vomiting and dehydration.

8.2.2 Perforation

When perforation occurs at the tumor site, the peritoneal contamination is usually localized. When perforation is located proximal of the tumor site, the fecal spread results in diffuse peritonitis, sometimes in septic shock.

In this case, physical examination reveals fever, tachypnea, tachycardia, and confusion; the abdomen may present a diffuse or a localized direct tenderness, guarding, or rebound tenderness. Bowel sounds are usually absent. Leukocytosis and neutrophilia, elevated amylase levels, and lactic acidosis are nonspecific indicators of perforation or necrosis [15].

8.2.3 Bleeding

Gastrointestinal (GI) bleeding from colonic tumors is manifested as hematochezia or melena or symptomatic anemia. Bleeding as a direct result of GI malignancy can vary in presentation from occult bleeding to massive hemorrhage, being the direct cause of death; anyhow, in spite of upper GI bleeding tumor, lower GI bleeding is generally less severe, with spontaneous cessation of bleeding in 80% of cases [16].

8.3 Imaging

Clinical evaluation and laboratory test are always the first step for evaluation in these patients, but they are not specific and variable. Nevertheless, clinical suspicion suggests which diagnostic tests are indicated to obtain a definitive diagnosis.

8.3.1 Occlusion

Abdominal plain X-ray is always the first radiologic diagnostic test, even if US bedside should be able to replace it, with the limit of operator expertise [17]. CT scan (with i.v. contrast) is the imaging test of referral for colorectal occlusion, because it offers absolute advantages in terms of neoplastic staging, cancer-related complications, and synchronous different diseases [18, 19].

When CT scan is not available, colonic enema is a valid alternative in identifying the site and the nature of obstruction.

In stable patients, colonoscopy should be considered for direct visualization of site of obstruction and to obtain biopsies, if an emergent surgical resection has not been planned or endoscopic stent placement can be performed [9, 20, 21].

8.3.2 Perforation

When the clinical scenario is suspected for bowel perforation, abdominal plain X-ray or abdominal US (even bedside) should be used as first screening tests; one of the limitations is the detection of small amount of free air as happens in case of perforation at the tumor site [22].

In stable patient, CT scan should be considered, in order to define the cause and the site of perforation (at the tumor or proximal to the tumor), despite free air in the peritoneal cavity leads to surgical exploration, because there are some cases of pneumoperitoneum not related to intestinal perforation [23, 24]. On the other hand, performing a CT scan never should expose the patient to unsafe delay with adjunctive risk for safety.

8.3.3 Bleeding

Colonscopy is the best option: in contrast to upper GI bleeding and in acute setting, it can be feasible although it requires rapid bowel preparation and may be poorly tolerated by the patient. Overall early colonoscopy appears to be safe [25].

CT angiography can give many information. Angiography is occasionally required to diagnose the site of bleeding (to obtain a positive test bleeding must be active at a rate of 0.5–1 mL/min) [26].

8.4 Treatment

Management of the complications of the primary colorectal cancer has the dual aim to come out from a critical clinical setting and to offer a good prognosis in terms of oncological outcome. The first is often time dependent.

8.4.1 Occlusion

8.4.1.1 Left Colon

To manage obstructive left colon cancer (OLCC), not only surgical solutions are available; most of the time, surgical and nonsurgical solutions are used together in two or three steps.

- Loop colostomy (as bridge to resection or palliation)
- Loop colostomy is reserved for severely ill patients who are too unfit for major surgical procedures and/or in case of unresectable tumors if self-expanding metallic stents (SEMS) are not feasible [27, 28].
- Primary resection with end colostomy (Hartmann's procedure—HP) or resection and primary anastomosis (RPA)
  In the absence of other risk factors, RPA is the best option for uncomplicated malignant left-sided large bowel obstruction [29]. There is no evidence that a covering stoma can reduce the risk of anastomotic leak and its severity [30]. Patients with high surgical risk, instead, are better managed with HP [31–33]. Only in case of cecal tears/perforation or evidence of bowel ischemia or synchronous right colonic cancers, a total colectomy is considered [20].
  Laparoscopy in emergency treatment of OLCC is not contraindicated but is reserved to selected favorable cases and in specialized centers [34].

- Tube decompression (TD)
  TD can be a valid alternative option in order to achieve a highly successful rate of elective surgery with RPA [35].
- Endoscopic colonic stenting by self-expanding metallic stents (SEMS)
  Endoscopic colonic stenting gives the same benefit in terms of resolution of occlusion for palliation since it is associated with similar mortality/morbidity rates but a shorter hospital stay [36]. SEMS as bridge to elective surgery offers a better short-term outcome than direct emergency surgery, the complications are comparable, but rate of stomas is significantly lower [36, 37].

Alternative treatments are preferred to SEMS in patients eligible for further bevacizumab-based therapy due to the high risk of perforation: that's why, early involvement of the oncologist in the decision is very important [38, 39].

8.4.1.2 Right Colon

- Resection and anastomosis with or without proximal stoma creation
  In right-sided colon cancer causing acute obstruction, right colectomy (RC) with primary anastomosis can be performed most of the time. Favorable anatomical and technical features and limitation of alternative to surgery make RC with primary anastomosis the option of choice. A terminal ileostomy associated with colonic fistula is an alternative when a primary anastomosis is considered unsafe [40].
- Intestinal internal bypass
  In case of unresectable right-sided colon cancer, a loop ileostomy or a side-to-side anastomosis between the terminal ileum and the transverse colon (the internal bypass).
- Decompressive cecostomy is abandoned for the high rate of malfunction and complication; only the percutaneous technique is reserved to very sick patients [41].
- Endoscopic stent placement for right colon obstruction is not recommended because of the high risk of migration and the technical difficulty to perform it; it's reserved for palliative management of inoperable proximal malignant occlusions [42].

8.4.2 Perforation

In case of cancer-related colon perforation, the priority is the control of sepsis source, combined with prompt medical treatment.

When free peritonitis occurs, usually related to perforation proximal to tumor site, patients are at higher risk for septic shock development compared to patients with contained collection usually related to perforation at the tumor site for necrosis; in the first case, mortality reaches rates of 19–65% and decreases to 0–24% in cases of localized peritonitis [3, 11].

Although the treatment of intra-abdominal infection is time dependent (the medical treatment and the source control must be started as soon as possible) [43, 44], whenever possible, oncological resection should be performed in order to obtain better oncological outcome. The patient clinical condition is the priority, and the performance of a standard oncological resection can lead to similar results of elective cases [3, 10].

In case of diastatic perforation (proximal to tumor site, generally the neoplasm is in the left and the perforation is in the cecum), simultaneous tumor resection and management of proximal perforation are indicated: depending on the colonic wall thickening, a subtotal colectomy may be required.

In case of perforation at the tumor site, it is indicated to perform a formal resection with or without anastomosis with or without stoma.

When the perforation site is the same of the tumor localization for a right side, a right colectomy can be performed. In case of poor general or "bad" local conditions, a resection without anastomosis and terminal ileostomy is performed.

When the perforation involves transverse and left side, usually a resection with anastomosis with or without ileostomy is attempted. Hartmann's procedure is performed, especially when clinical conditions require an immediate surgical control just keeping in mind that 50% of patients will have no reversal.

While a diastatic perforation is often a consequence of a distal occlusion, a perforation on at the tumor site is clearly an advanced-stage disease, and it represents an important issue for following therapy. The risk of peritoneal carcinomatosis in perforated colorectal cancer ranges between 14% and 54%, but further literature data is needed [45].

8.4.3 Bleeding

According to the hemodynamic status, the management of bleeding includes different and sequential steps. Blood transfusions and coagulation disorder treatment are often required [46].

8.4.3.1 Endoscopic Treatment

Once the patient is hemodynamically stable, colonoscopy can be performed after adequate colon cleansing. In patients with high-risk clinical features and signs or symptoms of ongoing bleeding, a rapid bowel purge should be initiated following hemodynamic resuscitation and a colonoscopy performed within 24 h of patient presentation after adequate colon preparation to potentially improve diagnostic and therapeutic yield.

Radiographic interventions can be considered in patients with high-risk clinical features and ongoing bleeding who have a negative upper endoscopy and do not respond adequately to hemodynamic resuscitation efforts and are therefore unlikely to tolerate bowel preparation and urgent colonoscopy.

Surgical treatment is required when ongoing bleeding is unresponsive to other measures. Early surgery provides no benefit when performed for minor indications.

Is reasonable to reserve surgery for those with evidence of continuous and severe bleeding. Accurate prior localization with colonoscopy or TC angiography of the site of bleeding is important for surgical management of lower GI bleeding.

8.5 Unstable Patients

Occlusion, perforation, or bleeding for CRC could bring to patient instability: in this case, patients are amenable for damage control treatment, if (at least one):

- pH <7.2
- Core temperature <35 °C
- BE <−8
- Laboratory/clinical evidence of coagulopathy
- Any sign of sepsis/septic shock which include the necessity of vasopressor

Acute bleeding causes hemodynamic instability, and this condition worsens in the condition of coronary artery disease, particularly in patients with heart failure, where antithrombotic and antiplatelet therapy need to medical and blood products support.

When facing clinical instability due to occlusion or perforation, the emergency physician, the surgeon, and the anesthesiologist should apply the damage control philosophy. Damage control (DC) should be started as soon as possible after resuscitation began.

Except in case of hemorrhagic shock, surgical emergency requires an initial period of resuscitation, before surgical intervention, in order to prevent hemodynamic collapse on induction of anesthesia. Few hours are necessary to re-establish adequate organ perfusion and to begin broad-spectrum antibiotic therapy.

In an operating theater of a septic shock due to a fecal peritonitis, the aim of DC is the prompt source control. Definitive treatment as anatomical reconstruction and abdominal closure is a secondary goal, and it's deferred eventually to secondary procedure after physiological normalization. If an open abdomen (OA) has to be considered, stoma creation is avoided, and bowel is left stapled inside the cavity.

The loop ileostomy is reserved for occlusion when the tumor is not easily resectable or in case of time-dependent surgical procedure, especially for left-sided lesions, where in an unstable patient, a single-stage procedure represents a time-consuming intervention, at high risk of anastomotic leak.

In those cases when planned re-laparotomy represents a necessity, a take back to operating theater is usually performed 24–48 h after the initial operation. The goal to be achieved after OA is the early and definitive closure of the abdominal wall as soon as possible in order to reduce complications associated with OA [47–49].

While in case of bleeding or occlusion, prophylaxis is enough to avoid bacterial translocation, in patients with colon carcinoma perforation, antibiotic therapy mainly targeting Gram-negative bacilli and anaerobic bacteria is always suggested. Furthermore, in critically ill patients with sepsis, early it's suggested using broader-spectrum antimicrobials.

8.6 Conclusions

Emergency related to a colorectal cancer gives two main problems: the first is related to the control of septic or hemorrhagic source, clinical instability, and metabolic disorders, and they are time dependent. The second issue is related to the oncological outcome.

Medical treatment and the source control should be started as soon as possible because the intra-abdominal infection can occur with septic shock or can early develop in it. While perforation may induce generalized peritonitis, colon obstruction causes volume depletion and electrolyte disorders; moreover, these factors coexist and together may faster lead to patient instability, represented by metabolic impairment, coagulopathy, and signs of shock. Even if less common, acute bleeding can occur directly as a cause of cardiovascular collapse, and also when it's associated with malignancy, it still represents a factor of an increased mortality rate [50].

The oncological outcome, instead, is strongly influenced by the advanced disease and by an incomplete preoperative treatment. That's why the surgeon, keeping in mind the septic status, should be aware to perform the best oncological resection giving to the patient the shorter postoperative recovery time and complication rate allowing to complete staging and chemotherapy programs.

References

1. Arnold M, et al. Global patterns and trends in colorectal cancer incidence and mortality. Gut. 2017;66(4):683–91.
2. Torre LA, et al. Global cancer incidence and mortality rates and trends--an update. Cancer Epidemiol Biomarkers Prev. 2016;25(1):16–27.
3. Zielinski MD, et al. Emergency management of perforated colon cancers: how aggressive should we be? J Gastrointest Surg. 2011;15(12):2232–8.
4. Alvarez JA, et al. Presentation, treatment, and multivariate analysis of risk factors for obstructive and perforative colorectal carcinoma. Am J Surg. 2005;190(3):376–82.
5. Gunnarsson H, et al. Emergency presentation of colon cancer is most frequent during summer. Colorectal Dis. 2011;13(6):663–8.
6. Barnett A, et al. Colorectal cancer emergencies. J Gastrointest Cancer. 2013;44(2):132–42.
7. Laine L, et al. Trends for incidence of hospitalization and death due to GI complications in the United States from 2001 to 2009. Am J Gastroenterol. 2012;107(8):1190–5. quiz 1196.
8. Pereira J, et al. Management of bleeding in patients with advanced cancer. Oncologist. 2004;9(5):561–70.
9. Frago R, et al. Current management of acute malignant large bowel obstruction: a systematic review. Am J Surg. 2014;207(1):127–38.
10. Biondo S, et al. Differences in patient postoperative and long-term outcomes between obstructive and perforated colonic cancer. Am J Surg. 2008;195(4):427–32.
11. Anwar MA, et al. Outcome of acutely perforated colorectal cancers: experience of a single district general hospital. Surg Oncol. 2006;15(2):91–6.
12. Markogiannakis H, et al. Acute mechanical bowel obstruction: clinical presentation, etiology, management and outcome. World J Gastroenterol. 2007;13(3):432–7.
13. Cappell MS, Batke M. Mechanical obstruction of the small bowel and colon. Med Clin North Am. 2008;92(3):575–97. viii.
14. Lopez-Kostner F, Hool GR, Lavery IC. Management and causes of acute large-bowel obstruction. Surg Clin North Am. 1997;77(6):1265–90.

15. Kahi CJ, Rex DK. Bowel obstruction and pseudo-obstruction. Gastroenterol Clin North Am. 2003;32(4):1229–47.
16. Marion Y, et al. The management of lower gastrointestinal bleeding. J Visc Surg. 2014;151(3):191–201.
17. Shelton BK. Intestinal obstruction. AACN Clin Issues. 1999;10(4):478–91.
18. Suri S, et al. Comparative evaluation of plain films, ultrasound and CT in the diagnosis of intestinal obstruction. Acta Radiol. 1999;40(4):422–8.
19. Frager D, et al. Prospective evaluation of colonic obstruction with computed tomography. Abdom Imaging. 1998;23(2):141–6.
20. Finan PJ, Campbell S, et al. The management of malignant large bowel obstruction: ACPGBI position statement. Colorectal Dis. 2007;9(Supp 4):17.
21. Gainant A, et al. Emergency management of acute colonic cancer obstruction. J Visc Surg. 2012;149(1):e3–e10.
22. Chen SC, et al. Ultrasonography is superior to plain radiography in the diagnosis of pneumoperitoneum. Br J Surg. 2002;89(3):351–4.
23. Mularski RA, Sippel JM, Osborne ML. Pneumoperitoneum: a review of nonsurgical causes. Crit Care Med. 2000;28(7):2638–44.
24. Tang A, et al. Clinical cases of nonsurgical pneumoperitoneum: categorizing the disease and treatment options. Am Surg. 2015;81(5):E206–8.
25. Werner DJ, et al. Endoscopic and angiographic management of lower gastrointestinal bleeding: review of the published literature. United Eur Gastroenterol J. 2018;6(3):337–42.
26. Nusbaum S, Baum S. Radiographic demonstration of unknown sites of gastrointestinal bleeding. Surg Forum. 1963;14:374–5.
27. De Salvo GL, Gava C, Pucciarelli S, Lise M. Curative surgery for obstruction from primary left colorectal carcinoma: primary or staged resection? Cochrane Database Syst Rev. 2004;(2):CD002101.
28. Krstic S, et al. Hartmann's procedure vs loop colostomy in the treatment of obstructive rectosigmoid cancer. World J Emerg Surg. 2014;9(1):52.
29. Fielding LP, Stewart-Brown S, Blesovsky L. Large-bowel obstruction caused by cancer: a prospective study. Br Med J. 1979;2(6189):515–7.
30. Kube R, et al. Surgical practices for malignant left colonic obstruction in Germany. Eur J Surg Oncol. 2010;36(1):65–71.
31. Trompetas V. Emergency management of malignant acute left-sided colonic obstruction. Ann R Coll Surg Engl. 2008;90(3):181–6.
32. Meyer F, et al. Emergency operation in carcinomas of the left colon: value of Hartmann's procedure. Tech Coloproctol. 2004;8(Suppl 1):s226–9.
33. Alves A, et al. Postoperative mortality and morbidity in French patients undergoing colorectal surgery: results of a prospective multicenter study. Arch Surg. 2005;140(3):278–83. discussion 284.
34. Ballian N, et al. Comparable postoperative morbidity and mortality after laparoscopic and open emergent restorative colectomy: outcomes from the ACS NSQIP. World J Surg. 2012;36(10):2488–96.
35. Araki Y, et al. Endoscopic decompression procedure in acute obstructing colorectal cancer. Endoscopy. 2000;32(8):641–3.
36. Harris GJ, et al. The management of neoplastic colorectal obstruction with colonic endoluminal stenting devices. Am J Surg. 2001;181(6):499–506.
37. Zhang Y, et al. Self-expanding metallic stent as a bridge to surgery versus emergency surgery for obstructive colorectal cancer: a meta-analysis. Surg Endosc. 2012;26(1):110–9.
38. Cennamo V, et al. Does stent placement for advanced colon cancer increase the risk of perforation during bevacizumab-based therapy? Clin Gastroenterol Hepatol. 2009;7(11):1174–6.
39. Manes G, et al. Endoscopic palliation in patients with incurable malignant colorectal obstruction by means of self-expanding metal stent: analysis of results and predictors of outcomes in a large multicenter series. Arch Surg. 2011;146(10):1157–62.

40. Faucheron JL, et al. Emergency surgery for obstructing colonic cancer: a comparison between right-sided and left-sided lesions. Eur J Trauma Emerg Surg. 2018;44(1):71–7.
41. Chang GJ, et al. Practice parameters for the management of colon cancer. Dis Colon Rectum. 2012;55(8):831–43.
42. Amelung FJ, et al. Emergency resection versus bridge to surgery with stenting in patients with acute right-sided colonic obstruction: a systematic review focusing on mortality and morbidity rates. Int J Colorectal Dis. 2015;30(9):1147–55.
43. Mazuski JE, et al. The surgical infection society revised guidelines on the management of intra-abdominal infection. Surg Infect (Larchmt). 2017;18(1):1–76.
44. Sartelli M, et al. Management of intra-abdominal infections: recommendations by the WSES 2016 consensus conference. World J Emerg Surg. 2017;12:22.
45. Honore C, et al. Definition of patients presenting a high risk of developing peritoneal carcinomatosis after curative surgery for colorectal cancer: a systematic review. Ann Surg Oncol. 2013;20(1):183–92.
46. Strate LL, Gralnek IM. ACG clinical guideline: management of patients with acute lower gastrointestinal bleeding. Am J Gastroenterol. 2016;111(4):459–74.
47. Person B, et al. Abbreviated emergency laparotomy in the non-trauma setting. World J Emerg Surg. 2009;4:41.
48. Weber DG, Bendinelli C, Balogh ZJ. Damage control surgery for abdominal emergencies. Br J Surg. 2014;101(1):e109–18.
49. Becher RD, et al. Damage control operations in non-trauma patients: defining criteria for the staged rapid source control laparotomy in emergency general surgery. World J Emerg Surg. 2016;11:10.
50. Kaya E, et al. Predictor of poor outcome in gastrointestinal bleeding in emergency department. World J Gastroenterol. 2016;22(16):4219–25.

9 Emergencies Related to Primary Rectal Cancer

Elisabeth Hain, Pénélope Raimbert, Magaly Zappa, and Yves Panis

9.1 Introduction

Colorectal cancer (CCR) is the third cause of cancer in Europe [1] and the second leading cause of cancer death in France [2]. CCR accounts for almost 12% of all cancer death, especially among patients aged 65 and over [3]. Although the widespread of CCR screening allows early management in a high proportion of patients, leading to a significant reduction of associated mortality, up to 15% of patients with CCR are still diagnosed as an urgent presentation that will require an emergency surgery in the majority of the cases [4–6]. Previous studies showed that emergency CCR presentation is associated with elderly, socially deprived, and comorbidities [7, 8]. Emergency presentations related to primary rectal cancer include digestive obstruction, rectal perforation, and severe hemorrhage. All of them remain rare and have been very few studied [9]. Despite improvements and advances in surgical techniques, when a surgery is required, CCR emergency presentations still have poor short-term outcomes as morbidity, mortality, and stoma creation rate remains higher than in elective procedure [10, 11]. Previous authors reported perioperative mortality rates between 5% and 34% for patients requiring an emergency resection of colorectal cancer versus only 4% for an elective surgery [4, 12]. Poor

E. Hain · P. Raimbert · Y. Panis (✉)
Department of Colorectal Surgery, Pôle des Maladies de l'Appareil Digestif (PMAD), Beaujon Hospital, Clichy Cedex, France

Assistance Publique-Hôpitaux de Paris (AP-HP), University Denis Diderot (Paris VII), Paris, France
e-mail: yves.panis@aphp.fr

M. Zappa
Department of Radiology, Beaujon Hospital, Clichy Cedex, France

Assistance Publique-Hôpitaux de Paris (AP-HP), University Denis Diderot (Paris VII), Paris, France

N. de'Angelis et al. (eds.), *Emergency Surgical Management of Colorectal Cancer*, Hot Topics in Acute Care Surgery and Trauma,
https://doi.org/10.1007/978-3-030-06225-5_9

postoperative outcomes can be explained by several reasons, including patient's physical status often altered and advanced tumor. Both frequently associated in the same patient can be responsible of hydroelectrolytic imbalance, malnutrition, and digestive obstruction. Furthermore, metabolic disorders can also acerbate underlying disease such as heart disease and diabetes. Finally, emergency CCR presentations are more associated with advanced stage tumor, higher histologic grade [13], and synchronous liver metastases. Finally, the emergency management of those frail patients with a complicated rectal cancer remains even more difficult because of the lack of information regarding the diagnosis and the accurate staging of the tumor at the time of management, especially if emergency surgery is needed.

While there is a general consensus concerning the management of patients with obstruction or perforation of the right or left colon [14], decision-making in emergencies related to primary rectal cancer is unclear, mainly because of the lack of studies devoted to this situation. This emergency management depends on several elements such as patients' general status, surgeon's experience, and type of complication. Although to date, the surgical approach for emergency presentation of rectal cancer is not standardized, two main principles should be theoretically respected: (1) if emergency proctectomy is indicated, the necessity of accurate lymphadenectomy during rectal resection in order to have good carcinologic resection at the first operation, which is crucial for optimal oncological treatment but also for both accurate staging and possible indication of adjuvant chemotherapy, and (2) best postoperative management in order to ensure short recovery to allow timely initiation of adjuvant treatment [15].

Previous studies reported poor long-term outcomes [16, 17], after emergency surgery for CRC. McArdle et al. reported an overall survival at 5 years of 58% after elective procedure versus 39% after emergency curative surgery ($p < 0.001$) [16]. However, in their study including 747 patients with CRC, Weixler et al. suggested that poor oncologic outcome was rather a consequence of the clinical presentation than to the emergency surgery itself [18]. Although this study included a large number of patients, only nine patients had an urgent surgery for rectal cancer. The accurate localization of the rectal tumor and the type of surgery are not specified [18]. The poor oncologic outcomes observed can be explained not only by the advanced stage of the tumor at the time of the treatment but also sometimes by the impossibility for the patients to receive neoadjuvant radiochemotherapy (if mid- or low-stage T3–T4 and/or N+ rectal cancer) [15, 19].

Thus, management of patients with an urgent symptomatic rectal cancer remains complex and requires the intervention of several specialists: surgeons, radiologists, intensivists, and oncologists. In this chapter, we will focus on three specific scenarios: obstructing rectal cancer, perforated rectal cancer, and bleeding rectal cancer.

9.2 Acute Lower Gastrointestinal Bleeding due to Rectal Cancer

Rectal bleeding is a common cause of consultation in emergency department [20] and has been reported to concern up to 50% of patients with CCR [21, 22]. Rectal bleeding with recent bowel movement modification associated with impaired general health and weight loss should be referred to CCR, and prompt endoscopy should be performed to locate the lesion and make some biopsies. The origin of rectal bleeding is erosion from the mucosal surface resulting in an occult hemorrhage, and it is rarely a cause of massive hemorrhage requiring emergency-specific treatment [23].

At admission of the patient, and before any attempt to stage the tumor, the priority is the assessment of the volemic status. In the presence of a hemodynamic unstable patient by acute massive rectal bleeding, the initial management is to restore normal blood pressure. Hemodynamic monitoring and large intravenous access have to be created for IV administration of crystalloid, before blood transfusion if needed. Management of electrolyte disturbances and underlying coagulopathy is also mandatory at the same time. As soon as hemodynamic status is stabilized, the priority is to try to localize the exact origin of bleeding and to precise the tumor stage before considering any surgical treatment [4]. For this reason, exact localization of the rectal bleeding by either endoscopy or angiography should be attempted before surgical treatment discussed.

The therapeutic management depends mainly on the hemodynamic status of the patients and is proposed on the algorithm on Fig. 9.1. After resuscitation measures, in case of a persistent hemodynamic instability with an active rectal bleeding diagnosed by angiography CT scan, embolization should be discussed as the first treatment. Although endoscopy has a better sensitivity to diagnose the origin of bleeding, for colonic and upper rectal bleeding lesions, active bleeding and the absence of bowel preparation can make this exam unfeasible [24–26]. Angiography CT scan

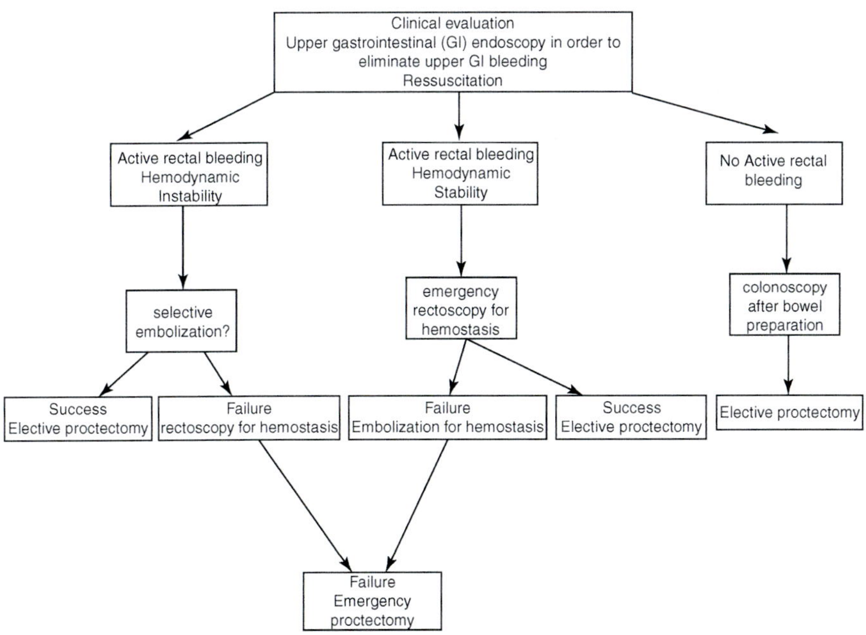

Fig. 9.1 Management of rectal cancer bleeding

and embolization has documented success rates of 42–86%; however, it carries the risk of worsening intestinal ischemia. In case of an active rectal bleeding with a hemodynamic stable patient, an urgent rectal endoscopy can also be performed. Rectal endoscopy is an important exam (1) which is known to identify the bleeding origin on the rectum in 74–89% of cases in the literature [24–26], (2) which permits to make efficient hemostasis, and (3) which allows tumor biopsies in order to have pathologic confirmation of the rectal cancer.

In case of failure of embolization or local hemostasis during rectal endoscopy, and in case of persistent severe bleeding and hemodynamic instability, emergency proctectomy should be discussed. Although no guidelines exist concerning the indications of emergency proctectomy for severe rectal bleeding, it includes hemodynamic instability despite vigorous resuscitation with more than six units of packed red blood cells, inability to stop hemorrhage with endoscopic techniques or embolization, recurrent bleeding after initial stabilization, recurrent hemorrhage associated with anemia, and ongoing slow bleeding requiring more than three units of blood products per day [27].

Very few data are available in the literature on emergency rectal resection. Although urgent proctectomy presents the advantage to be a definitive approach with the resection of the rectal tumor, the surgery is performed in difficult condition on a frail patient, and the risk is to perform a suboptimal lymphadenectomy, and the risk of a left colostomy with Hartmann's procedure is probably high especially in case of hemodynamic instability during operation. Furthermore, in case of large T3–T4 tumor, surgery without neoadjuvant radiochemotherapy exposes the patient to a higher risk of R1 or even R2 resection. For all these reasons, initial conservative management (rectoscopy or embolization) presents the advantages: (a) to avoid unnecessary emergency laparotomy, (b) to expose the patient to a too long recovery period during when adjuvant treatment cannot be initiated if indicated, and (c) to propose preoperatively neoadjuvant chemoradiation if indicated. The only debate is about the possible adverse effect of neoadjuvant radiation on a rectal tumor with a recent bleeding requiring local hemostasis, but no information has been reported to date about this problem. As pelvic irradiation for rectal cancer is known to have early toxicity leading sometimes to rectal bleeding [28], we can suppose that the risk of bleeding is probably increased in such patients with recent massive rectal tumor bleeding.

9.3 Acute Intestinal Obstruction by Rectal Cancer

Despite progress of colorectal cancer screening, still 8–29% of patients have at first presentation an intestinal obstruction due to CRC [29, 30]. In the most severe presentation, besides classical signs of intestinal obstruction (i.e., abdominal pain, no bowel movements, abdominal distention), the patient can also present medical complications such as dehydration, electrolytic disorders, respiratory impaired function secondary to abdominal distention, even sometimes surgical complications such as intestinal perforation either by the tumor itself or on a dilated colon above the tumor.

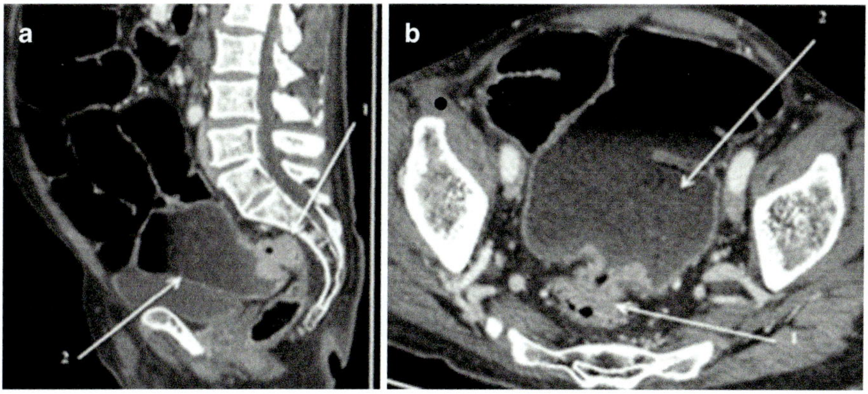

Fig. 9.2 (**a**) Sagittal CT scan with IV contrast: obstruction due to a rectal tumor. 1, rectal tumor; 2, dilated colon (**b**) axial CT scan

It can be diagnosed because of symptoms of diffuse peritonitis (in case of free perforation), or as a pelvic abscess.

CT scan is the gold standard imaging technique for patients presenting with suspicion of intestinal obstruction secondary to colorectal cancer: it can give the etiology and location of the obstruction and also possible complication. CT scan can make the correct diagnosis in nearly 89% of cases [31, 32] and allows accurate locoregional staging of the rectal tumor (Fig. 9.2). As patients presented with intestinal obstruction, colonoscopy is contraindicated. However, in some selected cases, rectosigmoidoscopy may be useful for placement of endoluminal stent, and this will be discussed later.

First of all, the management of patients with an obstruction due to rectal cancer should begin by resuscitation, rehydration, and correction of electrolytic disorders. Then, the decision-making for the treatment of the obstruction due to rectal cancer depends on the gravity of the obstruction. Except for the perforation cases, three main options remain for the treatment of the obstruction due to rectal cancer: the first two options can be defined as a "bridge to surgery", loop left colostomy and self-expandable metal stents. The third option is represented by proctectomy with or without anastomosis and includes Hartmann's procedure or a primary resection of the rectal tumor after intraoperative colonic irrigation with anastomosis, with or without a diverting ileostomy. The choice between those three strategies depends on the patient's general status, on the surgeon's expertise, and on the colonic dilation due to the rectal obstruction (Fig. 9.3).

9.3.1 Loop Left Colostomy

Proximal loop colostomy is an attractive option in emergency for the management of intestinal obstruction due to rectal cancer. The objective of the proximal colostomy (i.e., on the sigmoid) is to treat obstruction without performing resection which is delayed few days later. This operation presents many advantages:

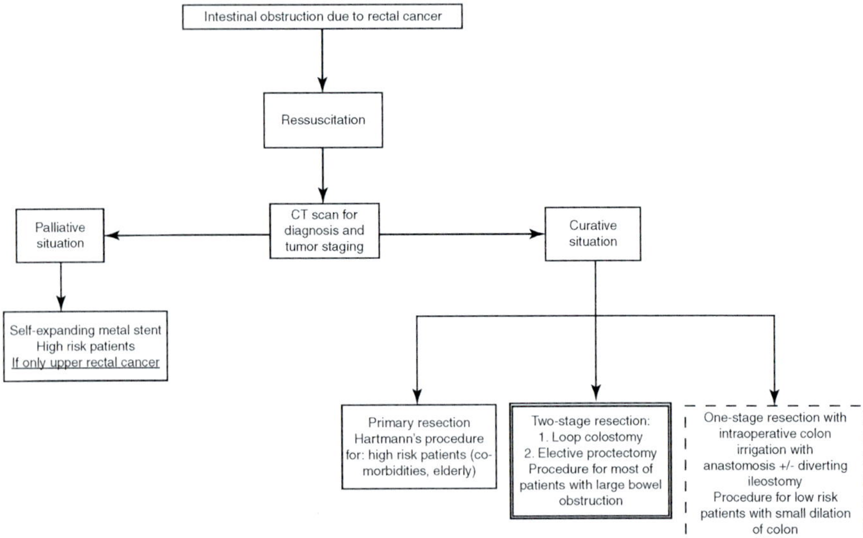

Fig. 9.3 Management of intestinal obstruction due to rectal cancer

- A short operative time which is a real benefit especially in frail patients with poor general status.
- An oncologic approach with a "bridge" to the resection of the tumor. The proximal loop colostomy will allow performing a complete staging of the tumor before the second step of proctectomy or neoadjuvant radiochemotherapy if indicated.

In order to facilitate the second step of proctectomy and colorectal or coloanal anastomosis, the colostomy must be fashioned on the distal part of the sigmoid, and not above.

Today, this left colostomy represents for many centers the first choice of treatment for patients presenting intestinal obstruction due to either rectal or sigmoid cancer.

9.3.2 Proctectomy with Hartmann's Procedure and Left Colostomy

Hartmann's procedure is the resection of the primary tumor with the creation of a left colostomy and the closure of the distal rectal stump below the tumor. It is today probably the most common operation performed in emergency in case of intestinal obstruction due to sigmoid or rectal cancer. This operation presents some advantages: (1) it allows to perform an oncologic resection of the rectum during the first operation, and (2) it eliminates the risk of postoperative leakage in case of risky low pelvic anastomosis which can delay the beginning of adjuvant treatment if persistent sepsis. However, Hartmann's procedure presents also some disadvantages: (1) risk of suboptimal lymphadenectomy due to technical difficulties during operation because of a dilated colon; (2) risk of R1 or even R2 resection in case of bulky tumor resected without neoadjuvant radiochemotherapy; and (3) finally, risk of definitive stoma in aged or high-risk patients for whom reoperation is thought to be risky or difficult. Indeed, the stoma reversal rate after Hartmann's procedure for CRC cancer remains close to 20% only [33, 34]. This low stoma closure rate can be easily explained by a poor general status at the time of surgery, the poor postoperative outcome with a higher mortality and morbidity than elective surgery. For these reasons, Hartmann's procedure should probably be restricted to elderly patients with underlying comorbidities and high American Society of Anesthesiologists (ASA) score and advanced obstruction with proximal distention on whom Hartmann's procedure is considered to be a definitive curative procedure.

9.3.3 Other Surgical Options

Although no recommendations have been established, single-stage primary resection of the rectal cancer and colorectal or anal anastomosis after intraoperative colonic irrigation with temporary ileostomy can also be proposed theoretically in this situation of intestinal obstruction due to rectal cancer. However, for most of the patients, it seems to be not a reasonable option. The main reasons are as follows: firstly, performing a colorectal or a coloanal anastomosis in a dilated and unprepared large bowel expose the patient to a high risk of leakage; secondly, as for Hartmann's procedure, risk of R1 or R2 resection if bulky tumor still exists if no neoadjuvant radiochemotherapy; and finally intraoperative colonic irrigation also includes risks as a longer operative time, a fecal spillage in the abdominal cavity which can increase the occurrence of an anastomotic leakage. Only selected patients with only partial intestinal obstruction and minor large bowel dilation can be proposed for such strategy.

Finally, in the rare case with massive dilatation of the whole colon due to obstruction by rectal cancer but with ischemia or even perforation of the caecum, the best option is probably an ileocecal resection with ileostomy and right colostomy which permit to treat obstruction and to have time for tumor staging and possible neoadjuvant radiochemotherapy.

9.3.4 Self-Expandable Metal Stents

Self-expandable metal stents (SEMS) were developed for the management of intestinal obstruction due to left colonic cancer, with two theoretical aims: curatively, as bridge to surgery before rectal resection and as a palliative procedure in patients with unresectable distant metastases [35–38]. SEMS has been widely studied for colonic obstruction rather than rectal obstruction in which placement of the stent can be impossible in case of too low tumor. However, it can be theoretically discussed in case of high rectal cancer. Although it seemed to be an attractive treatment of the obstruction allowing the correction of medical disorders and the complete tumor staging before treatment, this procedure is today known to be associated with a significant risk of perforation during the stent deployment, and also possible tumor cell dissemination, which can possibly jeopardize oncologic outcome [39, 40]. For these oncologic reasons, recent guidelines from several surgical and endoscopic societies have proposed to perform stent placement only as a palliative procedure bridge to surgery with curative intent.

9.4 Intestinal Perforation due to Rectal Cancer

Colorectal perforation is the second cause of surgical emergency in colorectal cancer. The incidence of perforation is estimated to be between 2.6% and 12% [41, 42]. The most frequent clinical symptom is abdominal pain. Perforation can be divided in two categories: free perforation, which causes diffuse peritonitis, and localized perforation which can be associated with a fistula between the rectum and a contiguity organ or only with a pelvic abscess.

Perforation due to rectal cancer commonly can occur (1) at the site of the primary tumor and can be due to a tumor lysis syndrome, sometimes facilitated by neoadjuvant radiochemotherapy, and (2) away from the tumor, on a dilated colon. The increasing pressure in the large bowel secondary to the rectal cancer obstruction can result to a localized ischemia of the large bowel and to a perforation according to the Laplace law. The most common site for a diastatic perforation is the cecum.

Perforation is associated with poor short-term outcome as it is known to be the most lethal complication of colorectal cancer with a mortality rate associated with peritonitis as high as 30–50% [4, 43]. Moreover, diastatic perforation of the cecum is an independent prognostic factor for morbi-mortality [44]. Very few information are reported about perforation due to rectal cancer, but this has been studied for colon cancer. It has been reported that colon cancer with perforation is considered as a poor prognostic factor along with T4 primary tumors [45, 46]. However, to the best of our knowledge, no studies have compared oncologic outcomes between patients with rectal cancer perforation and those with T4 rectal tumor.

9.4.1 Free Perforation

Free perforation with stool leak in the abdominal cavity leads to symptoms of diffuse peritonitis: major abdominal pain, fever, and generalized abdominal tenderness. CT imaging is generally performed (1) to confirm the diagnostic of perforation based on the presence of a pneumoperitoneum (Figs. 9.4 and 9.5a) and (2) to search some gravity signs such as pneumatosis and portal venous air. CT scan has a very good sensitivity and specificity to diagnose perforation from colorectal carcinoma (95–98% and 95–97%, respectively) [4]. A free perforation secondary from a colorectal tumor remains a surgical emergency responsible of poor short-term outcome.

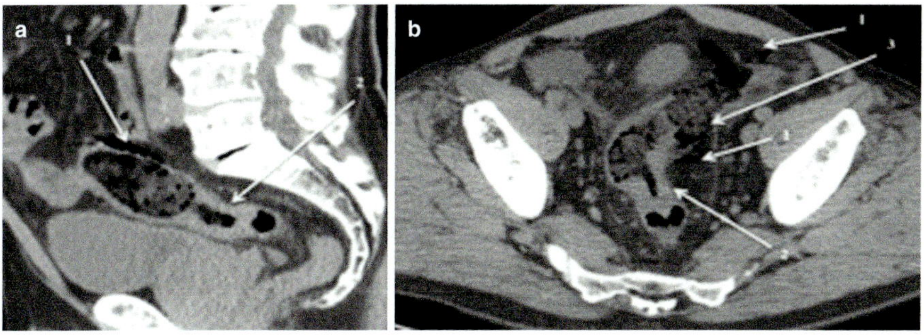

Fig. 9.4 (**a**) Sagittal CT scan with IV contrast: perforation due to a rectal tumor. 1, extra-digestive gas; 2, rectal tumor. (**b**) Axial CT scan. 3, site of the perforation

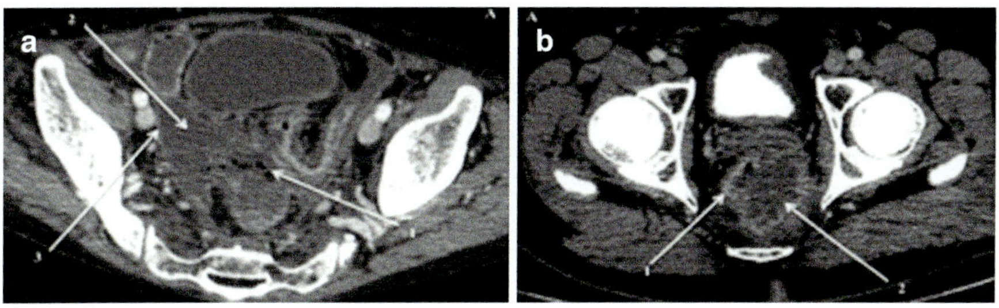

Fig. 9.5 (**a**) Axial CT scan with IV contrast: peritonitis secondary to an upper rectal tumor perforation. 1, extra-digestive gas; 2, peritoneal effusion; 3, peritoneum. (**b**) Axial CT scan 1, rectal tumor; 2, pelvic abscess

The surgical approach of this complication depends on the site of the perforation. In case of a perforation of the site of the rectal tumor associated with diffuse peritonitis, only a Hartmann procedure can be performed. In case of a diastatic perforation of the cecum, an ileocecal resection without rectal resection is the best option.

9.4.2 Pelvic Abscess

Contained perforation is diagnosed in a patient with localized abdominal pain, fever, and localized tenderness. CT scan confirms easily the diagnosis (Fig. 9.5b) which is more common than free perforation in colorectal cancer [47]. Treatment of pelvic abscess due to a rectal cancer perforation remains unclear and has to be discussed in multidisciplinary team meeting. For a small size abscess (<5 cm), IV antibiotics may probably be sufficient. For larger abscess, antibiotics associated with an ultrasound-guided or CT-guided percutaneous drainage can theoretically avoid the morbidity of an emergency proctectomy. Although percutaneous drainage presents many advantages as sparing the risk of a laparotomy, lower morbidity, and shorter length of hospital stay, drainage may result in spreading tumor cells along the drainage tract, in subcutaneous and skin plan which can lead to a metastatic disease [47]. For this reason, if the diagnosis of rectal is known, we prefer to avoid any percutaneous drainage if the aim is to treat the patient with curative intent. In these cases, if antibiotics fail to control sepsis, surgery with Hartmann's procedure is the only remaining option.

9.5 Conclusion

Emergencies related to primary rectal cancer remain rare and have been poorly reported in the literature. For this reason, it remains a subject of debate, and no guidelines have been proposed to date. The management of these patients needs most of the time a multidisciplinary team meeting with surgeons, intensivist, radiologists, and oncologists. The aim of the treatment is to try to avoid the high morbidity and the risk of suboptimal oncologic resection associated with emergency proctectomy.

References

1. Observatory IAfRoCEC. Available at http://eco.iarc.fr.
2. e-cancr. Projection d'incidence et de mortalité par localisation cancéreuse en 2017. Available at http://lesdonnees.e-cancer.fr/Themes/epidemiologie/Incidence-mortalite-nationale/Les-projections-2015-d-incidence-et-de-mortalite-par-cancer/Projection-d-incidence-et-de-mortalite-par-localisation-cancereuse-en-2017. 2017.
3. e-cancer. Le cancer colorectal. Available at http://lesdonnees.e-cancer.fr/Themes/Types-de-cancer/Le-cancer-colorectal. 2017.
4. Barnett A, Cedar A, Siddiqui F, et al. Colorectal cancer emergencies. J Gastrointest Cancer. 2013;44:132–42.
5. Gunnarsson H, Holm T, Ekholm A, Olsson LI. Emergency presentation of colon cancer is most frequent during summer. Colorectal Dis. 2011;13:663–8.
6. Abel GA, Shelton J, Johnson S, et al. Cancer-specific variation in emergency presentation by sex, age and deprivation across 27 common and rarer cancers. Br J Cancer. 2015;112(Suppl 1):S129–36.
7. Downing A, Aravani A, Macleod U, et al. Early mortality from colorectal cancer in England: a retrospective observational study of the factors associated with death in the first year after diagnosis. Br J Cancer. 2013;108:681–5.
8. McPhail S, Elliss-Brookes L, Shelton J, et al. Emergency presentation of cancer and short-term mortality. Br J Cancer. 2013;109:2027–34.
9. Baer C, Menon R, Bastawrous S, Bastawrous A. Emergency presentations of colorectal cancer. Surg Clin North Am. 2017;97:529–45.
10. Teixeira F, Akaishi EH, Ushinohama AZ, et al. Can we respect the principles of oncologic resection in an emergency surgery to treat colon cancer? World J Emerg Surg. 2015;10:5.
11. Chalieopanyarwong V, Boonpipattanapong T, Prechawittayakul P, Sangkhathat S. Endoscopic obstruction is associated with higher risk of acute events requiring emergency operation in colorectal cancer patients. World J Emerg Surg. 2013;8:34.
12. Panis Y, Maggiori L, Caranhac G, et al. Mortality after colorectal cancer surgery: a French survey of more than 84,000 patients. Ann Surg. 2011;254:738–43. discussion 743–734.
13. Kriwanek S, Armbruster C, Dittrich K, Beckerhinn P. Perforated colorectal cancer. Dis Colon Rectum. 1996;39:1409–14.

14. Goligher JC, Smiddy FG. The treatment of acute obstruction or perforation with carcinoma of the colon and rectum. Br J Surg. 1957;45:270–4.
15. Lakkis Z, Manceau G, Bridoux V, et al. Management of rectal cancer: the 2016 French guidelines. Colorectal Dis. 2017;19:115–22.
16. McArdle CS, Hole DJ. Emergency presentation of colorectal cancer is associated with poor 5-year survival. Br J Surg. 2004;91:605–9.
17. Bass G, Fleming C, Conneely J, et al. Emergency first presentation of colorectal cancer predicts significantly poorer outcomes: a review of 356 consecutive Irish patients. Dis Colon Rectum. 2009;52:678–84.
18. Weixler B, Warschkow R, Ramser M, et al. Urgent surgery after emergency presentation for colorectal cancer has no impact on overall and disease-free survival: a propensity score analysis. BMC Cancer. 2016;16:208.
19. van Gijn W, Marijnen CA, Nagtegaal ID, et al. Preoperative radiotherapy combined with total mesorectal excision for resectable rectal cancer: 12-year follow-up of the multicentre, randomised controlled TME trial. Lancet Oncol. 2011;12:575–82.
20. Ghassemi KA, Jensen DM. Lower GI bleeding: epidemiology and management. Curr Gastroenterol Rep. 2013;15:333.
21. Adelstein BA, Macaskill P, Chan SF, et al. Most bowel cancer symptoms do not indicate colorectal cancer and polyps: a systematic review. BMC Gastroenterol. 2011;11:65.
22. Korsgaard M, Pedersen L, Sorensen HT, Laurberg S. Reported symptoms, diagnostic delay and stage of colorectal cancer: a population-based study in Denmark. Colorectal Dis. 2006;8:688–95.
23. Rossini FP, Ferrari A, Spandre M, et al. Emergency colonoscopy. World J Surg. 1989;13:190–2.
24. Zuccaro G Jr. Management of the adult patient with acute lower gastrointestinal bleeding. American College of Gastroenterology. Practice Parameters Committee. Am J Gastroenterol. 1998;93:1202–8.
25. Davila RE, Rajan E, Adler DG, et al. ASGE Guideline: the role of endoscopy in the patient with lower-GI bleeding. Gastrointest Endosc. 2005;62:656–60.
26. Schuetz A, Jauch KW. Lower gastrointestinal bleeding: therapeutic strategies, surgical techniques and results. Langenbecks Arch Surg. 2001;386:17–25.
27. Tavakkolizadeh AAS. Acute gastrointestinal hemorrhage. In: Sabiston DC, Townsend Jr CM, editors. Sabiston text book of surgery: the biological basis of modern surgical practice. 19th ed. Philadelphia, PA: Elsevier; 2012. p. 1139–59.
28. Joye I, Haustermans K. Early and late toxicity of radiotherapy for rectal cancer. Recent Results Cancer Res. 2014;203:189–201.
29. Lee YM, Law WL, Chu KW, Poon RT. Emergency surgery for obstructing colorectal cancers: a comparison between right-sided and left-sided lesions. J Am Coll Surg. 2001;192:719–25.
30. Umpleby HC, Williamson RC. Survival in acute obstructing colorectal carcinoma. Dis Colon Rectum. 1984;27:299–304.
31. Frago R, Ramirez E, Millan M, et al. Current management of acute malignant large bowel obstruction: a systematic review. Am J Surg. 2014;207:127–38.
32. Frager D, Rovno HD, Baer JW, et al. Prospective evaluation of colonic obstruction with computed tomography. Abdom Imaging. 1998;23:141–6.
33. Zorcolo L, Covotta L, Carlomagno N, Bartolo DC. Safety of primary anastomosis in emergency colo-rectal surgery. Colorectal Dis. 2003;5:262–9.
34. Desai DC, Brennan EJ Jr, Reilly JF, Smink RD Jr. The utility of the Hartmann procedure. Am J Surg. 1998;175:152–4.
35. Karoui M, Charachon A, Delbaldo C, et al. Stents for palliation of obstructive metastatic colon cancer: impact on management and chemotherapy administration. Arch Surg. 2007;142:619–23. discussion 623.
36. Trompetas V. Emergency management of malignant acute left-sided colonic obstruction. Ann R Coll Surg Engl. 2008;90:181–6.
37. Kwak MS, Kim WS, Lee JM, et al. Does stenting as a bridge to surgery in left-sided colorectal cancer obstruction really worsen oncological outcomes? Dis Colon Rectum. 2016;59:725–32.

38. Dohmoto M, Hunerbein M, Schlag PM. Palliative endoscopic therapy of rectal carcinoma. Eur J Cancer. 1996;32A:25–9.
39. Maruthachalam K, Lash GE, Shenton BK, Horgan AF. Tumour cell dissemination following endoscopic stent insertion. Br J Surg. 2007;94:1151–4.
40. Sabbagh C, Browet F, Diouf M, et al. Is stenting as "a bridge to surgery" an oncologically safe strategy for the management of acute, left-sided, malignant, colonic obstruction? A comparative study with a propensity score analysis. Ann Surg. 2013;258:107–15.
41. Tsai HL, Hsieh JS, Yu FJ, et al. Perforated colonic cancer presenting as intra-abdominal abscess. Int J Colorectal Dis. 2007;22:15–9.
42. Lalani M, Rhee JC, Gutkin DW, et al. Uncommon presentations of some common malignancies: Case 3. Chronic lymphocytic leukemia involving the colon and presenting with perforation. J Clin Oncol. 2005;23:1315–7.
43. Langell JT, Mulvihill SJ. Gastrointestinal perforation and the acute abdomen. Med Clin North Am. 2008;92:599–625. viii–ix.
44. Alvarez JA, Baldonedo RF, Bear IG, et al. Presentation, treatment, and multivariate analysis of risk factors for obstructive and perforative colorectal carcinoma. Am J Surg. 2005;190:376–82.
45. Schmoll HJ, Van Cutsem E, Stein A, et al. ESMO Consensus Guidelines for management of patients with colon and rectal cancer. a personalized approach to clinical decision making. Ann Oncol. 2012;23:2479–516.
46. Benson AB III, Venook AP, Bekaii-Saab T, et al. Colon cancer, version 3.2014. J Natl Compr Canc Netw. 2014;12:1028–59.
47. Yeo ES, Ng KH, Eu KW. Perforated colorectal cancer: an important differential diagnosis in all presumed diverticular abscesses. Ann Acad Med Singapore. 2011;40:375–8.

Peritoneal Carcinomatosis and Other Emergencies Not Related to Primary Colorectal Cancer

10

Niccolò Petrucciani, Alexis Laurent, Francesco Brunetti, and Nicola de'Angelis

10.1 Introduction

Colorectal cancer emergencies may be related to the primary tumor, to liver metastases, or to other metastatic lesions, such as peritoneal disease. Peritoneal colorectal carcinomatosis requires medical and, in selected cases, surgical management that most of the times occurs in an emergency setting. In case of emergencies not related to the primary tumor, such as emergencies due to concomitant neutropenic, ischemic, and pseudomembranous colitis, the possibility of an incidental diagnosis of a colorectal neoplasm in patients presenting with a nonmalignant emergency diseases should be retained.

The aim of the present chapter is to discuss the incidence and risk factors of peritoneal carcinomatosis in patients with colorectal cancer, to examine the treatment modalities of emergency conditions related to peritoneal disease, and to discuss other emergencies not related to primary colorectal cancer or liver metastatic disease.

10.2 Colorectal Peritoneal Carcinomatosis: Pathophysiology, Incidence, and Risk Factors

Peritoneal carcinomatosis is due to the transcoelomic spread of colorectal cancer (CRC) in the peritoneal cavity. Several steps known as the "peritoneal metastatic cascade" are required for the development of peritoneal carcinomatosis, including

N. Petrucciani · A. Laurent · F. Brunetti · N. de'Angelis (✉)
Unit of Digestive, Hepato-Pancreato-Biliary Surgery and Liver Transplantation, Henri Mondor Hospital, AP-HP, Créteil, France

University of Paris Est, UPEC, Créteil, France

N. de'Angelis et al. (eds.), *Emergency Surgical Management of Colorectal Cancer*, Hot Topics in Acute Care Surgery and Trauma,
https://doi.org/10.1007/978-3-030-06225-5_10

the detachment of individual or clumps of tumor cells from the primary tumor, the attachment to the peritoneum, the peritoneal transport of tumor cells, the invasion of the subperitoneal space, and tumor cell proliferation and angiogenesis [1].

Intraperitoneal tumor spread may occur preoperatively as a result of full-thickness invasion of the colorectal wall by invasive cancer or may be induced iatrogenically during surgery, when tumor cells from the primary tumor and lymphatic or blood vessels may reach the peritoneal cavity consequently to surgical manipulations [2].

Synchronous peritoneal metastases occur in approximately 5% of patients with colorectal cancer, whereas metachronous carcinomatosis is reported in 5–19% of cases [3–5].

The peritoneal cavity may be the only site of recurrent disease in 25% of patients, which is one of the arguments in favor of aggressive treatment of peritoneal-only recurrence of CRC [2]. Risk factors for the development of peritoneal carcinomatosis include colonic cancer, high T-stage tumors (T3 and T4), N1–2 tumors, fewer than 12 harvested lymph nodes, emergency procedures, non-radical resection of the primary tumor, poor differentiation grade, and mucinous adenocarcinoma [3, 4, 6].

Predictive models have been validated to assess the risk of developing metachronous peritoneal carcinomatosis, in order to identify high-risk patients [7].

10.3 Staging of Peritoneal Carcinomatosis

The main used prognostic tool for peritoneal carcinomatosis is the Peritoneal Carcinomatosis Index (PCI), a scoring system that quantifies the extent of carcinomatosis, recognized as one of the most important prognostic indicators for the long-term outcomes of patients with peritoneal carcinomatosis [8]. The abdomen is divided into 13 regions: central region (0), right upper region (1), epigastrium region (2), left upper region (3), left blank region (4), left lower region (5), pelvis region (6), right lower region (7), right blank region (8), and the small bowel that is divided into four, upper jejunum region (9), lower jejunum region (10), upper ileum region (11), and lower ileum region (12). Each one is assigned a lesion-size (LS) score of 0–3, which would be representative of the largest implant lesion visualized. LS-0 stands for no tumor seen, LS-1 indicates implants <0.25 cm, LS-2 indicates implants between 0.25 and 5 cm, and LS-3 indicates implants >5 cm or a confluence of disease. PCI score is a final numerical score of 0–39. Several authors have demonstrated the relationship between PCI and overall survival [9]. In the study by Goere et al., patients with PCI below 10 had a 5-year OS of 53% versus 23% of those with PCI ranging from 10 to 20 and 12% for those with more than 20 [10]. Besides, Elias et al. [11] reported 5-year overall survival of 48% when the PCI was <15% vs. 12% when it was ≥15. PCI also influences the likelihood of complete cytoreduction [12].

10.4 Treatment Options and Survival Results

Treatment options of peritoneal carcinomatosis should ideally be discussed in a multidisciplinary oncologic team and range from systemic chemotherapy protocols, cytoreductive surgery with or without hyperthermic intraperitoneal chemotherapy, to palliative treatment [13, 14]. Even if randomized trials have suggested better survival outcomes in patients with peritoneal carcinomatosis treated with cytoreductive surgery and hyperthermic intraperitoneal chemotherapy (CRS/HIPEC), associated with systemic therapy compared to palliative management, treatment-related morbidity is higher in patients undergoing CRS/HIPEC [15, 16].

The majority of guidelines recommend the use of HIPEC as a potential curative treatment in selected patients; however the need of further randomized study to better explore benefits and risks has been highlighted by the NCCN group [5, 17].

Prognosis of colorectal carcinomatosis is poor, with median survival ranging from 6 months without chemotherapy, to 18 months with the use of chemotherapy combined with targeted therapy, to 22 months for patients undergoing complete cytoreductive surgery [18–22].

10.5 Emergency Related to Peritoneal Carcinomatosis

Among emergencies not related to primary colorectal cancer or liver metastases, emergencies related to peritoneal carcinomatosis represent complex and challenging clinical scenarios. Malignant bowel obstruction is a frequent complication, reported in 10–28% of all colorectal cancers, and it is common in patients with colorectal peritoneal carcinomatosis [23].

Clinical signs, as in bowel obstruction from other causes, include abdominal distension, pain, nausea and/or vomiting, and absence of gas or stool, with possible variations according to the level of the obstruction. Several etiologies are possible: mechanical obstruction may be caused by extrinsic bowel obstruction due to compression of the lumen by a tumoral mass (mesenteric, epiploic, parietal), by abdominal adhesions, or by radiation-induced fibrosis. Functional obstruction is possible, from impairment of intestinal motility due to mesentery or nervous infiltration, from secondary paralytic ileus due to intraperitoneal infection or ascites, or from high doses of opioid or anticholinergic drugs.

Diagnosis and optimal management of bowel obstruction in patients with peritoneal carcinomatosis are challenging and require the analysis of several variables including patient's performance status, treatment history, disease evolution, and mechanism of obstruction to define the optimal treatment. Etiological treatment, by means of relieving the obstruction, or symptomatic management only is possible. Multidisciplinary evaluation and consensus are recommended [23].

10.5.1 Diagnosis

It is crucial to obtain a correct diagnosis, in order to establish the best treatment. Computed tomography represents the main diagnostic tool, with specificity and sensitivity >90% [24]. Usually, bowel dilatation due to the obstruction allows the analysis of the bowel wall and the identification of a possible mechanical cause, without the need of gastrointestinal opacification. At CT scan, diagnosis of peritoneal carcinomatosis is based on the visualization of peritoneal masses, nodules or micronodules, thickening of the peritoneum, and/or ascites. Furthermore, CT scan can confirm the presence of mechanical obstruction by visualization of a transition zone between dilated and flat bowel. Bowel occlusion may be complicated by perforation, strangulation, or volvulus, identifying a potential indication for emergency surgery. Pneumoperitoneum represents a sign of bowel perforation, whereas specific signs help the diagnosis of volvulus (whirl sign) and bowel strangulation (bowel wall thickening, no enhancement of the intestinal wall). Parietal pneumatosis and portal vein pneumatosis represent late signs of ischemia. CT scan may also detect a nonmalignant cause of obstruction, which may be present in 15–30% of cases [25]. Adhesions represent a frequent cause of bowel obstruction even in patients with peritoneal carcinomatosis. Diagnosis of hernias is clinical, but CT scan may provide more information on the bowel segment affected. At least, diagnosis of radiation enteritis may be suggested by a regular thickening of the bowel wall.

10.5.2 Surgical Treatment

The treatment of bowel obstruction and related complications caused by carcinomatosis requires a complete evaluation of patients' condition, disease's features, and a precise diagnosis. Emergencies such as perforation, volvulus, and intestinal ischemia may be an indication for emergency surgery in these patients. However, patients' prognosis and condition should be carefully evaluated to avoid unnecessary surgery. Poor patient's condition or prognosis, or extended carcinomatosis, and massive infiltration of the root of the mesentery or of the mesocolon may represent relative contraindication to surgery. In case of operation, postoperative mortality and complications are not negligible, and results are better in patients having obstruction on a benign cause than on carcinomatosis [25]. In the series by Legendre et al., surgery improved the quality of life in 65% of patients, even if postoperative mortality was as high as 21% and the median survival was as low as 64 days [26, 27].

10.5.3 Medical Treatment

Medical management of peritoneal carcinomatosis is based on hydration, intestinal aspiration by nasogastric tube, steroids, and antisecretory and antiemetic drugs. Nasogastric tube is indicated for intractable vomiting and gastric distension, to relieve symptoms and avoid potential inhalation. Steroids have an anti-edematous effect on the obstructive mass and on the dilated bowel. They also have a central antiemetic effect. Administration of steroids such as methylprednisolone and dexamethasone is recommended for short periods (until approximately 10 days) at the time of the decision of medical management of the obstruction. Among the antisecretory drugs, the scopolamine and butylscopolamine have several effects, antispasmodic, antiemetic via vestibular centers, and antisecretory effect, and help in the management of vomiting and abdominal colic pain. They are contraindicated in case of glaucoma and urinary retention, and side effects include tachycardia, palpitations, and accommodation disorders. Proton-pump inhibitors inhibit hydrochloric acid secretion by blocking the HK-ATPase. Histamine antagonists block the H2 membrane receptor. Both drugs may be used to reduce acid secretion. PPIs are more effective in reduction of symptoms of bile reflux, esophagitis, and ulcers, whereas ranitidine is more effective in reducing the volume of gastric secretions [28, 29].

Somatostatin analogues (including octreotide and lanreotide) act in reducing splanchnic and portal blood flow, bowel secretions, and gastrointestinal motility and increasing gastrointestinal reabsorption. Somatostatin analogues are usually well tolerated with a few mild adverse events and no dropouts due to toxicity reported in a recent systematic review of RCTs. This study shows that results of RCTs are not concordant, with some showing significant reduction of nasogastric tube secretions or episodes of vomiting and other showing no difference comparing to placebo. However, the majority of authors support their use in this setting even in the need of higher evidence by further studies. Several classes of antiemetics, including metoclopramide, butyrophenones, haloperidol, and 5-HT3 receptor antagonists, are currently used to reduce vomiting induced by bowel obstruction, even if high-quality studies are lacking. Association of antiemetics is possible to obtain a clinical response [30, 31].

10.5.4 Endoscopic Treatments

Endoscopic treatment with placement of prosthesis is possible in selected cases of proximal or distal malignant bowel obstruction, even in the presence of carcinomatosis, as reported by a few studies [32]. A review concerning stent placement for malignant bowel obstruction found a clinical success of stenting in 81% of 116 patients with carcinomatosis, with reinterventions required in 17 of them for early (4) or late (13) stent failure. The results were comparable with those obtained in patients with malignant bowel obstruction without carcinomatosis [33].

Palliative gastrostomy is a therapeutic option in patients with high obstruction, suffering of intractable vomiting, not responders to medical treatment. Venting gastrostomy allows removal of nasogastric tube, and eating limited amount of food, which may be eliminated by the gastrostomy tube. The procedure may be performed radiologically or endoscopically in the majority of cases, with surgery reserved to those with history of previous partial gastrectomy or repeated surgery, adherences, or parietal masses not allowing gastric transillumination. Possible complications should be taken into account in the balance benefice risk, including surgical site infection, bleeding, and leakage around the tube [34–36].

10.6 Malignant Bowel Obstruction: Practical Points

Management of patients with malignant bowel requires careful evaluation of several aspects:

- Patients' and disease's characteristics: age; comorbidities; performance status; nutritional status; treatment; allergies; colorectal cancer history including staging and previous surgery, radiotherapy, or chemotherapy; extension of the peritoneal carcinomatosis; and possibility of a potentially curative treatment.
- Symptoms' evaluation: nausea, vomiting, fever, characteristics of the pain, sensation of abdominal distension, and gas and stool evacuation.
- Clinical examination: vital signs, performance status, nutritional status, research of signs of metastatic disease (superficial lymphadenopathy, parietal masses), and research of signs of peritonitis.
- Blood tests including white cell count, CRP, tumor markers, and nutritional markers.
- CT scan is recommended in the majority of cases to (1) identify the obstruction, the etiology, the characteristics, and the level of the stenosis; (2) differentiate benign from malignant cause (important for prognostic evaluation); (3) identify potential indication for emergency surgery (bowel perforation or ischemia for volvulus or strangulation); and (4) evaluate the extension of the disease.

In the light of these data, multidisciplinary evaluation including oncologists'/radiotherapists' and surgeons' advice is recommended. Assessing of patient's will is obviously fundamental. The decision should be individualized, case-by-case, and may consist in medical treatment, endoscopic/radiologic procedures or surgery.

Potential indications for surgery are nonneoplastic cause of obstruction (adherences, volvulus, hernias, incisional hernias) and bowel perforation and/or bowel ischemia.

However, surgery is generally contraindicated in case of:

1. Patient's disagreement
2. Poor patient's general condition
3. Very poor prognosis for extensive metastatic disease, multiple obstructions, and invasion of the root of mesentery

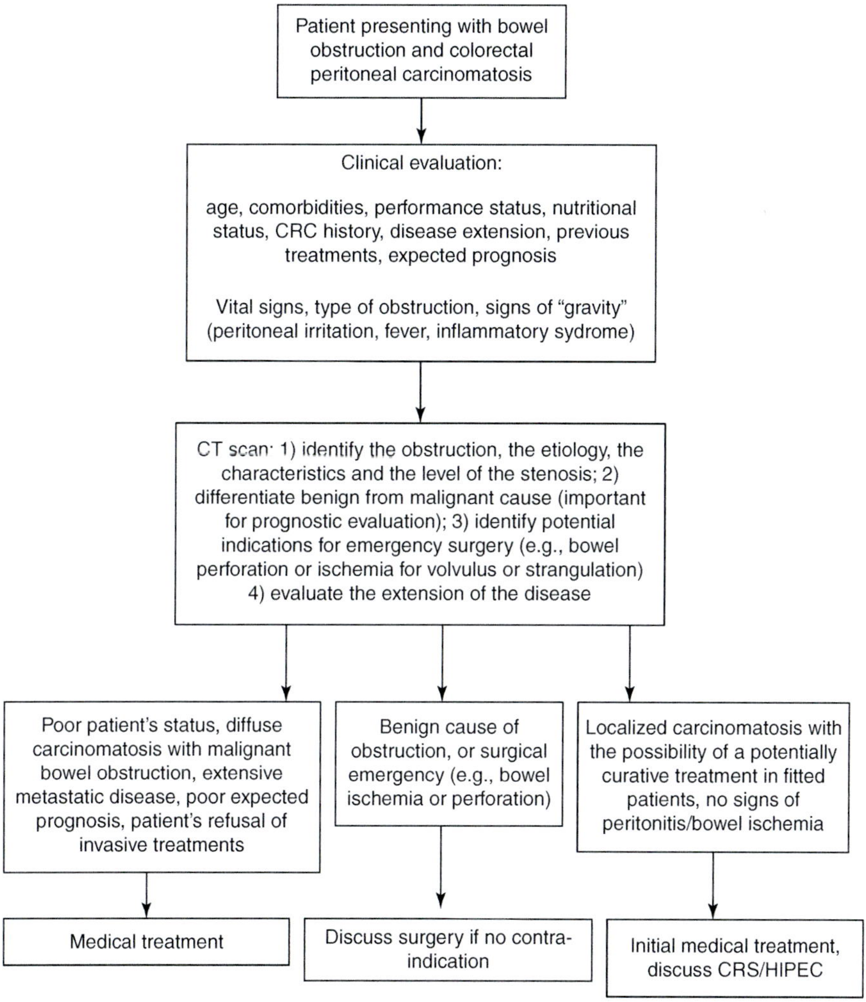

Fig. 10.1 Emergency management of bowel obstruction in patients with peritoneal carcinomatosis

A flowchart is proposed to show the possible clinical scenarios and the respective treatment options (Figs. 10.1 and 10.2).

In Figs. 10.3 and 10.4, the CT imaging of a patient with left colonic obstruction for peritoneal carcinomatosis (Fig. 10.3) complicated by colic perforation and peritonitis (Fig. 10.4) is shown.

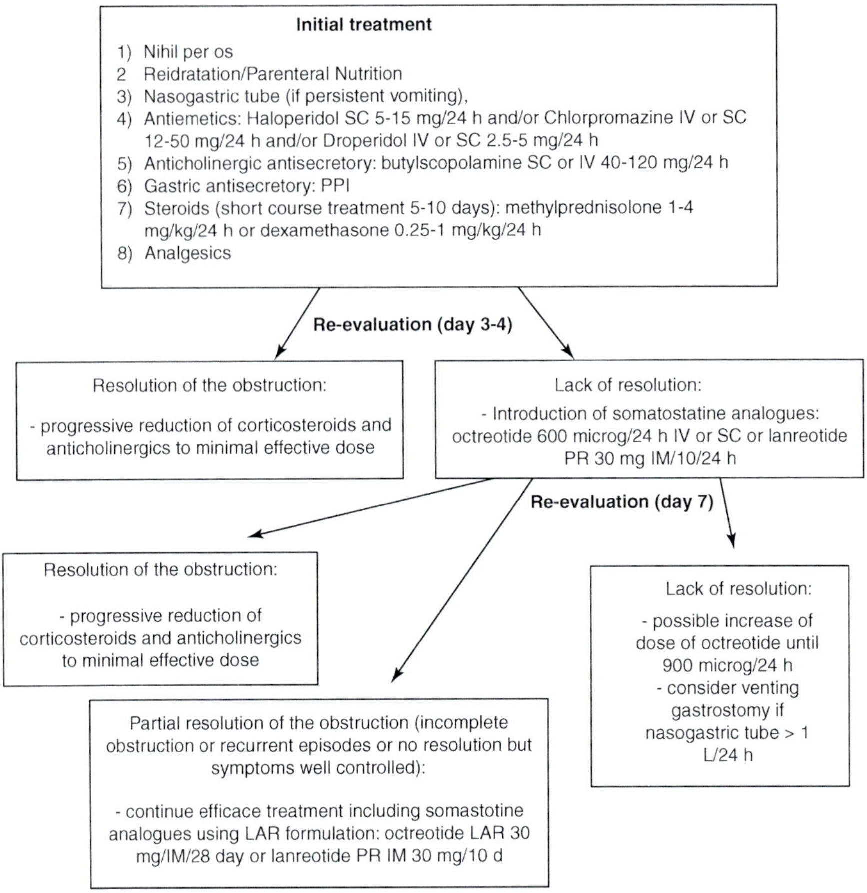

Fig. 10.2 Medical palliative management of bowel obstruction on peritoneal carcinomatosis

10.7 Emergency Related to Colitis (Ischemic, Neutropenic, and Pseudomembranous)

One percent to 11% of patients with obstructive colon cancer present with colonic wall thickening proximal to the colic tumor, for ischemic or obstructive colitis [37, 38]. Usually, bowel ischemia induced by bowel distention is regarded as the mechanism involved in colonic wall thickening. However, this finding can occur also in patients without colic obstruction. Furthermore, pathological examinations in these cases may show submucosal edema rather than frank bowel ischemia [37].

Ischemic colitis on CT scan appears as a smooth, annular wall thickening with a homogeneous or layered enhancement pattern. These areas are frequently contiguous with an irregularly thickened neoplastic segment. Occasionally, normal mucosa between the tumor and the ischemic segment may be present. Colonic wall

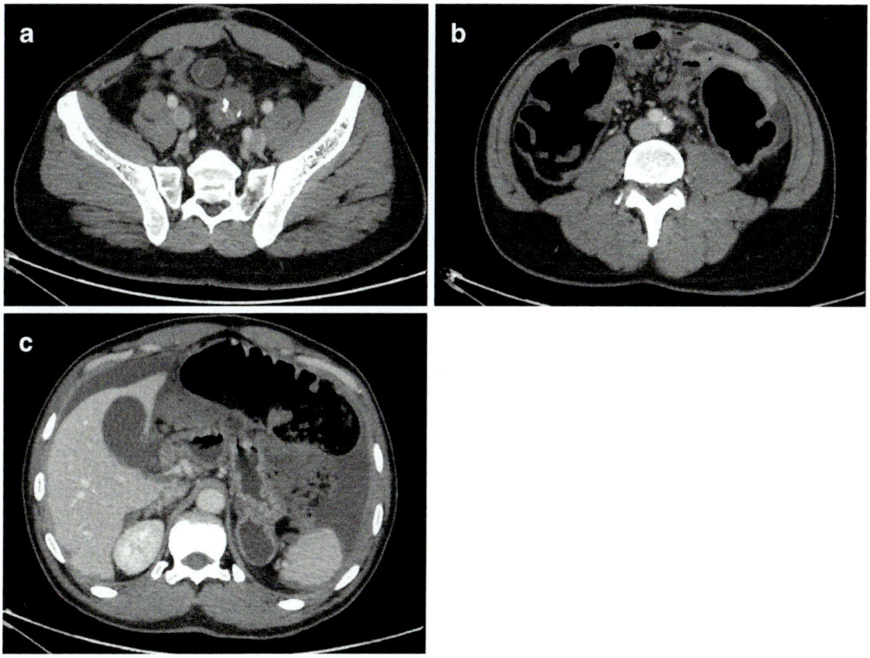

Fig. 10.3 (**a–c**) CT imaging of a patient with left colonic obstruction for peritoneal carcinomatosis. (**a**) Peritoneal carcinomatosis causing colic obstruction in a patient with previous left colectomy. (**b**) Cecum dilatation for colic obstruction. (**c**) Colic dilatation and ascites for colonic obstruction for peritoneal carcinomatosis

thickening distal to a large fungating mass may also be found corresponding to edema or colitis at pathological analysis [39, 40].

Neutropenic colitis is a clinical entity initially described in leukemic pediatric patients, which has been reported also in hematologic malignancies, solid tumors, immunosuppressive conditions as AIDS, and organ transplant [41]. It is a serious condition with mortality rates as high as 50% and a pooled incidence of 5.6% in patients with hematological malignancies, chemotherapy for solid tumors, and aplastic anemia [42]. Several chemotherapies and other drugs including taxane, cytosine arabinoside, gemcitabine, vincristine, doxorubicin, gemcitabine, cyclophosphamide, 5-fluorouracil, leucovorin, and daunorubicin, immunosuppressive therapy for organ transplant, antibiotics, and sulfasalazine for the treatment of rheumatoid arthritis have been associated with neutropenic colitis. Pathogenesis is not fully understood. Intestinal mucosal injury and neutropenia may lead to intestinal edema, engorged vessels, and a disrupted mucosal surface, with vulnerability to bacterial intramural invasion. Chemotherapeutic agents can cause direct mucosal injury (mucositis) or can predispose to distension and necrosis, thereby altering intestinal motility. The cecum is always affected by neutropenic colitis. The ascending and transverse colon may also be involved. Superimposed infections of the damaged mucosa may be caused by gram-negative rods, gram-positive cocci, enterococci,

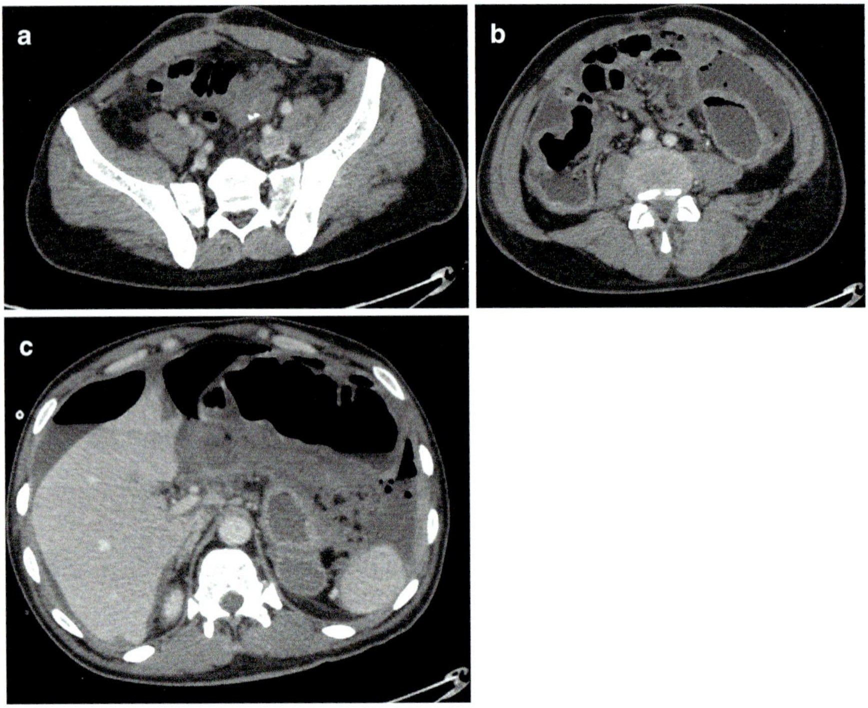

Fig. 10.4 (**a**–**c**) CT imaging of a patient (same patient shown in Fig. 10.3) with left colonic obstruction for peritoneal carcinomatosis, after colic perforation and peritonitis. (**a**) Peritoneal carcinomatosis causing colic obstruction in a patient with previous left colectomy. (**b**) Resolution of cecum dilatation after colic perforation. (**c**) Pneumoperitoneum and ascites after colic perforation due to colic obstruction due to peritoneal carcinomatosis

fungi, and virus have been implicated as causes. The most common symptoms are abdominal pain, diarrhea, fever, nausea, vomiting, and abdominal distension. Gastrointestinal bleeding is a less common symptom. Patients with colic necrosis or perforation present with signs of peritonitis, shock, and rapid clinical deterioration. Disease presentation usually occurs within 2 weeks following the completion of chemotherapy in the period of low leukocyte count. Diagnosis is based on clinical examination, laboratory findings (neutropenia, thrombocytopenia, electrolyte imbalance), and colonic aspect at CT scan (wall thickening, a dilated cecum or other colonic segment, an inflammatory mass, pericolonic inflammation, pneumatosis intestinalis). Conservative management of neutropenic colitis fluid resuscitation, with correction of electrolytes disorders, bowel rest, and broad-spectrum antibiotics. In critically ill patients, antibiotics should cover gram-positive, gram-negative, anaerobic pathogens and enterococci. Granulocyte colony-stimulating factors (G-CSF) have been recommended. Parenteral nutrition is used to maintain adequate caloric intake and avoid catabolism.

Among the differential diagnosis of colitis in patients treated for CRC, pseudomembranous colitis should be retained and ruled out. Pseudomembranous colitis is a colitis due to *Clostridium difficile* infection, with an incidence of 8.2 cases per 1000 discharges in 2010 and a mortality rate of around 7% [43]. Normal bacterial flora is disrupted, the colon is colonized with the *Clostridium difficile* bacteria, and toxins are released, causing mucosal damage and inflammation. Antibiotics but also chemotherapies may be at the origin of the initial modification of the flora. 5-FU is a chemotherapy agent commonly used for CRC. It causes diarrhea in 10–20% of cases and hematological toxicity in 10–45% of cases. The diarrhea is usually watery and generally of short duration. Pseudomembranous colitis has been associated with chemotherapy alone or antibiotics with chemotherapy regimens. Symptoms include profuse diarrhea (rarely bloody), abdominal pain and distension, and fever. At CT scan, thickening of the colic wall and the "double halo" sign may be found; however, the diagnosis is based on the detection of the B toxin in the stools, with a sensibility of 94–100% and a specificity of 99%. Possible complications include perforation, hemorrhage, toxic megacolon, dehydration, or sepsis. Initial treatment consists in antibiotics (metronidazole or vancomycin), whereas surgery is reserved to complicated cases (peritonitis) or to patients non-responding to medical treatment. Pseudomembranous colitis should be ruled out in CRC patients presenting with symptoms and signs of colitis [44].

10.8 Incidental Diagnosis of Colorectal Cancer During Emergency Treatment of Other Diseases

According to epidemiologic data by GLOBOCAN, colorectal cancer represents the third more frequent tumor worldwide with approximately 1,360,602 new cases/year and the second in Europe (excluding non-melanomas cutaneous tumors) with 447,136 new cases/year [45]. So, occasionally, incidental diagnosis of colorectal cancer may be done in patients presenting for other emergency conditions. Acute abdominal pain of other origins (cholecystitis, appendicitis, sigmoiditis) is usually investigated with CT scan with contrast enhancement, which may detect colorectal wall thickening or mesenteric or mesorectal lymphadenopathies [46]. Such patients should be stabilized and treated for the disease responsible of the emergency clinical scenario. In a second time, a colonoscopy with biopsies should be scheduled, along with tumor marker's dosage and a complete imaging staging, as indicated according to tumor localization and features (thoracic CT, MRI, echoendoscopy).

10.9 Conclusions

Among the emergency not related to the primary colorectal cancer, a relevant problem is malignant bowel obstruction in patients with peritoneal carcinomatosis. Management of these patients is complex and requires a multidisciplinary expertise and a complete evaluation of the patient's and disease status. If a benign cause (adherence, volvulus) is responsible of the obstruction or in case of bowel perforation, peritonitis, and bowel ischemia, surgery may be indicated. Medical management includes nasogastric aspiration, steroids, and antisecretory and antiemetic drugs, and it is appropriate in patients with obstruction and diffuse carcinosis. Endoscopic stenting may represent a less invasive option to relieve a proximal or distal obstruction, whereas venting gastrostomy is reserved to patients with intractable vomiting for high obstruction, not responsive to medical treatment and not tolerating nasogastric aspiration. Colitis associated with CRC may have different etiologies, ischemic, neutropenic, or pseudomembranous, and requires a prompt diagnosis and management.

References

1. Lemoine L, Sugarbaker P, Van der Speeten K. Pathophysiology of colorectal peritoneal carcinomatosis: role of the peritoneum. World J Gastroenterol. 2016;22:7692–707.
2. Koppe MJ, Boerman OC, Oyen WJ, Bleichrodt RP. Peritoneal carcinomatosis of colorectal origin: incidence and current treatment strategies. Ann Surg. 2006;243:212–22.
3. Lemmens VE, Klaver YL, Verwaal VJ, Rutten HJ, Coebergh JW, de Hingh IH. Predictors and survival of synchronous peritoneal carcinomatosis of colorectal origin: a population-based study. Int J Cancer. 2011;128:2717–25.
4. Segelman J, Granath F, Holm T, Machado M, Mahteme H, Martling A. Incidence, prevalence and risk factors for peritoneal carcinomatosis from colorectal cancer. Br J Surg. 2012;99:699–705.
5. Klaver CE, Groenen H, Morton DG, Laurberg S, Bemelman WA, Tanis PJ. Recommendations and consensus on the treatment of peritoneal metastases of colorectal origin: a systematic review of national and international guidelines. Colorectal Dis. 2017;19:224–36.
6. Sadahiro S, Suzuki T, Maeda Y, Tanaka A, Makuuchi H, Kamijo A, Haruki Y, Murayama C. Prognostic factors in patients with synchronous peritoneal carcinomatosis (PC) caused by a primary cancer of the colon. J Gastrointest Surg. 2009;13:1593–8.
7. Segelman J, Akre O, Gustafsson UO, Bottai M, Martling A. External validation of models predicting the individual risk of metachronous peritoneal carcinomatosis from colon and rectal cancer. Colorectal Dis. 2016;18:378–85.
8. Sugarbaker PH. Peritoneal surface oncology: review of a personal experience with colorectal and appendiceal malignancy. Tech Coloproctol. 2005;9:95–103.
9. Faron M, Macovei R, Goéré D, Honoré C, Benhaim L, Elias D. Linear relationship of peritoneal cancer index and survival in patients with peritoneal metastases from colorectal cancer. Ann Surg Oncol. 2016;23:114–9.
10. Goéré D, Malka D, Tzanis D, et al. Is there a possibility of a cure in patients with colorectal peritoneal carcinomatosis amenable to complete cytoreductive surgery and intraperitoneal chemotherapy? Ann Surg. 2013;257:1065–71.
11. Elias D, Mariani A, Cloutier AS, et al. Modified selection criteria for complete cytoreductive surgery plus HIPEC based on peritoneal cancer index and small bowel involvement for peritoneal carcinomatosis of colorectal origin. Eur J Surg Oncol. 2014;40:1467–73.
12. Glehen O, Kwiatkowski F, Sugarbaker PH, et al. Cytoreductive surgery combined with perioperative intraperitoneal chemotherapy for the management of peritoneal carcinomatosis from colorectal cancer: a multi-institutional study. J Clin Oncol. 2004;22:3284–92.
13. Mo S, Cai G. Multidisciplinary treatment for colorectal peritoneal metastases: review of the literature. Gastroenterol Res Pract. 2016;2016:1516259.
14. Wu W, Yan S, Liao X, et al. Curative versus palliative treatments for colorectal cancer with peritoneal carcinomatosis: a systematic review and meta-analysis. Oncotarget. 2017;8:113202–12.
15. Arjona-Sánchez A, Barrios P, Boldo-Roda E, et al. HIPECT4: multicentre, randomized clinical trial to evaluate safety and efficacy of Hyperthermic intra-peritoneal chemotherapy (HIPEC)

with Mitomycin C used during surgery for treatment of locally advanced colorectal carcinoma. BMC Cancer. 2018;18:183.
16. Avital I, Brücher BL, Nissan A, Stojadinovic A. Randomized clinical trials for colorectal cancer peritoneal surface malignancy. Surg Oncol Clin N Am. 2012;21:665–88.
17. NCCN. Clinical Practice Guidelines in Oncology, Colon Cancer, version 2.18, March 2018. https://www.nccn.org/professionals/physician_gls/pdf/colon.pdf. Accessed April 25, 2018.
18. Sadeghi B, Arvieux C, Glehen O, et al. Peritoneal carcinomatosis from non-gynecologic malignancies: results of the EVOCAPE 1 multicentric prospective study. Cancer. 2000;88:358–63.
19. Klaver YL, Leenders BJ, Creemers GJ, et al. Addition of biological therapies to palliative chemotherapy prolongs survival in patients with peritoneal carcinomatosis of colorectal origin. Am J Clin Oncol. 2013;36:157–61.
20. Verwaal VJ, Bruin S, Boot H, van Slooten G, van Tinteren H. 8-year follow-up of randomized trial: cytoreduction and hyperthermic intraperitoneal chemotherapy versus systemic chemotherapy in patients with peritoneal carcinomatosis of colorectal cancer. Ann Surg Oncol. 2008;15:2426–32.
21. Arakawa K, Kawai K, Ishihara S, et al. Prognostic significance of peritoneal metastasis in stage IV colorectal cancer patients with R0 resection: a multicenter, retrospective study. Dis Colon Rectum. 2017;60:1041–9.
22. Quere P, Facy O, Manfredi S, Jooste V, Faivre J, Lepage C, Bouvier AM. Epidemiology, management, and survival of peritoneal carcinomatosis from colorectal cancer: a population-based study. Dis Colon Rectum. 2015;58:743–52.
23. Laval G, Marcelin-Benazech B, Guirimand F, et al. Recommendations for bowel obstruction with peritoneal carcinomatosis. J Pain Symptom Manage. 2014;48:75–91.
24. Silva AC, Pimenta M, Guimarães LS. Small bowel obstruction: what to look for. Radiographics. 2009;29:423–39.
25. Woolfson RG, Jennings K, Whalen GF. Management of bowel obstruction in patients with abdominal cancer. Arch Surg. 1997;132:1093–7.
26. Legendre H, Vanhuyse F, Caroli-Bosc FX, Pector JC. Survival and quality of life after palliative surgery for neoplastic gastrointestinal obstruction. Eur J Surg Oncol. 2001;27:364–7.
27. Dalal KM, Gollub MJ, Miner TJ, et al. Management of patients with malignant bowel obstruction and stage IV colorectal cancer. J Palliat Med. 2011;14:822–8.
28. Clark K, Lam L, Currow D. Reducing gastric secretions--a role for histamine 2 antagonists or proton pump inhibitors in malignant bowel obstruction? Support Care Cancer. 2009;17:1463–8.
29. Ripamonti CI, Easson AM, Gerdes H. Management of malignant bowel obstruction. Eur J Cancer. 2008;44:1105–15.
30. Murray-Brown F, Dorman S. Haloperidol for the treatment of nausea and vomiting in palliative care patients. Cochrane Database Syst Rev. 2015;11(2):CD006271.
31. Obita GP, Boland EG, Currow DC, Johnson MJ, Boland JW. Somatostatin analogues compared with placebo and other pharmacologic agents in the management of symptoms of inoperable malignant bowel obstruction: a systematic review. J Pain Symptom Manage. 2016;52:901–919.e1.
32. Caceres A, Zhou Q, Iasonos A, Gerdes H, Chi DS, Barakat RR. Colorectal stents for palliation of large-bowel obstructions in recurrent gynecologic cancer: an updated series. Gynecol Oncol. 2008;108:482–5.
33. Mendelsohn RB, Gerdes H, Markowitz AJ, DiMaio CJ, Schattner MA. Carcinomatosis is not a contraindication to enteral stenting in selected patients with malignant gastric outlet obstruction. Gastrointest Endosc. 2011;73:1135–40.
34. Brooksbank MA, Game PA, Ashby MA. Palliative venting gastrostomy in malignant intestinal obstruction. Palliat Med. 2002;16:520–6.
35. Paul Olson TJ, Pinkerton C, Brasel KJ, Schwarze ML. Palliative surgery for malignant bowel obstruction from carcinomatosis: a systematic review. JAMA Surg. 2014;149:383–92.
36. Shariat-Madar B, Jayakrishnan TT, Gamblin TC, Turaga KK. Surgical management of bowel obstruction in patients with peritoneal carcinomatosis. J Surg Oncol. 2014;110:666–9.

37. Ko GY, Ha HK, Lee HJ, et al. Usefulness of CT in patients with ischemic colitis proximal to colonic cancer. AJR Am J Roentgenol. 1997;168:951–6.
38. Xiong L, Chintapalli KN, Dodd GD, et al. Frequency and CT patterns of bowel wall thickening proximal to cancer of the colon. AJR Am J Roentgenol. 2004;182:905–9.
39. Jang HJ, Lim HK, Park CK, Kim SH, Park JM, Choi YL. Segmental wall thickening in the colonic loop distal to colonic carcinoma at CT: importance and histopathologic correlation. Radiology. 2000;216:712–7.
40. Chiu HH, Chen CM, Mo LR, Chao TJ. Gastrointestinal: ischemic colitis associated with colon cancer. J Gastroenterol Hepatol. 2005;20:1458.
41. Rodrigues FG, Dasilva G, Wexner SD. Neutropenic enterocolitis. World J Gastroenterol. 2017;23:42–7.
42. Gorschlüter M, Mey U, Strehl J, et al. Neutropenic enterocolitis in adults: systematic analysis of evidence quality. Eur J Haematol. 2005;75:1–13.
43. Ong GK, Reidy TJ, Huk MD, Lane FR. Clostridium difficile colitis: a clinical review. Am J Surg. 2017;213:565–71.
44. Morales Chamorro R, Serrano Blanch R, Méndez Vidal MJ, Gómez España MA, Rubio Pérez MJ, de la Haba Rodríguez JR, Aranda Aguilar E. Pseudomembranous colitis associated with chemotherapy with 5-fluorouracil. Clin Transl Oncol. 2005;7:258–61.
45. GLOBOCAN 2012. Estimated cancer incidence, mortality and prevalence worldwide in 2012. http://globocan.iarc.fr/Pages/fact_sheets_cancer.aspx. Accessed April 25, 2018.
46. Mangat S, Kozoriz MG, Bicknell S, Spielmann A. The accuracy of colorectal cancer detection by computed tomography in the unprepared large bowel in a community-based hospital. Can Assoc Radiol J. 2018;69:92–6.

Emergencies Related to Advanced Metastatic Colorectal Cancer

11

Riccardo Memeo, Alessandro Verbo, Patrick Pessaux, and Emanuele Felli

11.1 Introduction

Oncologic patient with advanced metastatic liver cancer is exposed to life-threatening complications. The origins and management of these complications could be different and request a multidisciplinary management in order to reduce the risk of uneventful events and continue cancer management. This kind of complication can origin from tumor bleeding or rupture, biliary obstruction due to mass compression or intraductal metastasis, hemobilia, liver abscess and infection, portal vein thrombosis and stenosis, and hepatic vein compression. The aim of this chapter is to identify the best therapeutic strategy for each of these complications.

11.2 Bleeding

In 1844 Abercrombie first described spontaneous liver bleeding [1], and still today it globally remains a rare complication, even when all the possible etiologies are considered. Liver bleeding secondary to colorectal liver metastasis is extremely rare. Symptoms and signs are often non-specific, but as any hemorrhagic episode, it

R. Memeo (✉)
Department of Emergency and Organ Transplantation, Institute of General Surgery and Liver Transplantation, University of Bari, Bari, Italy

A. Verbo
Hepato-Biliary and Pancreatic Surgical Unit, Miulli Hospital, Bari, Italy

P. Pessaux · E. Felli
Hepato-Biliary and Pancreatic Surgical Unit, General, Digestive, and Endocrine Surgery, IRCAD, Strasbourg's IHU (Institute for Minimally Invasive Image-Guided Surgery), University of Strasbourg, Strasbourg, France

N. de'Angelis et al. (eds.), *Emergency Surgical Management of Colorectal Cancer*, Hot Topics in Acute Care Surgery and Trauma,
https://doi.org/10.1007/978-3-030-06225-5_11

can be a life-threatening condition. Treatment is variable, from a conservative approach to more invasive procedures such as percutaneous trans-arterial embolization, explorative laparotomy for arterial ligation, hepatectomy, or packing; ideally, the treatment strategy should always be secondary to a multidisciplinary team discussion, according to the patient clinical status and the prognosis of the disease. Battula and colleagues [2] reported over a 16 single-center experience and a cohort of 4271 malignant and 2275 benign hepatobiliary patients referred to the unit in the study period and 67 patients with spontaneous liver bleeding. Two of these (2.9%) were secondary to non-resectable colorectal liver metastasis. One of the two patients was managed conservatively and the other with packing. In the same period, a total of 1884 patients have been diagnosed of metastatic colorectal cancer; considering this, we can assume that the incidence of spontaneous bleeding secondary to colorectal liver metastasis is about 0.1%. Different types of bleeding can be present (arterial or venous); number and localization of liver metastasis are important to consider the treatment of choice. In the case of spontaneous liver hemorrhage and good general conditions, detailed history, past medical history, careful physical examination, blood tests, and contrast-enhanced CT scan are mandatory to establish a correct diagnosis and plan the best treatment. The CT finding in the acute setting is the presence of an arterial blush secondary to contrast extravasation. If blood loss is not associated with active bleeding, a conservative treatment with blood transfusions or simple fluid resuscitation can be made, monitoring vital signs and blood cell count. When active arterial bleeding is present, a trans-arterial embolization is the treatment of choice. Sometimes after a percutaneous embolization bleeding can persist, reserving a subsequent explorative laparotomy in better conditions. In case of hemodynamic instability and without the possibility of performing a CT scan, an explorative laparotomy is mandatory. If local control is not possible, ligation of an arterial branch may be an option, with consequent possible biliary tree ischemia. Hepatectomy is rarely needed because of the frequent context of advanced, non-resectable disease. If no mean of bleeding control is present, packing is the last resource.

11.3 Rupture and Hemoperitoneum

Spontaneous hepatic tumor rupture secondary to metastatic liver disease is a rare event. Liver metastases are usually less vascularized than primary liver tumors and have a more fibrous component. In the literature many reports are present concerning spontaneous hepatic rupture from different sites, including the lung, esophagus, stomach, gallbladder, pancreas, colon, kidney, prostate, and others [3–6]. Clinical presentation is variable and often associated with advanced metastatic disease. Abdominal pain or discomfort, fever, nausea, or vomiting is frequently present. In case of bleeding, hypotension, tachycardia, or hemorrhagic shock is frequent. Careful clinical examination, complete blood exams, and contrast-enhanced CT scan are the first step in order to make the diagnosis, to evaluate the extension of liver metastasis and other possible localizations of the disease, and to choose the best treatment. In case of rupture associated with active bleeding and hemoperitoneum, in a patient hemodynamically stable, trans-arterial embolization should be the first treatment. Once the hemorrhage has been controlled, and in the presence of huge hemoperitoneum, a peritoneal lavage made by laparoscopy or laparotomy can be associated to avoid fluid collection and infection. When active bleeding cannot be controlled, or in case of hemodynamic instability, urgent laparotomy associated with local control, hepatic arterial ligation, or packing may be an option. Hepatectomy can be considered if metastasis is localized and if the prognosis of the disease justifies an additional operative risk. As for the perforated colorectal primary tumors, metastatic rupture has a poor outcome because of the diffusion of neoplastic cells in the peritoneum.

11.3.1 Biliary Obstruction

Jaundice in oncological patient can arise from different causes. Most of the time, neoplastic mass could cause a mechanic compression of a bile duct (extrinsic compression, invasion, or intraluminal metastatic obstruction) or be caused by terminal liver dysfunction due to neoplastic invasion of liver parenchyma.

It is usually identified with upper quadrant abdominal pain, dark urine, and acholic stools, and often itch is present. Blood test is characterized by augmented bilirubin, associated with augmented transaminases and alkaline phosphatase. The easiest way to comprehend if jaundice is caused by mechanical obstacle [7, 8] or liver dysfunction is to perform a Doppler ultrasound of the liver. In case of biliary dilatation and obstruction, it could be useful to complete diagnosis with a CT scan or a magnetic resonance cholangiopancreatography, to stage the liver invasion of the biliary tree. In case of jaundice, a biliary decompression could be necessary, due to the high risk of cholangitis and sepsis. This decompression could be achieved either endoscopically or percutaneously [9]. Usually, endoscopic decompression is preferred, allowing a biliary drainage in the duodenum with an augmented comfort for the patient. Plastic or metal stent [10] could be used, depending on the possibility or not to have a surgical treatment of the liver mass. Metal stent is often chosen in case of palliative cases, in which a longer drainage should be guaranteed. In case of impossibility to have an endoscopic stent placement, percutaneous drainage could be used to treat the emergency and to achieve a rapid decompression of structures. Once emergency is treated, the involved area could be passed through, and an internal-external drainage [11] could be placed. Biliary obstruction treatment could be necessary to start chemotherapy, which is contraindicated in case of severe jaundice.

11.4 Hemobilia

Hemobilia is a rare cause of digestive tract hemorrhage, and it is secondary to iatrogenic injury in about 70% of cases [12–14]. Other causes of hemobilia are rare and include malignancy, gallstones, and vascular and inflammatory diseases.

Colorectal liver metastases are a very rare cause of spontaneous hemobilia. The historical triad described by Heinrich Quincke in 1871 including gastrointestinal hemorrhage, pain, and jaundice is present only in 22% of cases [12]. Most of the time, any of these symptoms and signs can be present independently and in variable chronologic order. Anemia may be mild and can be the only finding in case of minor bleeding secondary to invasion or erosion of the bile duct walls. More consistent bleeding is usually associated with cholestasis, often already present in case of diffuse metastatic liver invasion. When active arterial bleeding is massive, hematemesis, rectal bleeding, and hemorrhagic shock are the commonest clinical presentation. Diagnosis is usually made looking for active bleeding in contrast-enhanced CT scan; most of the time, bleeding is seen as a blush in the arterial phase. Fluid resuscitation, blood transfusion when required, and careful monitoring are the common treatments to any other cause of hemorrhagic shock. Percutaneous arterial embolization or stenting is the treatment of choice in most of the cases, reaching nearly 100% of success in selected series [15]. Once the bleeding has been controlled, the clots present in the biliary tract may cause obstructive jaundice, needing endoscopic treatment or bile duct surgical exploration. In the rare cases of percutaneous treatment failure, surgery may be a last resource, with the hepatic artery branch ligation and biliary drainage or decompression to treat the obstruction caused by clots in the main bile duct.

11.4.1 Liver Abscess and Infection

Liver abscess can be defined as an infected cavity caused by bacteria via arterial, portal vein, bile duct, or blood stream. In the case of advanced oncologic patient, liver metastasis could cause an alteration in liver parenchyma due to the presence of metastatic mass [16]. Clinical signs include abdominal pain, fever, and an inflammatory syndrome. Liver function tests could be more or less abnormal, depending on the extent of the abscess and degree of sepsis. In particular, oncologic patients, who are immunosuppressed and often fragilized by antitumoral therapies, are considered at higher risk of complication and mortality.

A liver abscess is often diagnosed by ultrasound or in more than 90% of patients by CT scan.

The management varies in function of clinical condition of the patient and on size of abscess. In some cases, rupture of abscess could create intra-abdominal collection with sepsis. In case of advanced metastatic malignancy [17], abscess should be treated as "benign" abscess, with the priority to reduce sepsis and allow the systemic treatment of cancer.

The management of liver abscess less than 3 cm can be treated via antibiotic based on culture. Larger abscess could be drained with percutaneous technique, even if failure of drainage could be caused by yeast, multiloculated abscess, or the communication with biliary tree, which could be frequent in advanced metastatic liver disease.

It is extremely important to treat the origin of abscess, in order to reduce the risk of recurrence. In case of non-resolutive percutaneous treatment, surgical treatment could be necessary to reduce the risk of sepsis.

11.5 Portal and Hepatic Vein Thrombosis/Stenosis

Colorectal liver metastases are rarely responsible of portal and hepatic vein, direct invasion, or compression. Usually macrovascular invasion is typically seen in hepatocellular carcinoma, and colorectal liver metastases are usually responsible of microscopic tumor invasion of the vein, with a reported incidence of 22.5% [18]. Macroscopic neoplastic thrombosis in the main trunk of the portal vein has a reported incidence of approximately 2.8% [19], and few reports are present [20, 21]. Exceptionally, portal tumor thrombosis is not associated with liver metastasis [22]. More frequently liver pedicle nodal metastases are responsible of portal compression, infiltration, and/or occlusion. Treatment is not standardized and firstly is directed to restore the portal flow in order to avoid splanchnic congestion and hepatic failure. In case of portal vein main trunk partial thrombosis, non-resectable disease, and concomitant comorbidities that do not allow any invasive treatment, simple continuous heparin vein infusion may be an option to avoid the extension of the tumor thrombus with additional clots. Percutaneous treatment can be tailored regarding the type and localization of the thrombus. In case of branch (right or left) complete thrombosis, near the portal bifurcation, a plug or coils can be used to stop the tumor progression to the other side or to the main portal trunk. Percutaneous thrombus aspiration can be proposed but has a temporary effect. Venous stent is indicated in case of compression or partial occlusion, and it can be used for the main trunk but also in the portal bifurcation to prevent the progression on the other side or to maintain one side of the liver perfused by the portal flow. Continuous heparin infusion may reduce the risk of additional thrombosis. When none of these possibilities can be considered, surgical exploration with direct thrombectomy is the last option. Proximal control of the main portal trunk is mandatory to control possible massive hemorrhage; lateral incision on the portal vein with possible repermeabilization of the round ligament can be associated, to pass a blunt instrument to remove the thrombus.

References

1. Abercrombie J. Hemorrhage of the liver. Lond Med Gaz. 1844;34:792–4.
2. Battula N, Tsapralis D, Takhar A, et al. Aetio-pathogenesis and the management of spontaneous liver bleeding in the West: a 16-year single-centre experience. HPB. 2012;14:382–9.
3. Schoedel KE, Dekker A. Hemoperitoneum in the setting of metastatic cancer to the liver. A report of two cases with review of the literature. Dig Dis Sci. 1992;37:153–4.
4. Tung CF, Chang CS, Chow WK, Peng YC, Hwang JI, Wen MC. Hemoperitoneum secondary to spontaneous rupture of metastatic epidermoid carcinoma of liver: case report and review of the literature. Hepatogastroenterology. 2002;49:1415–7.

5. Sohda T, Hanano T, Miyamoto H, Kitano Y, Iwata K, Yokoyama M, Irie M, Takeyama Y, Shakado S, Sakisaka S. Spontaneous rupture of metastatic alpha-fetoprotein-producing gastric cancer of the liver. Hepatol Int. 2008;2:258–61.
6. Duan Y, et al. Spontaneous rupture of hepatic metastasis from small cell neuroendocrine carcinoma of maxillary sinus. World J Surg Oncol. 2014;12:126.
7. Quinn L, Bagia S. Effective palliation of obstructive jaundice due to colorectal cancer liver metastasis. ANZ J Surg. 2014;84(6):493–4. Available from: https://www.ncbi.nlm.nih.gov/pubmed/24168172.
8. Traeger L, Kiroff G. Intrabiliary obstruction by colorectal metastases. J Surg Case Rep. 2018;2018(1):rjx259. Available from: https://www.ncbi.nlm.nih.gov/pubmed/29383240.
9. Kim KM, Park JW, Lee JK, Lee KH, Lee KT, Shim SG. A comparison of preoperative biliary drainage methods for perihilar cholangiocarcinoma: endoscopic versus percutaneous transhepatic biliary drainage. Gut Liver. 2015;9(6):791. Available from: https://www.ncbi.nlm.nih.gov/pubmed/26087784.
10. Sawas T, Al Halabi S, Parsi MA, Vargo JJ. Self-expandable metal stents versus plastic stents for malignant biliary obstruction: a meta-analysis. Gastrointest Endosc. 2015;82(2):256–267.e7. Available from: https://www.ncbi.nlm.nih.gov/pubmed/25982849.
11. Niu H, Gao W, Cheng J, Liu B, Li Y, Huang K, et al. Improvement of percutaneous transhepatic biliary internal-external drainage and its initial experience in patients with malignant obstruction of the upper biliary tree. Hepatogastroenterology. 2011;59(117):1368–73. Available from: https://www.ncbi.nlm.nih.gov/pubmed/22115804.
12. Green MH, Duell RM, et al. Comprehensive summary of case series reports on presentation, etiology, evaluation, and management of hemobilia. Br J Surg. 2001;88:773–86.
13. Zaydfudim VM, Angle JF, et al. Current management of hemobilia. Curr Surg Rep. 2014;2:54.
14. Chin MW, Enns R. Hemobilia. Curr Gastroenterol Rep. 2010;12:121–9.
15. Defreyne L, Vanlangenhove P, De Vos M, et al. Embolization as a first approach with endoscopically unmanageable acute nonvariceal gastrointestinal hemorrhage. Radiology. 2001;218:739–48.
16. Lardière-Deguelte S, Ragot E, Amroun K, Piardi T, Dokmak S, Bruno O, et al. Hepatic abscess: diagnosis and management. J Visc Surg. 2015;152(4):231–43. Available from: https://www.ncbi.nlm.nih.gov/pubmed/25770745.
17. Law S-T, Li KK. Is hepatic neoplasm-related pyogenic liver abscess a distinct clinical entity? World J Gastroenterol. 2012;18(10):1110–6. Available from: http://www.wjgnet.com/1007-9327/full/v18/i10/1110.htm.
18. Yamamoto J, Sugihara K, et al. Pathologic support for limited hepatectomy in the treatment of liver metastasis from colorectal cancer. Ann Surg. 1995;221:74–8.
19. Tada K, Kokudo N, Seki M, et al. Hepatic resection for colorectal metastasis with macroscopic tumor thrombus in the portal vein. World J Surg. 2003;27:299–303.
20. Shintani D, Tajima Y, Baba H, et al. Colon cancer with portal vein tumor thrombosis-a case report and review of the literature. Gan To Kagaku Ryoho. 2012;39(2):2243–5.
21. Furuyama H, Fuji H, Okumura S, et al. A case of recurrent colon cancer developed thrombus in superior mesenteric vein after chemotherapy. Gan To Kagaku Ryoho. 2013;40:659–61.
22. Yamamoto N, et al. Massive portal vein tumor thrombus from colorectal cancer without any metastatic nodules in the liver parenchyma. Rare Tumors. 2011;3(4):e47.

Multidisciplinary Management of Postoperative Complications

12

Massimo Sartelli

12.1 Introduction

The most frequent postoperative surgical complications after colorectal resections are surgical site infection, anastomotic leakage, and postoperative (localized or diffuse) peritonitis.

Surgical site infections (SSIs) are consistently associated with significant morbidity and mortality and prolonged hospitalization. Colorectal surgery is, at best, clean-contaminated procedures, and sometimes there may be contamination of both the peritoneal cavity and the surfaces of the surgical wound. The development of SSIs is related to four factors: (a) the degree and type of microbial contamination of the wound during surgery; (b) the duration of the procedure; (c) host factors such as age, diabetes, malnutrition, obesity, and immune suppression; and (d) external factors such as skin preparation, contamination of instruments, and inadequate antibiotic prophylaxis. Surgical site infection in patients undergoing colorectal resection has been specifically studied because it is a frequent cause of morbidity with an incidence of 3–30% [1].

Although it may complicate all gastrointestinal anastomosis, anastomotic leak is most frequent after rectal resection [2]. The prevalence of anastomotic leak has been reported to be between 0.5% and 21% after colon and rectal resections, although there is lack of a clear definition for what constitutes an anastomotic leak [3]. Bruce et al. [4] published a systematic review of studies on the definition and measurement of anastomotic leak after gastrointestinal surgery; in the 97 studies reviewed, there were a total of 56 separate definitions of anastomotic leak. A leak was defined by the need for reoperation, clinical findings, or radiologic criteria, making comparisons between studies difficult or impossible [4].

M. Sartelli (✉)
Department of Surgery, Macerata hospital, Macerata, Italy

N. de'Angelis et al. (eds.), *Emergency Surgical Management of Colorectal Cancer*, Hot Topics in Acute Care Surgery and Trauma,
https://doi.org/10.1007/978-3-030-06225-5_12

Extensive literature is available on the topic of risk factors for anastomotic leakage. Risk factors for anastomotic dehiscence have traditionally been stratified into three categories, patient, operative, and disease-related factors [5], but consensus is lacking on their independent role due to their mutual interdependency [6].

The role of protective stoma has been controversially discussed. The use of a protective stoma is an effective application that can reduce the rate of anastomotic leakage in patients who receive low anterior resection for rectal cancer. The morbidity associated with protective stomas and the complications of stoma closure are negligible compared with the reoperations required for anastomosis leakage in the absence of a protective stoma. Results from recent meta-analysis suggest that a defunctioning stoma could effectively reduce the clinical consequences of anastomotic leakage and reoperation and should be recommended in patients undergoing low rectal anterior resection for rectal cancer [7].

In minor leaks with subclinical forms, conservative management with antibiotics may be an acceptable treatment option. In stable patients, a localized peritoneal abscess cavity can be generally drained under radiological guidance. Patients with diffuse postoperative peritonitis should undergo an early surgical source control and appropriate antimicrobial therapy.

In few instances, the anastomosis may be intact; however, the patient may present a residual peritonitis. The cause may be the inadequate intraoperative drainage of an intraoperative contamination, with concomitant insufficient defense capacity to control the bacterial contamination. In any cases postoperative collections may be the results of infected hematomas.

A correct management of postoperative localized and diffuse peritonitis when it occurs always needs a multidisciplinary approach.

12.2 Multidisciplinary Management of Patients with Postoperative Localized and Diffuse Peritonitis

The diagnosis of postoperative peritonitis may be difficult because there are no specific clinical signs and laboratory tests to reject or confirm the diagnosis. The atypical clinical presentation may be responsible for a delay in treatment. Moreover, in patients already stressed by the previous operation, sepsis can precipitate quickly to septic shock. These patients may present with inadequate perfusion, leading to global tissue hypoxia. Fluid support should be initiated as early as possible in patients with sepsis or septic shock [8]. It is a major component of cardiovascular support in early sepsis. When fluid challenge fails to restore adequate arterial pressure and organ perfusion, clinicians should resort to vasopressor agents. Vasopressor drugs maintain adequate blood pressure and preserve perfusion pressure, thereby optimizing blood flow in various organs. They should be administered early in patients with severe sepsis or septic shock to restore organ perfusion [9].

Source control encompasses all measures undertaken to eliminate the source of infection, reduce the bacterial inoculum, and correct or control anatomic derangements to restore normal physiologic function.

Percutaneous drainage should be considered the optimal means of treating postoperative localized abscesses in stable patients.

Conversely the timing and adequacy of source control are of outmost importance in the management of diffuse postoperative, as late and/or incomplete procedures may have severely adverse consequences on outcome.

The primary objectives of surgical intervention include (a) determining the cause of peritonitis, (b) draining fluid collections, and (c) controlling the origin of the abdominal sepsis.

Surgical options for anastomotic leak after low rectal resection are well codified and include either fecal diversion with a diverting loop ileostomy or colostomy or resection of the anastomosis and creation of an end colostomy (Hartmann's resection) [10, 11]. The first strategy requires less operative stress and allows a convenient restoration of intestinal continuity at a later stage. However, it leaves *in the source of infection* and predisposes the patients to bowel stenosis and chronic fistula. Hartmann's procedure is more radical and effective at controlling the source of infection, but restoring intestinal continuity can be challenging.

In patients with postoperative peritonitis, the normal flora may be modified, and intra-abdominal infections may be caused by several unexpected pathogens and by more resistant flora, which may include enterococci, extended-spectrum β-lactamases-producing *Enterobacteriaceae* (ESBLs), and *Candida* spp.

Antimicrobial therapy between initial intervention and reoperation seems to be a significant risk factor for emergence of multidrug-resistant (MDR) pathogens in patients with PP. Therefore a correct antimicrobial prophylaxis is mandatory to limit the spread of MDR in operated patients [12, 13].

In these infections empiric antimicrobial regimens with broad spectrum of activity are recommended with the intent to cover the most likely pathogens, basing on local surveillance data and risk factors for resistant microorganisms.

All patients with postoperative peritonitis require culture and drug susceptibility testing to guide targeted antibiotic therapy.

Subsequent modification (de-escalation) of the initial regimen becomes possible later, when culture results are available and clinical status can be better assessed, 24–72 h after initiation of empiric therapy.

12.3 Conclusions

Postoperative peritonitis (PP) is a life-threatening hospital-acquired intra-abdominal infection with high rates of morbidity and mortality.

The complication itself does not frequently represent a problem but is more likely a consequence of late diagnosis and therefore of insufficient and too late therapy. The use of a protective stoma is an effective application that can reduce the rate of anastomotic leakage in patients who receive low anterior resection for rectal cancer. The morbidity associated with protective stomas and the complications of stoma closure are negligible compared with the reoperations required for anastomosis leakage in the absence of a protective stoma.

A correct management of postoperative localized and diffuse peritonitis when it occurs always needs a multidisciplinary approach.

References

1. Smith RL, Bohl JK, McElearney ST, et al. Wound infection after elective colorectal resection. Ann Surg. 2004;239(5):599–605.
2. Daams F, Luyer M, Lange JF. Colorectal anastomotic leakage: aspects of prevention, detection and treatment. World J Gastroenterol. 2013;19(15):2293–7229.
3. Trencheva K, Morrissey KP, Wells M, Mancuso CA, Lee SW, Sonoda T, Michelassi F, Charlson ME, Milsom JW. Identifying important predictors for anastomotic leak after colon and rectal resection: prospective study on 616 patients. Ann Surg. 2013;257(1):108–13.
4. Bruce J, Krukowski ZH, Al-Khairy G, Russel EM, Park KG. Systematic review of the definition and measurement of anastomotic leak after gastrointestinal surgery. Br J Surg. 2001;88:1157–68.
5. Hirst NA, Tiernan JP, Millner PA, Jayne DG. Systematic review of methods to predict and detect anastomotic leakage in colorectal surgery. Colorectal Dis. 2014;16(2):95–109.
6. Schrock TR, Deveney CW, Dunphy JE. Factor contributing to leakage of colonic anastomosis. Ann Surg. 1973;177:513–8.
7. Gu WL, Wu SW. Meta-analysis of defunctioning stoma in low anterior resection with total mesorectal excision for rectal cancer: evidence based on thirteen studies. World J Surg Oncol. 2015;13:9.
8. Moore LJ, Moore FA. Epidemiology of sepsis in surgical patients. Surg Clin North Am. 2012;92(6):1425–43.
9. Dellinger RP, Levy MM, Carlet JM, Bion J, Parker MM, Jaeschke R, Reinhart K, Angus DC, Brun-Buisson C, Beale R, Calandra T, Dhainaut JF, Gerlach H, Harvey M, Marini JJ, Marshall J, Ranieri M, Ramsay G, Sevransky J, Thompson BT, Townsend S, Vender JS, Zimmerman JL, Vincent JL, Emergency Physicians Canadian Critical Care Society European Society of Clinical Microbiology and Infectious Diseases European Society of Intensive Care Medicine European Respiratory Society International Sepsis Forum Japanese Association for Acute Medicine Japanese Society of Intensive Care Medicine Society of Critical Care Medicine Society of Hospital Medicine Surgical Infection Society World Federation of Societies of Intensive and Critical Care Medicine. Surviving sepsis campaign: international guidelines for management of severe sepsis and septic shock: 2018. Crit Care Med. 2008;36(1):296–327.
10. Sartelli M, Catena F, Di Saverio S, Ansaloni L, Malangoni M, Moore EE, Moore FA, Ivatury R, Coimbra R, Leppaniemi A, Biffl W, Kluger Y, Fraga GP, Ordonez CA, Marwah S, Gerych I, Lee JG, Tranà C, Coccolini F, Corradetti F, Kirkby-Bott J. Current concept of abdominal sepsis: WSES position paper. World J Emerg Surg. 2014;9(1):22.
11. Marshall JC. Principles of source control in the early management of sepsis. Curr Infect Dis Rep. 2010;12(5):345–53.
12. Augustin P, Kermarrec N, Muller-Serieys C, Lasocki S, Chosidow D, Marmuse JP, Valin N, Desmonts JM, Montravers P. Risk factors for multidrug resistant bacteria and optimization of empirical antibiotic therapy in postoperative peritonitis. Crit Care. 2010;14(1):R20.
13. Lee DS, Ryu JA, Chung CR, Yang J, Jeon K, Suh GY, Lee WY, Park CM. Risk factors for acquisition of multidrug-resistant bacteria in patients with anastomotic leakage after colorectal cancer surgery. Int J Colorectal Dis. 2015;30(4):497–504.

13 Enhanced Recovery After Emergency Colorectal Surgery

Meara Dean and R. Justin Davies

13.1 Background

ERAS programmemes were first described for elective colorectal surgery [1] and have been validated in the elective setting, with benefits of reduced length of hospital stay, perioperative morbidity and mortality, healthcare costs [2] and improved patient satisfaction [3]. These benefits have been described in both open and laparoscopic colorectal surgery [4]. These programmes have also been shown to be feasible and effective in elderly patients undergoing colorectal surgery [5].

At the outset, these programmes aimed to reduce the variability of perioperative management, which was traditionally ad hoc, day by day decisions by the patients' surgical team, often based on the individual surgeons' experience. ERAS protocols were based on established practice guidelines and evidence-based literature. Varied interventions are usually provided in a "bundle", commencing in the weeks before elective surgery and continuing intraoperatively and in the postoperative period (see Table 13.1) [7].

As most programmes implement these varied interventions simultaneously, it is difficult to determine which components are the most beneficial. A retrospective review based on 8 years of experience with ERAS found that the strongest predictors of reduced hospital stay were early mobilisation, early oral nutrition, early removal of urinary catheter, early removal of epidural, lack of nasogastric tube and non-opioid analgesia [8]. ERAS interventions involve a multidisciplinary team including physicians, surgeons, nurses, physiotherapists and anaesthetists.

M. Dean (✉) · R. J. Davies
Cambridge Colorectal Unit, Addenbrooke's Hospital, Cambridge University Hospitals NHS Foundation Trust, Cambridge, UK
e-mail: meara.dean@addenbrookes.nhs.uk

N. de'Angelis et al. (eds.), *Emergency Surgical Management of Colorectal Cancer*, Hot Topics in Acute Care Surgery and Trauma,
https://doi.org/10.1007/978-3-030-06225-5_13

Table 13.1 Potential ERAS interventions for colon and rectal surgery[a]

Pre-op	Intra-op	Post-op
• Preadmission education and counselling (including milestones, discharge criteria) • Preoperative stoma education and marking • Preadmission optimisation • Preoperative nutrition: clear fluids <2 h pre-op, carbohydrate loading • Preoperative antibiotics • Consider mechanical bowel preparation	• Prevention of surgical site infection • Minimally invasive surgery where possible • Consider addition of regional anaesthesia, e.g. epidural/spinal for open surgery • Avoiding nasogastric tubes • Avoidance of intra-abdominal drain • Fluid management (avoiding volume excess)	• Early mobilisation • Immediate post-op diet • Ileus prevention • Consider gum chewing • Early discontinuation of IV fluids • Early removal of urinary catheter • Standardised venous thromboembolism prophylaxis • Multimodal, opioid-sparing pain control • Prevention of perioperative nausea and vomiting

[a]Based on the 2017 ASCRS guidelines [6]

13.2 Reducing Surgical Trauma

Surgical trauma refers to both the effects of the systemic stress response and local tissue damage that occurs in response to surgery. The magnitude of this response is proportional to the severity of the surgical trauma and differs between open and laparoscopic surgery [9]. Longer operating times induce a larger peritoneal inflammatory response [10, 11]. ERAS interventions aim to minimise the stress response and improve the metabolic response to surgery.

13.2.1 Markers of Surgical Trauma

CRP is an acute phase reactant protein that increases during periods of inflammation and tissue damage. It is synthesised by hepatocytes upon stimulation with interlekin-6 (IL-6) [12]. The use of ERAS protocols is associated with decreased levels of CRP and IL-6 postoperatively [13]. A recent meta-analysis concluded the most likely intervention to account for this observation is the use of minimally invasive surgery, as there is convincing evidence that laparoscopic surgery is associated with decreased postoperative CRP [14]. A persistently elevated CRP beyond Day 5 and rising CRP on Day 3 may be predictive of infective complications and prolonged hospital stay after colorectal resection [15], including anastomotic leak [16]. Following on, CRP level may be a useful negatively predictive tool to facilitate early discharge following colorectal surgery [17].

13.2.2 General Measures to Reduce the Surgical Stress Response

A clear liquid diet up to 2 h before surgery is associated with a smaller gastric volume and higher gastric pH at the time of surgery and an improved sense of patient wellbeing [18, 19]. Excessive provision or restriction of fluids can impair organ function and increase morbidity [20, 21], so close attention to appropriate fluid replacement is vital. Furthermore intravenous fluids should be ceased as soon as possible postoperatively to avoid fluid overload and resulting tissue oedema. Fluid type is also important, with the use of balanced chloride-restricted crystalloid solutions being preferred to normal saline to decrease the risk of hyperchloraemic metabolic acidosis [22]. Nasogastric tubes should be avoided where possible, as their routine use has been associated with delayed resumption of oral intake, without benefit in terms of prevention of nausea or vomiting or return of bowel function [23, 24]. Early removal of urinary catheters is preferable to reduce the risks of postoperative urinary tract infection and improve patient mobility [25]. While it can be assumed these measures would reduce surgical stress, there are few studies examining the effect of these individual ERAS components on the surgical stress response in colorectal surgery [14].

13.2.3 Operative Interventions to Reduce Surgical Trauma

"The cleaner and gentler the act of operation, the less the patient suffers, the smoother and quicker his convalescence (and) the more exquisite his healed wound."
Lord Moynihan

The importance of minimising surgical trauma has been long recognised, and there are many time-honoured techniques that are described. In open and laparoscopic surgery, these include:

- Reducing unnecessary handling of tissues
- Minimising contamination
- Avoiding introduction of foreign material into the peritoneal cavity
- Avoiding tissue exposure to a dry environment
- Judicious use of heat-emitting devices to avoid thermal injury
- Avoiding tumour spillage
- Mobilisation of colon along bloodless planes

Laparoscopic colorectal resection has been shown to be beneficial in terms of quicker return of bowel function, less blood loss, reduced narcotic use, less postoperative pain, reduced length of hospital stay, reduced overall morbidity and improved short-term quality of life [26–31]. The laparoscopic approach has been associated with a shorter hospital stay and reduced postoperative mortality in emergency colorectal cancer resections [32].

Surgical techniques that can reduce surgical trauma in minimally invasive surgery include:

1. Insertion and removal of instruments under vision
2. Avoiding peritoneal injury during lavage
3. Using lower intra-abdominal pressure settings for pneumoperitoneum
4. Avoid gas leaks where possible
5. The use of wound protectors and non-traumatic retraction systems [33]

13.2.4 Surgical Trauma and Tumour Biology

Complex relationships exist between surgical trauma, inflammation and tumour biology in colorectal cancer progression, metastasis and survival. Growth factors and cytokines play an important role in normal tissue healing but also have an essential role in tumour recurrence and formation of metastases. The most potent factor for angiogenesis is vascular endothelial growth factor (VEGF), which has several subtypes [34]. VEGF-D promotes cancer spread via the lymphatic system, a crucial step in metastasis [35]. Serum VEGF is elevated after open and laparoscopic surgery and remains so for as long as 4 weeks postoperatively [36, 37].

These complex relationships remain unclear and require further investigation. However as the metastatic process can be enhanced by the surgical procedure itself, potential oncological advantage exists in using surgical techniques that minimise surgical trauma and its resultant immunological impact. This is especially important in colorectal cancer patients, who are prone to be immunosuppressed for a variety of reasons including age, nutritional status, recent neoadjuvant chemoradiotherapy and the direct immunosuppressive effect of the tumour itself, which increases with stage of disease and is reversible after tumour resection [38–40].

13.3 ERAS Protocols in Emergency Colorectal Surgery

Data from the American College of Surgeons (ACS) National Surgical Quality Improvement Project (NSQIP) reported patients undergoing emergency colorectal resection had the worst outcomes of all emergency general surgical patients, with an overall 30-day morbidity of 46.74% [41]. The application of ERAS interventions to this patient group may improve outcomes. Furthermore, patients undergoing emergency abdominal surgery may benefit from additional evidence-based measures to improve outcomes. Expediting resuscitation, early identification of sepsis, early administration of antibiotics and admission to an intensive care environment postoperatively have been shown to reduce mortality in patients undergoing emergency laparotomy [42].

Published studies exploring the use of ERAS in emergency surgery have adjusted common ERAS protocols, as not all interventions are possible or appropriate in more time critical situations. Depending on the urgency of surgery, preoperative education/counselling or medical optimisation may not be possible. Emergency surgical patients may experience a delay in diagnosis and/or resuscitation and may require large volume fluid resuscitation due to SIRS/sepsis-related hypotension. Many emergency surgical patients will have co-existing bowel obstruction or ileus, requiring prolonged preoperative fasting and/or nasogastric tube insertion. In this context early feeding is also not appropriate. Intraoperative findings of purulent or faeculent peritonitis may prompt the use of intra-abdominal drains or even laparostomy with re-laparotomy. Patients having emergency colorectal surgery are more likely to have formation of a stoma, which is associated with higher rates of readmission [43]. Emergency surgery patients are more likely to be cared for in an intensive care unit postoperatively, where many ERAS interventions may not be possible. Emergency surgery is more likely to occur after hours, when less staff are available to implement interventions.

13.3.1 Outcomes of ERAS Protocols in Emergency Colorectal Surgery

The evidence for the use of ERAS protocols in emergency colorectal surgery is limited to cohort studies with low patient numbers. Table 13.2 provides a summary of reporting outcomes in emergency colorectal surgery.

Retrospective cohort studies have assessed the use of ERAS in emergency surgery patients undergoing major abdominal surgery (colorectal resections, adhesiolysis, small bowel resection, Hartmann's procedure and appendicectomies [44, 46]), reporting equivalent outcomes compared to the pre-ERAS period and to elective patients.

The only study that exclusively examined emergency colon resection reported a reduced median length of hospital stay (ERAS (5.5 days, range 3–16) vs. the non-ERAS group (7.5 days, range 5–25)), a shorter time to first flatus (1.6 days vs. 2.8 days) and earlier resumption of normal diet (3.5 days vs. 5.5 days) [45]. Patients in this group were operated for the indication of colorectal cancer, and authors reported the interval from operation to initiation of adjuvant chemotherapy was significantly shorter in the ERAS group (37 days vs. 49 days) [45].

The risk calculator CR-POSSUM score has been used to predict the failure of ERAS in patients undergoing elective colorectal surgery [47]. It is likely patients undergoing emergency colorectal surgery have higher CR-POSSUM scores, which may be useful for assessing suitability for inclusion in ERAS programmes.

Ideally an evidence-based ERAS protocol tailored to the needs of patients having emergency colorectal surgery should be developed. In particular, evidence for diet strategy in emergency surgery requires adequately powered randomised controlled trails [48].

Table 13.2 Literature review: ERAS in emergency colorectal surgery

Author	Year	Country	Description	Outcome
Wisely [44]	2016	Australia	Retrospective cohort: 370 emergency abdominal surgeries (159 colorectal resections)	No change in outcomes including major and minor complications, unplanned readmission, length of stay or inpatient mortality
Lohsiriwat [45]	2014	Thailand	Case matched cohort: 20 ERAS compared with 40 conventional postoperative cares after emergency colorectal surgery	Reduced hospital stay and faster return of bowel function
Roulin [46]	2014	Switzerland	Prospective cohort: 28 urgent colectomies vs. 63 elective colectomies, all ERAS	Similar outcomes in emergency vs. elective setting

13.4 Implementing ERAS Protocols

Implementing ERAS programmes poses many challenges due to their complex, multicomponent structure. Barriers to implementation include patient-, staff- and organisation-related factors, in addition to limitations of resources (including financial, staffing, space restrictions and education). Quality evaluation and monitoring is a vital aspect of ERAS programmes, particularly at implementation.

As these programmes were implemented worldwide, early experience was assessed using qualitative process evaluations [49–51]. This has helped to identify enablers and also potential barriers to implementation (see Table 13.3). Knowledge of enablers and barriers at the planning stage can assist practitioners to develop strategies that address potential issues and so more effectively enable successful programme implementation.

Different strategies can be used to increase the effectiveness of introducing new interventions. These include audit and feedback, reminders, education workshops and meetings, opinion leaders and written educational material [52]. Of these, appointing opinion leaders or "local champions" is the most effective intervention [53]. Ideally identifying an opinion leader for each discipline (e.g. nursing, physiotherapy, anaesthesia and surgery) should be selected to lead implementation. Having a dedicated implementation team who are able to meet regularly is ideal, as is a dedicated ERAS nurse. Specialist nurses are vital to providing education (including presentations, in-services), perioperative care and postoperative evaluation [54]. Furthermore, engaging nursing staff is essential to enabling the successful and continued use of the pathways. In the era of electronic medical records, the use of patient care templates for orders ("order sets") has assisted teams to establish ERAS protocols. An example is having the postoperative order set linked to the operation note, with specific orders for each ERAS intervention.

Audit and feedback is a vital component of implementation. Results of audit should be fed back to the team, along with any data regarding an individual hospital performance against benchmark data. To support efficient and successful implementation, measures need to be taken on a national or regional level to support caregivers to create necessary changes to improve healthcare provision.

Table 13.3 Enablers and barriers to ERAS implementation

Enablers	Barriers
• Good teamwork and communication • Consistency across the team • Stakeholder engagement • Normalisation of ERAS into everyday practice • Effective integration with existing systems • Audit and feedback	• Lack of communication and/or collaboration between departments • Need to change attitudes and behaviour • Limited resources • Limited access to stoma care nurses • Lack of patient support on discharge • Special needs of highly co-morbid patients

13.5 Conclusion

Reducing the morbidity and mortality of emergency surgery remains a key priority in general surgical practice. Early studies suggest ERAS is safe and feasible in the emergency colorectal surgery setting, with potential benefits when compared to conventional care. Further studies are required to better define these benefits and to determine the precise interventions that should be used in the emergency setting.

References

1. Kehlet H, Wilmore DW. Multimodal strategies to improve surgical outcome. Am J Surg. 2002;183:630–41.
2. Hjort Jakobsen D, Sonne E, Basse L, Bisgaard T, Kehlet H. Convalescence after colonic resection with fast track versus conventional care. Scand J Surg. 2002;93:24–8.
3. Thiele RH, Rea KM, Turrentine FE, Friel CM, Hassinger TE, McMurry TL, Goudreau BJ, Umapathi BA, Kron IL, Sawyer RG, Hedrick TL. Standardization of care: impact of an enhanced recovery protocol on length of stay, complications, and direct costs after colorectal surgery. J Am Coll Surg. 2015;220:430–43.
4. Currie AC, Malietzis G, Jenkins JT, Yamada T, Ashrafian H, Athanasiou T, Okabayashi K, Kennedy RH. Network meta-analysis of protocol driven care and laparoscopic surgery for colorectal cancer. Br J Surg. 2016;103:1783–94.
5. Launay-Savary MV, Mathonnet M, Theissen A, Ostermann S, Raynaud-Simon A, Slim K. GRACE (Groupe francophone de Rehabilitation Amelioree apres Chirurgie). Are enhanced recovery programmes in colorectal surgery feasible and useful in the elderly? A systematic review of the literature. J Visc Surg. 2017;154(1):29–35.
6. Carmichael JC, Keller DS, Baldini G, Bordeianou L, Weiss E, Lee L, Boutros M, McClane J, Feldman LS, Steele SR. Clinical practice guidelines for enhanced recovery after colon and rectal surgery from the American Society of Colon and Rectal Surgeons and Society of American Gastrointestinal and Endoscopic Surgeons. Dis Colon Rectum. 2017;60(8):761–84.
7. Nygren J, Thacker J, Carli F, Fearon KC, Norderval S, Lobo DN, Ljungqvist O, Soop M, Ramirez J. Guidelines for perioperative care in elective rectal/pelvic surgery: enhanced recovery after surgery society recommendations. Clin Nutr. 2012;31:801–6.
8. Bakker N, Cakir H, Dooderman HJ, Houdijk AP. Eight years of experience with enhanced recovery after surgery in patients with colon cancer: impact of measures to improve adherence. Surgery. 2015;157(6):1130–6.
9. Baigrie RJ, Lamont PM, Kwiatkowski D, Dallman MJ, Morris PJ. Systemic cytokine response after major surgery. Br J Surg. 1992;79(8):757–60.
10. Badia JM, Whawell SA, Scott-Coombes DM, Abel PD, Williamson RC, Thompson JN. Peritoneal and systemic cytokine response to laparotomy. Br J Surg. 1996;83(3):347–8.
11. Sammour T, Kahokehr A, Chan S, Booth RJ, Hill AG. The humoral response after laparoscopic versus open colorectal surgery: a meta-analysis. J Surg Res. 2010;164(1):28–37.
12. Peppys MB, Hirschfield GM. C-reactive protein: a critical update. J Clin Invest. 2003;111:1805–12.
13. Mari G, Crippa J, Costanzi A, Mazzola M, Rossi M, Maggioni D. ERAS protocol reduces IL-6 secretion in colorectal laparoscopic surgery: results from a randomized clinical trial. Surg Laparosc Endosc Percutan Tech. 2016;26(6):444–8.
14. Watt DG, McSorley ST, Horgan PG, McMillan DC. Enhanced recovery after surgery: which components, if any, impact on the systemic inflammatory response

following colorectal surgery?: A systematic review. Medicine. 2015;94(36):e1286. https://doi.org/10.1097/MD0000000000001286.
15. Lane JC, Wright S, Burch J, Kennedy RH, Jenkins JT. Early prediction of adverse events in enhanced recovery based upon the host systemic inflammatory response. Colorectal Dis. 2013;15(2):224–30.
16. MacKay GJ, Molloy RG, O'Dwyer PJ. C-reactive protein as a predictor of postoperative infective complications following elective colorectal resection. Colorectal Dis. 2011;13:583–7.
17. Reynolds IS, Boland MR, Reilly F, Deasy A, Majeed MH, Deasy J, Burke JP, McNamara DA. C-reactive protein as a predictor of anastomotic leak in the first week after anterior resection for rectal cancer. Colorectal Dis. 2017;19(9):812–8.
18. McGrady EM, Macdonald AG. Effect of the preoperative administration of water on gastric volume and pH. Br J Anaesth. 1988;60(7):803–5.
19. Read MS, Vaughan RS. Allowing pre-operative patients to drink: effects on patients' safety and comfort of unlimited oral water until 2 hours before anaesthesia. Acta Anaesthesiol Scand. 1991;35(7):591–5.
20. Chappell D, Jacob M, Hofmann-Kiefer K, Conzen P, Rehm M. A rational approach to perioperative uid management. Anesthesiology. 2008;109(4):723–40.
21. Boland MR, Reynolds I, McCawley N, Galvin E, El-Masry S, Deasy J, McNamara DA. Liberal perioperative fluid administration is an independent risk factor for morbidity and is associated with longer hospital stay after rectal cancer surgery. Ann R Coll Surg Engl. 2017;99(2):113–6.
22. Burdett E, Dushianthan A, Bennett-Guerrero E, Cro S, Gan TJ, Grocott MP, James MF, Mythen MG, O'Malley CM, Roche AM, Rowan K. Perioperative buffered versus non-buffered fluid administration for surgery in adults. Cochrane Database Syst Rev. 2012;12:CD004089. https://doi.org/10.1002/14651858.CD004089.pub2.
23. Li K, Zhou Z, Chen Z, Zhang Y, Wang C. "Fast Track" nasogastric decompression of rectal cancer surgery. Front Med. 2011;5(3):306–9.
24. Ortiz H, Armendariz P, Yarnoz C. Is early postoperative feeding feasible in elective colon and rectal surgery? Int J Colorectal Dis. 1996;11:119–21.
25. Wald HL, Ma A, Bratzler DW, Kramer AM. Indwelling uri-nary catheter use in the postoperative period: analysis of the national surgical infection prevention project data. Arch Surg. 2008;143:551–7.
26. Hewett PJ, Allardyce RA, Bagshaw PF, Frampton CM, Frizelle FA, Reiger NA, Smith JA, Solomon MJ, Stephens JH, Stevenson AR. Short-term outcomes of the Australasian randomized clinical study comparing laparoscopic and conventional open surgical treatments for colon cancer: the ALCCaS trial. Ann Surg. 2008;248:728–38.
27. Veldkamp R, Kuhry E, Hop WC, Jeekel J, Kazemier G, Bonjer HJ, Haglind E, Pahlman L, Cuesta MA, Msika S, Morino M, Lacy AM, COlon Cancer Laparoscopic or Open Resection Study Group (COLOR). Laparoscopic surgery versus open surgery for colon cancer: short-term outcomes of a randomised trial. Lancet Oncol. 2005;6(7):477–84.
28. Stage JG, Schulze S, Møller P, Overgaard H, Andersen M, Rebsdorf-Pedersen VB, Neilsen HJ. Prospective randomized study of laparoscopic versus open colonic resection for adenocarcinoma. Br J Surg. 1997;84(3):391–6.
29. Weeks JC, Nelson H, Gelber S, Sargent D, Schroeder G. Clinical Outcomes of Surgical Therapy (COST) Study Group. Short-term quality-of-life outcomes following laparoscopic-assisted colectomy vs open colectomy for colon cancer: a randomized trial. JAMA. 2002;287:321–8.
30. Schwenk W, Haase O, Neudecker J, Muller JM. Short term benefits for laparoscopic colorectal resection. Cochrane Database Syst Rev. 2005;(3):CD003145.
31. Kuhry E, Schwenk WF, Gaupset R, Romild U, Bonjer HJ. Long-term results of laparoscopic colorectal cancer resection. Cochrane Database Syst Rev. 2008;(2):CD003432. https://doi.org/10.1002/14651858.CD003432.pub2.
32. Vallance AE, Keller DS, Hill J, Braun M, Kuryba A, van der Meulen J, Walker K, Chand M. Role of emergency laparoscopic colectomy for colorectal cancer: a population-based study in England. Ann Surg. 2018; https://doi.org/10.1097/SLA.0000000000002752.

33. Cheng KP, Roslani AC, Sehha N, Kueh JH, Law CW, Chong HY, Arumugam K. ALEXIS O-Ring wound retractor vs conventional wound protection for the prevention of surgical site infections in colorectal resections. Colorectal Dis. 2012;14(6):e346–51. https://doi.org/10.1111/j.1463-1318.2012.02943.
34. Hansen E, Wolff N, Knuechel R, Ruschoff J, Hofstaedter F, Taeger K. Tumor cells in blood shed from the surgical field. Arch Surg. 1995;130(4):387–93.
35. Kamezis T, Shayan R, Caesar C, Roufail S, Harris NC, Ardipradja K, Zhang YF, Williams SP, Farnsworth RH, Chai MG, Rupasinghe TW, Tull DL, Baldwin ME, Sloan EK, Fox SB, Achen MG, Stacker SA. VEGF-D promotes tumour metastasis by regulating prostaglandins produces by the collecting lymphatic endothelium. Cancer Cell. 2012;21:181–95.
36. Futami R, Miyashita M, Nomura T, Makino H, Matsutani T, Sasajima K, Tajiri T. Increased serum vascular endothelial growth factor following major surgical injury. J Nippon Med Sch. 2007;74(3):223–9.
37. Belizon A, Balik E, Horst P, Feingold D, Arnell T, Azarani T, Cekic V, Skitt R, Kumara S, Whelan RL. Persistent elevation of plasma vascular endothelial growth factor levels during the first month after minimally invasive colorectal resection. Surg Endosc. 2008;22(2):287–97.
38. Heriot AG, Marriott J, Cookson S, Kumar D, Dalgleish AG. Reduction in cytokine production in colorectal cancer patients: association with stage and reversal by resection. Br J Cancer. 2000;82(5):1009–12.
39. Galizia G, Lieto E, De Vita F, Romano C, Orditura M, Castellano P, Imperatore V, Infusino S, Catalano G, Pignatelli C. Circulating levels of interleukin 10 and interleukin 6 in gastric and colon cancer patients before and after surgery: relationship with radicality and outcome. J Interferon Cytokine Res. 2002;22(4):473–82.
40. Evans CFM, Galustian C, Bodman-Smith M, Dalgleish AG, Kumar D. The effect of colorectal cancer upon host peripheral immune cell function. Colorectal Dis. 2010;12(6):561–9.
41. Ingraham AM, Cohen ME, Bilimoria KY, Raval MV, Ko CY, Nathens AB, Hall BL. Comparison of 30 day outcomes after emergency general surgery procedures: potential for targeted improvement. Surgery. 2010;148(2):217–38.
42. Huddart S, Peden CJ, Swart M, McCormick B, Dickinson M, Mohammed MA, Quiney N, ELPQuiC Collaborator Group; ELPQuiC Collaborator Group. Use of a pathway quality improvement care bundle to reduce mortality after emergency laparotomy. Br J Surg. 2015;102(1):57–66.
43. Shah PM, Johnston L, Sarosiek B, Harrigan A, Friel CM, Thiele RH, Hedrick TL. Reducing readmissions while shortening length of stay: the positive impact of an enhanced recovery protocol in colorectal surgery. Dis Colon Rectum. 2017;60(2):219–27.
44. Wisely JC, Barclay KL. Effects of an Enhanced Recovery After Surgery programmeme on emergency surgical patients. ANZ J Surg. 2016;86(11):883–8.
45. Lohsiriwat V. Enhanced recovery after surgery vs conventional care in emergency colorectal surgery. World J Gastroenterol. 2014;20(38):13950–5.
46. Roulin D, Blanc C, Muradbegovic M, Hahnloser D, Demartines N, Hubner M. Enhanced recovery pathway for urgent colectomy. World J Surg. 2014;38(8):2153–9.
47. Renz BW, Kasparek MS, Seeliger H, Worthley DL, Jauch KW, Kreis ME, Smith MJ, Mueller MH. The CR-POSSUM risk calculator predicts failure of enhanced recovery after colorectal surgery. Acta Chir Belg. 2015;115(1):20–6.
48. Le Guen M, Fessler J, Fischler M. Early oral feeding after emergency abdominal operations: another paradigm to be broken? Curr Opin Clin Nutr Metab Care. 2014;17(5):477–82.
49. Gotlib Conn L, McKenzie M, Pearsall EA, McLeod RS. Successful implementation of an enhanced recovery after surgery programmeme for elective colorectal surgery: a process evaluation of champions' experiences. Implem Sci. 2015;10:99. https://doi.org/10.1186/s13012-015-0289-y.
50. Alawadi ZM, Leal I, Phatak UR, Flores-Gonzalez JR, Holihan JL, Karanjawala BE, Millas SG, Kao LS. Facilitators and barriers of implementing enhanced recovery in colorectal surgery at a safety net hospital: a provider and patient perspective. Surgery. 2016;159(3):700–12.

51. Pearsall EA, Meghji Z, Pitzul KB, Aarts MA, McKenzie M, McLeod RS, Okrainec A. A qualitative study to understand the barriers and enablers in implementing an Enhanced Recovery After Surgery programme. Ann Surg. 2014;261(1):92–6.
52. Feldman L, Delaney C, Ljungqvist, O, Carli F. 2015 The SAGES/ERAS® Society Manual of enhanced recovery programmes for gastrointestinal surgery. Springer, Cham. 978-3-319-20364-5.
53. Flodgren G, Parmelli E, Doumit G, Gattellari M, O'Brien MA, Grimshaw J, Eccles MP. Local opinion leaders: effects on professional practice and health care outcomes. Cochrane Database Syst Rev. 2011;(8):CD000125. https://doi.org/10.1002/14651858.CD000125.pub4.
54. Brady KM, Keller DS, Delaney CP. Successful implementation of an enhanced recovery pathway: the nurse's role. AORN J. 2015;102(5):469–81.

On the Immune Status of Patients with Colorectal Carcinoma

14

Pim P. Edomskis, Daniël P. V. Lambrichts, and Johan F. Lange

14.1 Introduction

This chapter emphasizes the consequences of an immunocompromised status in patients with colorectal malignancies. Focus will be put on the origin of the different colorectal segments, ranging from the cecum up to and including the anal sphincter, in order to get a better understanding of the pathophysiological mechanisms of colorectal carcinoma. For comprehension of immunological mechanisms, a clear understanding of colorectal anatomy, embryology, and physiology is also needed. Furthermore, a closer look into the immunocompromised status and relevant immune deficiencies will be provided. More specifically, pathophysiological mechanisms, genetic mutations, immunosuppressant drugs, and underlying immunodeficiencies are of interest. Lastly, specific immunosuppressive diseases that are related to an immunocompromised status will be discussed together with their relationship to colorectal surgery.

P. P. Edomskis (✉) · D. P. V. Lambrichts
Department of Surgery, Erasmus University Medical Center Rotterdam, Rotterdam, The Netherlands
e-mail: p.edomskis@erasmusmc.nl

J. F. Lange
Department of Surgery, Erasmus University Medical Center Rotterdam, Rotterdam, The Netherlands

Department of Surgery, IJsselland Ziekenhuis, Capelle aan den IJssel, The Netherlands

N. de'Angelis et al. (eds.), *Emergency Surgical Management of Colorectal Cancer*, Hot Topics in Acute Care Surgery and Trauma,
https://doi.org/10.1007/978-3-030-06225-5_14

14.2 Differences in Colorectal Neoplasms

The terminology used in literature regarding colonic, rectal, and anal neoplasms to indicate malignancies of the large intestine is heterogeneous, so uniformity is required in order to correctly compare and interpret results from different studies. There is a complex interplay of anatomical, histological, chromosomal, and molecular factors that suggests there is a spectrum of different diseases that are presently labeled as colorectal cancer [1]. In general, one can differentiate between the types of neoplasms through their location, genesis, as well as their specific cell structures and characteristics. Differentiation between these entities is meaningful, since it provides insights into the pathogenesis of colorectal neoplasms.

14.2.1 Location

Traditionally, neoplasms of the colon and rectum are classified by their anatomic location. At first, support came for a hypothesis that suggested two different types of colon cancer [2, 3]. Later on, more support arrived to divide the large intestine into three segments. Herein, the proximal colon extends from cecum to splenic flexure, the distal colon arising distally from this site and extending to the rectum. The rectum itself can be considered a distinct entity as well [4]. Additionally, rectal neoplasms can also be surgically classified into four different groups categorized to their lowest, most distal, part of the tumor. Type I rectal cancers are supra-anal, which is defined as >1 cm from the anal ring. Type II are juxta-anal tumors, that is, lesions ≤1 cm from the anal ring. Type III are intra-anal tumors, that is, lesions with internal anal sphincter invasion. Lastly, type IV transanal tumors are defined by the invasion of the external anal sphincter or levator ani muscle [5]. Clinically, it is important to classify rectal neoplasms correctly, since it provides guidance in choosing the right intervention, which is paramount to optimize outcomes, e.g., preservation of anal sphincter, bladder, and sexual organ functions.

14.2.2 Embryology and Vascularization

From an embryological standpoint, the proximal (ascending and transverse) part of the colon originates from the midgut, whereas the distal (descending) part of the colon starts at the splenic flexure, the rectum arises from the hindgut. Anatomically, the proximal colon is supplied by branches of the superior mesenteric artery, the inferior mesenteric artery supplies the descending colon, sigmoid, and rectum. The capillary network of the proximal colon has a greater total microvascular volume compared to that of the distal colon [6].

In addition to the aforementioned circulation, colic collateral arterial circulation between the superior and inferior mesenteric arteries through the marginal artery of Drummond and possibly through the ascending branch of the left colic artery must be considered [7]. In clinical practice, the latter is especially relevant with regard to surgical resection of a part of the colon. Furthermore, increased blood flow is important in regard to nourishment of the tumor. During tumor progression neoangiogenesis plays a central role in tumor growth and survival. The angiogenic activity of a tumor does not necessarily correlate with tumor aggressiveness. Nonetheless, it can be a prognostic factor for certain tumor types [8]. Various antiangiogenic therapies were tested with the idea to starve tumors of necessary oxygen and nutrients. These therapies demonstrated strong heterogeneity in reaction with activity in some and inactivity or toxicity in others with tumor adaptation and acceleration of metastatic tumor growth [9]. The immune system regulates angiogenesis in cancer with both pro- and antiangiogenic activities. The induction of angiogenesis is mediated by tumor-associated macrophages and myeloid-derived suppressor cells which produce proinflammatory cytokines, endothelial growth factors, and protease implicated in neoangiogenesis [10].

Moreover, it is important to consider the venous outflow of the colon. The ascending and transverse colon drain into the superior mesenteric vein, whereas the descending and sigmoid colon empty into the inferior mesenteric vein. The superior mesenteric and inferior mesenteric veins ultimately empty into the hepatic portal vein. This allows toxins absorbed from the colon to be processed by the liver for detoxification. Not only toxins can pass, but also hematological metastatic spread might take place via this route. Hence, when metastatic spread is suspected, blood flow drainage must be considered to make sure not to overlook metastasis.

14.2.3 Clinical Presentation

Differences in clinical presentation between proximal and distal colon cancer are well known; it is safe to state that neoplasms of the proximal and distal colon (right- and left-sided) can be considered two entities exhibiting clinically different features. In general, symptoms tend to be more subtle in the proximal colon with microcytic anemia and weight loss in contrast to the distal colon where alteration in bowel habit and rectal bleeding are more apparent.

Furthermore, features of carcinomas of the proximal colon express a more aggressive pathological course with regard to TNM-stage and morphological characteristics [11]. Distal colon cancer more often presents as early-stage disease as compared to proximal cancer, which also causes disparity in prognosis according to tumor site [12]. Subsequently, differences in survival can be observed overall survival being worse in right- versus left-sided colorectal cancer independent of disease stage (HR 1.14, 95% CI [1.06, 1.22], $p < 0.01$) [13].

14.2.4 Morphology and Histology

Neoplasms can be classified by their specific cell morphology and histopathological features. The defining feature of colorectal carcinoma is invasion through the muscularis mucosae into the submucosa. The vast majority (>95%) of colorectal carcinoma are adenocarcinomas, which arise from epithelial cells related to glandular formation [14]. Glandular formation is the basis of histologic tumor grading: in well-differentiated adenocarcinoma, >95% of the tumor is gland forming; in moderately differentiated adenocarcinoma, this percentage is 50–95%; and in poorly differentiated carcinoma, the tumor is mostly solid with <50% gland formation [15]. Other, more rare variants of colorectal carcinomas include neuroendocrine, mucinous, signet ring cell, squamous cell, adeno-squamous, spindle cell, and undifferentiated carcinomas.

Mucinous adenocarcinoma is a distinct form of colorectal cancer found in approximately 10% of colorectal cancer patients, the tumor by definition being composed of >50% extracellular mucin [16, 17]. Mucinous cancer is more often found in female patients and is predominantly located in the proximal colon, usually diagnosed at a higher stage [18].

It is widely accepted that mucinous cancer constitutes a different pathological entity, but mechanisms that are herein involved are still not completely elucidated. Although mucinous cancer is found at a higher stage, the literature remains divided about the prognostic value in comparison with typical adenocarcinomas of the colon [19, 20].

Other types of carcinoma are rare to extremely rare. Signet ring cell carcinoma represents <1% of all colorectal carcinomas, and, similar to mucinous carcinoma, they are defined by >50% of cancer cells showing signet ring cell features, characterized by a prominent intracytoplasmic mucin vacuole pushing the nucleus to the periphery of the cell [21]. Moreover, signet ring cell carcinomas are defined by poor cell differentiation and behold an infiltrative growth pattern being associated with a worse prognostic outcome compared to conventional adenocarcinomas [22, 23].

Additionally, neuroendocrine carcinomas are rare and highly aggressive colon tumors accounting for <1% of colorectal malignancies [24]. At a clinical level, patients with poorly differentiated neuroendocrine carcinoma have a significantly worse overall survival rate compared to patients with conventional colorectal adenocarcinoma (HR 7.7 95% CI [2.6–22.6], $p < 0.001$) [25]. Moreover, patients appear to have a marginally better prognosis if they present without metastatic spread [26].

Morphological differentiation in carcinoma, e.g. adenocarcinoma, mucinous adenocarcinoma, signet ring cell, or neuroendocrine carcinoma, does not seem to represent consecutive steps of tumor development but rather constitute different genetic pathways [27, 28]. In order to fully understand and describe the mechanisms that are involved in immunocompromised patients, differences of each specific characterization and classification must be taken into account, since prognosis is correlated with these features. Despite all this, classifications into groups also have its limits due to widespread inter-individual heterogeneity. Although classification is getting more refined, ideal classification has not been found up until this day.

14.3 Tumor Biology and Immunological Response

During the development of adenocarcinoma, several molecular, cellular, and histological alterations give rise to the transition from normal epithelium to adenoma and eventually to cancer. Multiple differences in colon carcinomas have been discussed in the previous part of this chapter, starting from anatomical classification to clinical presentation, morphology, and histopathological features. Nevertheless, tumors with similar features and histological profile tend to have important differences in response to treatment. Nowadays, it is well known that the most plausible explanation for these differences may be due to the strong heterogeneity around and inside of tumors cells, thus specific tumor biology is also linked to immunologic response.

The formation of an inflammatory microenvironment also plays a pivotal role in colorectal cancer development and progression [29]. Colorectal malignancies contain a mix of malignant epithelial cells and benign stroma, e.g., fibroblasts, lymphatic and vascular structures, and inflammatory cells. The portion of malignant cells within a tumor area is an independent prognostic marker in colorectal cancer, the relevance of this marker increasing with tumor stage [30, 31].

In addition, the tumor microenvironment is important in tumor progression during the course of malignancy. Initially, the microenvironment will mainly suppress spread of malignant cells, as, for example, macrophages are able to remove neutrophils and control the inflammatory activity [32].

Other stromal cells like fibroblasts will also inhibit tumor spread by healing the mucosa through migration to the extracellular matrix where they appear to be a fundamental component in wound contraction [33]. Eventually, these stromal cell defense mechanisms develop differently. Regardless of its origin, "smoldering" inflammation in the tumor microenvironment has many tumor-promoting effects [29]. In a state of permanent activation, fibroblasts can, for example, cultivate elevated levels of growth factor, thereby supporting tumor growth.

Evenly important, tumor growth and consequent start of metastatic spread are supported by the stromal cells. Herein, the extracellular matrix gets dysregulated by proteolysis, which is a strictly controlled process in normal tissue, but is apparent in carcinoma. Matrix metalloproteinases (MMPs) are the enzymes responsible for this interference, since they are responsible for degradation of the extra cellular matrix. These enzymes are found to be crucial in cancer development and metastatic spread and are often upregulated, particularly in left-sided tumors. Therefore, MMP inhibitors could be a potential therapeutic target in prevention of distant metastasis prolonging overall survival [34, 35].

Duplicates of tumor cells exhibit different alterations, which allow selection of cells that are resistant to immunological clearance being called immune selection. The development of immune selection is crucial in tumor progression. The mechanisms by which the immune system is alerted to the presence of a developing tumor are not fully understood. This process where susceptible tumor cells are being removed by the immune system is called immunoediting [36]. It is hypothesized that tumor cells do have these immunoediting qualities and innate and adaptive immune systems work together to detect the presence of a developing tumor in order to eliminate the tumor cells, before they become clinically apparent [37]. However, hereafter, a selected group of tumor cells, not susceptible for clearance of the immune system, remain present. Subsequent escape mechanisms might help tumor cells to evade immunological control to start metastatic spread.

14.4 Genetic Expression

Not only a differentiation in tumor biology can be made, but also a distinction in gene expression is of importance. Gene expression helps to better understand etiology, immunological escape, and metastatic spread of colorectal carcinoma, something that is of paramount importance in the development of new therapies. Glebov et al. [38] distinguished gene expression profiles in normal mucosal epithelium of adults, and comparing the ascending to the descending colon, they found over 200 genes showing a significant difference in expression. When the same comparison was made in fetal genes, only 87 genes of the mucosal epithelium expressed differently. This indicates that, although anatomically relevant differences are already established in the embryonic colon, additional changes in gene expression occur during postnatal development [38].

Besides different gene expression in normal mucosal epithelium, different gene expression profiles in proximal and distal adenocarcinomas have also been assessed. Out of a selected 186 genes, Birkenkamp-Demtroder et al. [39] identified only 30 common genes in adenocarcinomas of both the left and right side of the colon, which could be regarded as general tumor markers.

Furthermore, enzymes that are active during inflammation can be upregulated over specific parts of the colon. During inflammation in the proximal colon, there normally is more expression of COX-2, an enzyme responsible for prostaglandin production, compared to expression levels in the distal colon. Elevated levels of COX-2 are present in the majority of colorectal carcinoma and in a subset of adenomas [40, 41]. However, increased expression of COX-2 in adenocarcinoma was found to be higher in left-sided compared with right-sided adenocarcinoma [39]. Possibly, as a result of this phenomenon COX-2, overexpression in adenocarcinoma is associated with worse survival among colon cancer patients (HR 1.37; 95% confidence interval (CI), 0.87–2.14) [42]. Naturally this can be explained by lower initial levels of expression, but still it can be a viable marker and possible therapeutic target.

In conclusion, not only anatomy but also distinction in gene expression profiles and pathway activity can help to determine cancer-specific tumor progression and clinical outcome facilitating the development of new therapeutic targets.

14.5 Microbiome

Although many features of the colon have been studied, the intestinal microbiome (microbial population, structure, and function) has often not been taken into account in the past, but there is a growing interest for the role of the microbiome in carcinogenic development and immunologic condition. Baxter et al. [43] analyzed if tumor growth had a correlation with the intestinal microbiota of germ-free mice after they had fecal transplantation from healthy humans or a patient with colorectal cancer. In this model, the presence of the *Clostridium* genus had a negative correlation with tumor cell count. On the contrary, the abundance of *Fusobacterium nucleatum* DNA has been correlated positively with advanced disease stage and higher colorectal cancer-specific mortality [44]. *Bacteroides fragilis* is another bacterium that has been studied being associated with poor disease-free survival in patients with colorectal cancer [45]. Although these studies do not cover the whole microbiome, they show that the intestinal microbiota may modulate local immune responses and therewith affect disease stage and mortality.

14.6 Immunocompromised Status in Patients

A person who has an immunodeficiency of any kind is said to be immunocompromised. Evidently there could be many and various reasons for an impaired immune system. Normally, a healthy immune system possesses the ability to recognize altered cells and promotes an effective immunologic reaction to neoantigens on the cellular surface of tumor cells. Often the immunologic response will eliminate developing cancer cells before they become clinically apparent, this ability being called immunosurveillance. In humans immunosurveillance has long been questioned but was suspected with the observation of an increase in carcinoma occurrence in patients with immunodeficiency. Particularly in HIV-infected persons, as well as in solid organ transplant patients, increased rates of cancer were found [46, 47].

Also, immunocompromised conditions are well known to be associated with a higher risk of developing de novo cancers in lymphoproliferative diseases and skin cancers. However, this association for intestinal cancer is still controversial [48, 49]. A person who has an immunodeficiency may be vulnerable to opportunistic infections but also be prone to cancer development, since immunosurveillance can be decreased. Immunodeficiency disorders can be congenital or acquired, and a distinction is necessary to comprehend the underlying etiology.

Congenital immunodeficiency disorders are a rare group of chronic disorders, also known as primary immunodeficiency. Examples of congenital immunodeficiencies are X-linked agammaglobulinemia and CVID (common variable immunodeficiency), where low levels of immunoglobulins are cause for infections. Syndromes can also be the cause of an immunodeficiency; velocardiofacial or DiGeorge syndrome, for example, is a syndrome where the thymus and thyroid are not developed properly, initiating immunodeficiency as well [50]. All of these diseases are extremely rare, and their relationship with colorectal malignancies is largely unclear; hence, this specific group will not be covered in detail in this chapter.

Acquired immunodeficiencies, also known as secondary immunodeficiencies, occur more frequently and can be a result of various causes. Well-known causes for acquired immunodeficiencies include environmental stress, age, genetic and metabolic diseases, immunosuppressive drugs, surgery or trauma, malnutrition, and infectious diseases [51]. Since the literature on the relationship between primary immunodeficiency disorders and colorectal cancer is scarce, the next paragraphs will further focus on acquired immunodeficiency disorders.

14.6.1 Metabolic Diseases

A metabolic disease can also inflict alterations or have a deleterious effect on immunity. One of the most common examples is diabetes mellitus type II. Herein, factors that contribute to immunodeficiency are impaired glucose metabolism, insufficient blood flow, and denervation, which increase susceptibility to infections in these patients. Moreover, diabetic patients are known for their poor lymphoproliferative response to mitogens (chemical substance to commence cell division) as well as defective phagocytosis and cell chemotaxis (cell movement in response to chemical stimulus) [52], which also adds to an impaired immunosurveillance.

14.6.2 Age

Moreover, age has its influence on immunosurveillance and can contribute to a diminished immune status. Newly born prematures, for example, are well known for their high susceptibility to infections. The reason to this impaired immunity is to be found in the secondary lymphoid organs (spleen, lymph nodes, tonsils, Peyer's patches, mucosa-associated lymphoid tissue) that have not been matured properly. In combination with the absence of maternal IgG (main antibody for humoral immunity) transferred by the placenta, this will cause impaired immunity [53].

Elderly people can have equal problems with adequate immunization. Loss of T-cell function in elderly, and thereby lacking cellular immunity, can be caused via two pathways. Naive T-cell production capacity can be restricted, and oligoclonal T-cell expansion occurs, meaning that both T-cell count and diversity decrease, due to these phenomena.

As well as cellular immunity, B-cell secretion capacity of hematopoietic growth factors is also diminished in the elderly, which results in poor ability to upregulate the production of neutrophils [54].

14.6.3 Environmental Stress

Chronic adverse environmental stress, too, can affect the immune system. Exposure to radiation eventually weakens all immune functions. Radiation can be used in cancer treatment, forming ions in the cells of the tissues it passes through as it dislodges electrons from atoms. Besides, radiation has been shown to induce endothelial cell dysfunction, marked by increased permeability, detachment from the underlying basement membrane, and apoptosis [55]. This can kill cells or change genes inhibiting the cells to grow. Other known mutagenic and carcinogenic effects of radiation are seen in UV light and can be attributed to the induction of DNA damage and errors [56]. However, linkage to colorectal malignancies due to this mechanism seems far-fetched. Consequences of radiotherapy are undeniable; therefore another exclusive chapter will be dealing with this topic in detail.

14.6.4 Surgery and Spleen Injury

After surgery or trauma, an inflammatory response gets triggered due to the disruption of epithelial barriers. This response is followed by a release of inflammatory cytokines, nitric oxide, and reactive oxygen species that disintegrates the vascular barrier, and as a consequence leakage of molecules become apparent. The occurrence of leakage of these molecules results in a stress response with edema, inflammation, and often disease progression [57]. Eventually the loss of epithelial barriers combined with elevated levels of cortisol, due to stress, contributes to overall impaired immunosuppression in patients who had a traumatic event or elective surgery.

Substantially different from standard traumatized patients are patients with injury to the spleen or prior history of splenectomy. This group deserves special consideration, while they are particularly susceptible to infections by encapsulated bacteria such as *Streptococcus pneumoniae* or *Haemophilus influenzae*. In order to prevent an overwhelming postsplenectomy infection after surgery, potentially with severe sepsis and septic shock, active vaccination should be given before any surgical intervention takes place [58].

14.6.5 Malnutrition

Malnutrition is another key element of functional and immunological compromise that is associated with poor clinical outcome [59]. It could be hypothesized that malnutrition reflects a state of prolonged catabolism impairing host immune function and leading to an inadequate response to inflammatory stimuli. Sarcopenia can be considered the syndrome of loss of muscle mass, quality, and strength and is more common in older adults. This syndrome can be seen as a precursor syndrome or the physical manifestation of frailty [60]. Frailty is especially important in the perioperative period, during which patients are subject to high levels of physiologic stress and inflammation [61].

In elderly patients, preoperative malnutrition is common and worsens the condition of this already vulnerable population [62]. Many nutritional assessments are used in daily clinical practice, compared with body weight loss, low BMI, and low serum albumin providing more accuracy in predicting postoperative morbidities [63]. Preoperative albumin level is an objective, simple, and qualified nutritional assessment method for the evaluation of surgical risks in colorectal cancer patients [63]. Nutritional assessment at the outpatient department makes it possible to use the time lapse between examination and surgery to improve the nutritional status. Therefore, routine nutritional assessment is highly advisable so that appropriate measures may be taken to minimize potential postoperative complications.

14.6.6 Immunosuppressive Medication

The effect of chronic immunosuppression or immunomodulation has often been topic of discussion, since the effect on long-term oncologic outcomes for patients undergoing surgery is not well known. To make sure to draw the right conclusions on this topic, it is necessary to evaluate immunosuppressive drugs one by one.

Firstly, corticosteroids will be the topic of discussion, which is one of the most evaluated group of drugs regarding this topic. For ethical reasons, it is very hard to conduct a randomized controlled trial of patients receiving either corticosteroids or placebo for a longer period of time, while corticosteroids are known to increase the risk on anastomotic leakage [64]. Therefore, the effect of chronic corticosteroid use in colorectal surgery is still more or less under debate. Ostenfeld et al. [65] conducted a nested case-control study to examine the effect of systemic glucocorticoids. They concluded that frequent use of glucocorticoids was not associated with an overall increased risk for colorectal cancer [65]. Several other studies have looked at the effect of preoperative corticosteroid use in colorectal surgery. A study by Ziegler et al. [66] included 5123 patients who underwent a colectomy of whom 214 were treated with corticosteroids. In their study they found a significant higher anastomotic leakage rate in diabetic patients who received corticosteroids preoperatively. Another study by Slieker et al. [64] reported an increased risk for anastomotic leakage in patients taking corticosteroids as long-term medication and those taking steroids perioperatively. Conversely, several other studies evaluating corticosteroid use, with dispersed ranges of time of usage preoperatively, failed to show a significantly increased risk of anastomotic leakage [67–69]. A possible explanation for these outcomes could be the relative small number of patients in these studies [67, 69], these studies probably being underpowered. Also, lower overall survival was observed in rectal cancer patients given dexamethasone perioperatively compared with patients not given dexamethasone [70], this finding suggests that rectal cancer patients may get a survival benefit from avoiding perioperative dexamethasone. An explanation to the decreased survival with corticosteroids may be represented by an inadequate immune response that withholds cleaning up cancerous cells. In conclusion, treatment with corticosteroids may increase the risk of anastomotic leakage in patients undergoing colorectal surgery, although further studies are necessary before a final conclusion can be made.

In addition, purine analogues such as azathioprine, thiopurine, and 6-mercaptopurine have been widely debated in literature for their immunosuppressive features especially in inflammatory bowel disease [71]. Purine analogues are antimetabolite immunosuppressive agents that mimic the structure of endogenous metabolic purines and interfere with the synthesis of nucleic acid. By preventing the clonal expansion of lymphocytes in the induction phase of the immune response, they affect both cellular and humoral immunity.

Thiopurines are frequently being used in organ transplantation and autoimmune diseases, such as rheumatoid arthritis, systemic vasculitis, SLE, and inflammatory bowel disease. Myrelid et al. [72] examined the risk of anastomotic leakage after resection in patients with Crohn's disease and found a significant increased rate in patients who received azathioprine or mercaptopurine. The clinical implication of this finding is that patients having only purine analogues (or more additional risk factors) may potentially benefit from having a deviating stoma, since their risk for anastomotic complications is already increased. Although purine analogues can reduce the risk for colorectal cancer in severe colitis patients [73], usage of purine analogues should be extensively overthought.

14.6.7 Human Immunodeficiency Virus

Acquired immunodeficiency syndrome (AIDS)-defining cancers (e.g., Kaposi sarcoma, non-Hodgkin lymphoma, cervical cancer) have long been associated with human immunodeficiency virus (HIV) infection. The introduction of highly active antiretroviral therapy (HAART) for HIV in the late 1990s has led to improved immunocompetence and lower AIDS-related mortality. A trend toward an increasing cumulative incidence of colorectal cancer among HIV-positive patients was observed, in contrast to significantly decreased cumulative incidence and hazard rates among uninfected persons [74]. Studies evaluating screening options for colorectal cancer in HIV/AIDS patients have traditionally been ignored due to historical high mortality rates in AIDS. Nevertheless, HIV-infected patients not only have a higher prevalence of colonic neoplasms, but adenocarcinomas also develop at a younger age being more advanced than in uninfected patients [75]. This finding suggests that screening colonoscopy should be offered to HIV-infected patients.

The relative risk of surgical management for colorectal cancer in people with HIV remains uncertain. However, treatment for colorectal carcinoma in HIV-infected patients is associated with a fall in the median CD4 cell count [76], which makes them especially vulnerable to opportunistic infections. As a consequence surgeons should be aware of the profound immunological effects in this specific group of patients with colorectal carcinoma and should be considering antibiotic prophylaxis to a lower threshold to avoid opportunistic infections.

Previously in this chapter, the origin and definition of anatomic location in rectal cancer has been discussed. The anatomic continuity of the anal canal and the rectum gives reason to consider the etiology of anal cancer as well. In HIV-infected patients, three major histological subtypes of malignant neoplasms of the colon can be distinguished, (adenocarcinoma, mucinous adenocarcinoma, signet ring cell carcinoma); besides the abovementioned three major subtypes, risk for anal or rectal squamous cell carcinoma is elevated in the HIV-infected populations. Site misclassification was present, and detailed information on tumor location is needed to prove that rectal squamous cell carcinoma is a distinct entity [77].

Not all anal cancers in HIV-infected people can directly be attributed to HIV infection. Anal cancer, unlike colon and rectal cancer, is caused by oncogenic subtypes of HPV. Both anal and cervical cancers share similar histological and pathological characteristics and are both associated with HPV infection. However, in the general population, anal cancer is quite uncommon and comprises only a small portion of all gastrointestinal malignancies. Subsequently, anal cancer risk associated with HIV infection is particularly high in men having sex with men, with an estimated 37-fold increased risk compared with the general population [46].

Anal Pap smear is currently the best studied screening method for anal cancer, results being reported as atypical squamous cells, low-grade anal intraepithelial neoplasia, and high-grade anal intraepithelial neoplasia [78].

In conclusion, the rectal and anal regions are continuous, and tumors can span both regions, which make it difficult to distinguish. Prophylaxis for opportunistic infections should be considered, especially when CD4 cell count drops. Anal cancer has a different etiology compared to colon and rectal originated cancers.

14.7 Conclusion

Differentiation between the types of neoplasms through their location, genesis, and clinical presentation, as well as their specific cell structures and characteristics, is meaningful. Subdivision will provide more insight into the pathogenesis and therapeutic options of colorectal cancer. Heterogeneity between and inside tumor cells can be a good explanation for capricious behavior of the tumor and leads to divergence in response to therapy. Other distinct endogenous factors as patients' genetic background and immunodeficiency, together with exogenous factors as lifestyle and dietary intake exposure to environmental stress, determine the immunological status of a colorectal cancer patient. In order to get a clear view on the complex factors that contribute to tumor development, progression and metastasis immunological aspects must certainly not be ignored.

References

1. Yamauchi M, et al. Assessment of colorectal cancer molecular features along bowel subsites challenges the conception of distinct dichotomy of proximal versus distal colorectum. Gut. 2012;61(6):847–54.
2. Beart RW, et al. Trends in right and left-sided colon cancer. Dis Colon Rectum. 1983;26(6):393–8.
3. Bufill JA. Colorectal cancer: evidence for distinct genetic categories based on proximal or distal tumor location. Ann Intern Med. 1990;113(10):779–88.
4. Li FY, Lai MD. Colorectal cancer, one entity or three. J Zhejiang Univ Sci B. 2009;10(3):219–29.
5. Rullier E, et al. Low rectal cancer: classification and standardization of surgery. Dis Colon Rectum. 2013;56(5):560–7.
6. Skinner SA, O'Brien PE. The microvascular structure of the normal colon in rats and humans. J Surg Res. 1996;61(2):482–90.
7. Lange JF, et al. Riolan's arch: confusing, misnomer, and obsolete. A literature survey of the connection(s) between the superior and inferior mesenteric arteries. Am J Surg. 2007;193(6):742–8.
8. Bergers G, Benjamin LE. Tumorigenesis and the angiogenic switch. Nat Rev Cancer. 2003;3(6):401–10.
9. Ebos JM, et al. Accelerated metastasis after short-term treatment with a potent inhibitor of tumor angiogenesis. Cancer Cell. 2009;15(3):232–9.
10. Tartour E, et al. Angiogenesis and immunity: a bidirectional link potentially relevant for the monitoring of antiangiogenic therapy and the development of novel therapeutic combination with immunotherapy. Cancer Metastasis Rev. 2011;30(1):83–95.

11. Snaebjornsson P, et al. Colon cancer in Iceland—a nationwide comparative study on various pathology parameters with respect to right and left tumor location and patients age. Int J Cancer. 2010;127(11):2645–53.
12. Hansen IO, Jess P. Possible better long-term survival in left versus right-sided colon cancer - a systematic review. Dan Med J. 2012;59(6):A4444.
13. Benedix F, et al. Colon carcinoma—classification into right and left sided cancer or according to colonic subsite?—Analysis of 29,568 patients. Eur J Surg Oncol. 2011;37(2):134–9.
14. American Cancer Society. What is colorectal cancer? 2018 [cited 2018 01-08-2018]. Available from: https://www.cancer.org/cancer/colon-rectal-cancer/about/what-is-colorectal-cancer.html.
15. Fleming FJ, Gillen P. Reversal of Hartmann's procedure following acute diverticulitis: is timing everything? Int J Colorectal Dis. 2009;24(10):1219–25.
16. Ferlay J, et al. Estimates of worldwide burden of cancer in 2008: GLOBOCAN 2008. Int J Cancer. 2010;127(12):2893–917.
17. Bosman FT, Carneiro F, Hruban RH, Theise ND. WHO classification of tumours of the digestive system. 4th ed. Minnesota: International Agency for Research on Cancer, University of Minnesota; 2010.
18. Hyngstrom JR, et al. Clinicopathology and outcomes for mucinous and signet ring colorectal adenocarcinoma: analysis from the National Cancer Data Base. Ann Surg Oncol. 2012;19(9):2814–21.
19. Kang H, et al. A 10-year outcomes evaluation of mucinous and signet-ring cell carcinoma of the colon and rectum. Dis Colon Rectum. 2005;48(6):1161–8.
20. Verhulst J, et al. Mucinous subtype as prognostic factor in colorectal cancer: a systematic review and meta-analysis. J Clin Pathol. 2012;65(5):381–8.
21. Fleming M, et al. Colorectal carcinoma: pathologic aspects. J Gastrointest Oncol. 2012;3(3):153–73.
22. Chen JS, et al. Clinical outcome of signet ring cell carcinoma and mucinous adenocarcinoma of the colon. Chang Gung Med J. 2010;33(1):51–7.
23. Leopoldo S, et al. Two subtypes of mucinous adenocarcinoma of the colorectum: clinicopathological and genetic features. Ann Surg Oncol. 2008;15(5):1429–39.
24. Bernick PE, et al. Neuroendocrine carcinomas of the colon and rectum. Dis Colon Rectum. 2004;47(2):163–9.
25. Olevian DC, et al. Colorectal poorly differentiated neuroendocrine carcinomas frequently exhibit BRAF mutations and are associated with poor overall survival. Hum Pathol. 2016;49:124–34.
26. Smith JD, et al. A retrospective review of 126 high-grade neuroendocrine carcinomas of the colon and rectum. Ann Surg Oncol. 2014;21(9):2956–62.
27. Kelemen LE, Kobel M. Mucinous carcinomas of the ovary and colorectum: different organ, same dilemma. Lancet Oncol. 2011;12(11):1071–80.
28. Borger ME, et al. Signet ring cell differentiation in mucinous colorectal carcinoma. J Pathol. 2007;212(3):278–86.
29. Mantovani A, et al. Cancer-related inflammation. Nature. 2008;454(7203):436–44.
30. Tsujino T, et al. Stromal myofibroblasts predict disease recurrence for colorectal cancer. Clin Cancer Res. 2007;13(7):2082–90.
31. Hutchins GGA, et al. Intratumoral stromal morphometry predicts disease recurrence but not response to 5-fluorouracil-results from the QUASAR trial of colorectal cancer. Histopathology. 2018;72(3):391–404.
32. Koh TJ, DiPietro LA. Inflammation and wound healing: the role of the macrophage. Expert Rev Mol Med. 2011;13:e23.
33. Gabbiani G, Hansson GK. ATVB in focus: smooth muscle cells. Arterioscler Thromb Vasc Biol. 2003;23(3):379.
34. Aparicio T, et al. Matrix metalloproteinase inhibition prevents colon cancer peritoneal carcinomatosis development and prolongs survival in rats. Carcinogenesis. 1999;20(8):1445–51.

35. Jensen SA, et al. Expression of matrix metalloproteinase 9 (MMP-9) and tissue inhibitor of metalloproteinases 1 (TIMP-1) by colorectal cancer cells and adjacent stroma cells—associations with histopathology and patients outcome. Eur J Cancer. 2010;46(18):3233–42.
36. Garrido F, et al. Implications for immunosurveillance of altered HLA class I phenotypes in human tumours. Immunol Today. 1997;18(2):89–95.
37. Schreiber RD, Old LJ, Smyth MJ. Cancer immunoediting: integrating immunity's roles in cancer suppression and promotion. Science. 2011;331(6024):1565–70.
38. Glebov OK, et al. Distinguishing right from left colon by the pattern of gene expression. Cancer Epidemiol Biomark Prev. 2003;12(8):755–62.
39. Birkenkamp-Demtroder K, et al. Differential gene expression in colon cancer of the caecum versus the sigmoid and rectosigmoid. Gut. 2005;54(3):374–84.
40. Elder DJ, et al. Human colorectal adenomas demonstrate a size-dependent increase in epithelial cyclooxygenase-2 expression. J Pathol. 2002;198(4):428–34.
41. Eberhart CE, et al. Up-regulation of cyclooxygenase 2 gene expression in human colorectal adenomas and adenocarcinomas. Gastroenterology. 1994;107(4):1183–8.
42. Ogino S, et al. Cyclooxygenase-2 expression is an independent predictor of poor prognosis in colon cancer. Clin Cancer Res. 2008;14(24):8221–7.
43. Baxter NT, et al. Structure of the gut microbiome following colonization with human feces determines colonic tumor burden. Microbiome. 2014;2:20.
44. Kostic AD, et al. Fusobacterium nucleatum potentiates intestinal tumorigenesis and modulates the tumor-immune microenvironment. Cell Host Microbe. 2013;14(2):207–15.
45. Wei Z, et al. Could gut microbiota serve as prognostic biomarker associated with colorectal cancer patients' survival? A pilot study on relevant mechanism. Oncotarget. 2016;7(29):46158–72.
46. Frisch M, Biggar RJ, Goedert JJ. Human papillomavirus-associated cancers in patients with human immunodeficiency virus infection and acquired immunodeficiency syndrome. J Natl Cancer Inst. 2000;92(18):1500–10.
47. Penn I, Starzl TE. Malignant tumors arising de novo in immunosuppressed organ transplant recipients. Transplantation. 1972;14(4):407–17.
48. Merchea A, et al. Outcomes of colorectal cancer arising in solid organ transplant recipients. J Gastrointest Surg. 2014;18(3):599–604.
49. Lee HS, et al. Is a stricter colonoscopy screening protocol necessary in liver transplant recipients? Comparison with an average-risk population. Dis Colon Rectum. 2014;57(8):976–82.
50. Ming JE, Stiehm ER, Graham JM Jr. Syndromic immunodeficiencies: genetic syndromes associated with immune abnormalities. Crit Rev Clin Lab Sci. 2003;40(6):587–642.
51. Chinen J, Shearer WT. 6. Secondary immunodeficiencies, including HIV infection. J Allergy Clin Immunol. 2008;121(2. Suppl):S388–S392; quiz S417.
52. Delamaire M, et al. Impaired leucocyte functions in diabetic patients. Diabet Med. 1997;14(1):29–34.
53. Fouda GG, et al. The impact of IgG transplacental transfer on early life immunity. Immunohorizons. 2018;2(1):14–25.
54. Pawelec G, et al. Human immunosenescence: does it have an infectious component? Ann N Y Acad Sci. 2006;1067:56–65.
55. Langley RE, et al. Radiation-induced apoptosis in microvascular endothelial cells. Br J Cancer. 1997;75(5):666–72.
56. Matsumura Y, Ananthaswamy HN. Toxic effects of ultraviolet radiation on the skin. Toxicol Appl Pharmacol. 2004;195(3):298–308.
57. Giannoudis PV. Current concepts of the inflammatory response after major trauma: an update. Injury. 2003;34(6):397–404.
58. Theilacker C, et al. Overwhelming postsplenectomy infection: a prospective multicenter cohort study. Clin Infect Dis. 2016;62(7):871–8.
59. Covinsky KE, et al. The relationship between clinical assessments of nutritional status and adverse outcomes in older hospitalized medical patients. J Am Geriatr Soc. 1999;47(5):532–8.
60. Wilson D, et al. Frailty and sarcopenia: the potential role of an aged immune system. Ageing Res Rev. 2017;36:1–10.

61. Walston J, et al. Research agenda for frailty in older adults: toward a better understanding of physiology and etiology: summary from the American Geriatrics Society/National Institute on Aging Research Conference on Frailty in Older Adults. J Am Geriatr Soc. 2006;54(6):991–1001.
62. Mudge AM, et al. Helping understand nutritional gaps in the elderly (HUNGER): a prospective study of patient factors associated with inadequate nutritional intake in older medical inpatients. Clin Nutr. 2011;30(3):320–5.
63. Hu WH, et al. Preoperative malnutrition assessments as predictors of postoperative mortality and morbidity in colorectal cancer: an analysis of ACS-NSQIP. Nutr J. 2015;14:91.
64. Slieker JC, et al. Long-term and perioperative corticosteroids in anastomotic leakage: a prospective study of 259 left-sided colorectal anastomoses. Arch Surg. 2012;147(5):447–52.
65. Ostenfeld EB, et al. Use of systemic glucocorticoids and the risk of colorectal cancer. Aliment Pharmacol Ther. 2013;37(1):146–52.
66. Ziegler MA, et al. Risk factors for anastomotic leak and mortality in diabetic patients undergoing colectomy: analysis from a statewide surgical quality collaborative. Arch Surg. 2012;147(7):600–5.
67. Lake JP, et al. Effect of high-dose steroids on anastomotic complications after proctocolectomy with ileal pouch-anal anastomosis. J Gastrointest Surg. 2004;8(5):547–51.
68. Tresallet C, et al. Effect of systemic corticosteroids on elective left-sided colorectal resection with colorectal anastomosis. Am J Surg. 2008;195(4):447–51.
69. Vignali A, et al. Effect of prednisolone on local and systemic response in laparoscopic vs. open colon surgery: a randomized, double-blind, placebo-controlled trial. Dis Colon Rectum. 2009;52(6):1080–8.
70. Yu HC, et al. Avoiding perioperative dexamethasone may improve the outcome of patients with rectal cancer. Eur J Surg Oncol. 2015;41(5):667–73.
71. Gong J, et al. Use of thiopurines and risk of colorectal neoplasia in patients with inflammatory bowel diseases: a meta-analysis. PLoS One. 2013;8(11):e81487.
72. Myrelid P, et al. Thiopurine therapy is associated with postoperative intra-abdominal septic complications in abdominal surgery for Crohn's disease. Dis Colon Rectum. 2009;52(8):1387–94.
73. Actis GC, et al. Azathioprine, mucosal healing in ulcerative colitis, and the chemoprevention of colitic cancer: a clinical-practice-based forecast. Inflamm Allergy Drug Targets. 2010;9(1):6–9.
74. Silverberg MJ, et al. Cumulative incidence of cancer among persons with HIV in North America: a cohort study. Ann Intern Med. 2015;163(7):507–18.
75. Bini EJ, Green B, Poles MA. Screening colonoscopy for the detection of neoplastic lesions in asymptomatic HIV-infected subjects. Gut. 2009;58(8):1129–34.
76. Alfa-Wali M, et al. Colorectal cancer in HIV positive individuals: the immunological effects of treatment. Eur J Cancer. 2011;47(16):2403–7.
77. Coghill AE, et al. Rectal squamous cell carcinoma in immunosuppressed populations: is this a distinct entity from anal cancer? AIDS. 2016;30(1):105–12.
78. Scott H, et al. Routine anal cytology screening for anal squamous intraepithelial lesions in an urban HIV clinic. Sex Transm Dis. 2008;35(2):197–202.

Medical and Surgical Management of Colorectal Cancer Patients Presenting with Haemostatic Disorders

15

Valerio Celentano

15.1 Introduction

Haemostasis is a complex process whose function is to limit blood loss from an injured vessel and to maintain normal blood flow in the circulation [1].

Maintaining haemostasis during surgery is essential [2] to preserve physiologic functions for the patient, provide the surgeon with the ability to see the operative field and promote successful wound management and patient outcomes. In addition, effective surgical haemostasis also results in fewer blood transfusions, decreased operating time and reduced morbidity and mortality for patients.

Proper haemostasis is a function of balance between procoagulant systems (platelets, coagulation cascade) and anticoagulant systems (APC/protein S, fibrinolysis). If haemostasis is out of balance due to a defect in one of these systems, then either thrombosis or bleeding may occur [3]. The coagulation system is exquisitely regulated: in addition to clot formation that must occur to prevent bleeding at the time of vascular injury, two related processes must exist to prevent propagation of the clot beyond the site of injury. First, there is a feedback inhibition on the coagulation cascade, which deactivates the enzyme complexes leading to thrombin formation. Second, mechanisms of fibrinolysis allow for breakdown of the fibrin clot and subsequent repair of the injured vessel with deposition of connective tissue [4].

Normal coagulation pathway represents a balance between the procoagulant pathway that is responsible for clot formation and the mechanisms that inhibit the same beyond the injury site. Imbalance of the coagulation system may occur in the perioperative period or during critical illness, which may be secondary to numerous factors leading to a tendency of either thrombosis or bleeding [5].

V. Celentano (✉)
Department of Colorectal Surgery, Queen Alexandra Hospital, Portsmouth Hospitals NHS Trust, Portsmouth, UK

University of Portsmouth, Portsmouth, UK

N. de'Angelis et al. (eds.), *Emergency Surgical Management of Colorectal Cancer*, Hot Topics in Acute Care Surgery and Trauma,
https://doi.org/10.1007/978-3-030-06225-5_15

Bleeding disorders are characterized by defects in haemostasis that lead to an increased susceptibility to bleeding. They are caused either by platelet disorders (primary haemostasis defect), coagulation defects (secondary haemostasis defect), or a combination of both. In people with congenital or acquired bleeding disorders undergoing surgical interventions, haemostatic treatment is needed in order to correct the underlying coagulation abnormalities and minimize the bleeding risk. This treatment varies according to the specific haemostatic defect, its severity and the type of surgical procedure. Ideally, surgical interventions in patients with bleeding disorders should be performed as elective procedures, following careful pre-, intra- and postoperative planning. Unfortunately, not uncommonly patients with diagnosed bleeding disorders or on anticoagulation therapy present with acute surgical conditions requiring emergency surgery. A multidisciplinary approach is essential, and the surgical team must closely liaise with the haematology and anaesthetic team. The need for massive transfusion should be anticipated, and guidelines should be in place to provide the simultaneous administration of blood, plasma, and platelets.

A basic understanding of haemostasis is necessary for properly interpreting laboratory studies in order to accurately diagnose the disorder and ensure appropriate treatment.

15.2 Physiology of Haemostasis

Haemostasis is the physiological process that stops bleeding at the site of an injury while maintaining normal blood flow elsewhere in the circulation. The endothelium in blood vessels maintains an anticoagulant surface that serves to maintain blood in its fluid state, but if the blood vessel is damaged, components of the subendothelial matrix are exposed to the blood [6].

There are two main components of haemostasis. Primary haemostasis refers to platelet aggregation and platelet plug formation. Platelets are activated in a multifaceted process, and as a result they adhere to the site of injury and to each other [7], plugging the injury. Secondary haemostasis refers to the deposition of insoluble fibrin, which is generated by the proteolytic coagulation cascade [8]. This insoluble fibrin forms a mesh that is incorporated into and around the platelet plug. This mesh serves to strengthen and stabilize the blood clot.

Under physiologic conditions, haemostasis is accomplished by a complex sequence of interactions between platelets, the endothelium, and multiple circulating or membrane-bound coagulation factors. Four major physiologic events participate in the haemostatic process: vascular constriction, platelet plug formation, fibrin formation, and fibrinolysis [9]. Although each tends to be activated in order, the four processes are interrelated so that there is a continuum and multiple reinforcements (Table 15.1).

Table 15.1 Schematically, after a loss of vascular integrity (e.g. an injury to a vessel), four major events occur in the following sequence

1. Vasoconstriction This is the initial response to vessel injury which limits the flow of blood to the area. Vasoconstriction is subsequently linked to platelet plug formation. Thromboxane A2 (TXA2) is produced locally at the site of injury via the release of arachidonic acid from platelet membranes and is a potent constrictor of smooth muscle. Similarly, endothelin synthesized by injured endothelium and serotonin (5-hydroxytryptamine) released during platelet aggregation are potent vasoconstrictors. The extent of vasoconstriction varies with the degree of vessel injury. A small artery with a lateral incision may remain open due to physical forces, whereas a similarly sized vessel that is completely transected may contract to the extent that bleeding ceases spontaneously.
2. Platelet plug formation Platelets have a pivotal role in haemostasis by forming the initial haemostatic plug that provides a surface for the assembly of activated coagulation factors leading to the formation of fibrin-stabilized platelet aggregates and subsequent clot retraction. In a healthy blood vessel, and under normal blood flow, platelets do not adhere to surfaces or aggregate with each other. However, in the event of injury, platelets are exposed to subendothelial matrix, and adhesion and activation of platelets begins. After vasoconstriction, platelets are activated by thrombin and aggregate at the site of injury to form a temporary, loose platelet plug. This clumping activity is stimulated by the protein fibrinogen and by platelets binding to collagen exposed following rupture of the endothelial lining of vessels when injured. This process requires von Willebrand's factor (VWF), a protein in the subendothelium which binds to glycoprotein I/IX/V on the platelet membrane. After adhesion, platelets initiate a release reaction that recruits other platelets from the circulating blood to seal the disrupted vessel; up to this point, this process is known as primary haemostasis.
3. Fibrin clot formation To stabilize the initially loose platelet plug, a fibrin clot or mesh forms to trap the plug. This process called secondary haemostasis consists of the cascade of coagulation serine proteases that culminates in cleavage of soluble fibrinogen by thrombin to form a crosslinked fibrin mesh at the site of an injury. Most of the clotting factors are proteins that are synthesized in the liver and circulate in an inactive form. Many of the proteins have protease capability, thereby allowing them to cleave their target beneath them in the cascade and activate it by exposing its own protease site. The elements of the coagulation cascade are designated by Roman numerals; an 'a' suffix denotes the active form of the factor. There are two pathways involved with the clotting cascade that meet at a certain point to become a common pathway. The intrinsic pathway is activated by damage directly to the blood vessel and the exposure of collagen to the circulating platelets within the blood. The extrinsic pathway is activated by tissue damage outside of the blood vessel, hypoxia, sepsis, malignancy and inflammation. The common point in both pathways is the activation of factor X to factor Xa. Factor Xa activates prothrombin (factor II) to thrombin (factor IIa). Thrombin, in turn, converts fibrinogen to fibrin. One convenient feature of depicting the coagulation cascade with two merging arms is that commonly used laboratory tests segregate abnormalities of clotting to one of the two arms. An elevated activated partial thromboplastin time (aPTT) is associated with abnormal function of the intrinsic arm of the cascade, whereas an elevated prothrombin time (PT) is associated with the extrinsic arm.

(continued)

Table 15.1 (continued)

4. Fibrinolysis The role of the fibrinolytic system is to dissolve blood clots during the process of wound healing and to prevent blood clots in healthy blood vessels. This occurs through the action of plasmin. The fibrinolytic system is a parallel system which is activated along with activation of coagulation cascade and serves to limit the size of clot. Fibrinolysis is an enzymatic process that dissolves the fibrin clot into fibrin degradation products (FDPs) by plasmin originating from fibrin-bound plasminogen in the liver.

15.3 Clinical Assessment of Patients with Haemostatic Disorders

A good detailed comprehensive history is the best predictor of a bleeding problem [10]. Questions should be asked to assess the type and sites of bleeding, whether it involves the cutaneous and mucous membranes (i.e. petechiae, purpura bruises, epistaxis, gingival bleeding, menorrhagia and/or haematuria). Bleeding from skin and mucous membranes tends to occur with platelet disorders, while bleeding into deep tissue, joints and muscles suggest a coagulation factor defect.

Questions on whether the bleeding is spontaneous or follows trauma must also be asked. Any history of blood transfusion or other blood components is very important. Information on all surgeries including tooth extractions and any history of abnormal bleeding during or after surgery should be evaluated. Any patient who has had major surgery, a tonsillectomy or dental extractions, without unusual bleeding has had the best evaluation of their coagulation system possible [11].

Excessive bleeding in response to circumcision or from the umbilical stump is common in patients with haemophilia A or B [12]. Patients with vascular disorders secondary to connective tissue abnormalities such as Ehlers-Danlos syndrome may give a history of easily distensible skin or extraordinary ligament laxness. Drug history is of extreme importance since a wide variety of drugs affect haemostasis, and recent treatment with aspirin and antiaggregants, heparin, and oral anticoagulants should be noted.

Family history can be relevant in case of congenital disorders: haemophilia follows a pattern of X-linked recessive inheritance. However, up to 30% of case of haemophilia A are spontaneous mutations with no family history. Von Willebrand's disease is difficult to diagnose because of the variability in inheritance [13], autosomal dominant and recessive and the variability among patients in the level of von Willebrand factor present.

The history should include information on diseases and organs that may also affect haemostasis, such as liver and renal disease, essential thrombocythaemia, systemic lupus erythematosus, haematological malignancies, myeloproliferative disease and solid organ malignancies. Abnormal haemostasis should be anticipated in patients with short bowel or malabsorption syndromes, who may have impaired coagulation secondary to vitamin K deficiency. Surgical haemostasis may prove difficult in patients with vascular and connective tissue disorders, such as

Ehlers-Danlos syndrome, or in patients under chronic steroids treatment or with prior radiation therapy to the abdomen, in whom careful tissue handling is mandatory.

On physical examination one should look for signs of bleeding or their sequelae and for signs of a possible underlying disorder that can cause the haemostatic derangement. Careful examination of the skin is essential for the detection of petechiae and ecchymoses. These signs may be prominent on the legs, where the hydrostatic pressure is greatest. Hematomas, ecchymoses, and protracted oozing should be looked for at sites of venipunctures, injections and arterial and venous catheter insertion sites. Joint deformities and limited joint mobility are suggestive of severe deficiency of factor VII, VIII, IX or X or severe von Willebrand disease. Weight and body mass index must be measured.

The immediate clinical history of hospitalized patients should focus on recent surgeries, blood losses and blood products transfusions, the physiological status (vital parameters, temperature, and pH) and extent of previous resuscitation to suspect and identify the presence of a coagulopathy.

15.4 Laboratory Assessment

First-line investigations [14] can include a full blood count (FBC) to assess platelet count, peripheral blood smear examination, prothrombin time (PT), fibrinogen, activated partial thromboplastin time (APTT), a thrombin time (TT), bleeding time (BT) and D-dimer.

Platelets play an integral role in haemostasis by forming a haemostatic plug and by contributing to thrombin formation. The normal circulating number of platelets ranges from 150,000 to 450,000 platelets per microliter of blood, and if not consumed in a clotting reaction, platelets are normally removed by the spleen and have an average life span of 7–10 days.

The FBC will reveal abnormalities in platelet numbers, and the blood film will show platelet morphology, excluding the possibility of a systemic illness and other haematological disorders. The intrinsic pathway of coagulation is assessed by aPTT (normal value 25–38 s) so that any abnormalities are detected. Prothrombin time (normal value 10–14 s) assesses the extrinsic coagulation pathway and the generation of fibrin, detected by the thrombin time (normal value 15–19 s).

Other necessary blood tests include haemoglobin level and group and safe in case a transfusion of blood products is needed. Calcium, liver electrolytes and renal function tests are necessary not only to replace deficits but also to determine the appropriate dose of treatments in patients with acute or chronic kidney injury.

The activated partial thromboplastin time (aPTT) evaluates the function of fibrinogen, prothrombin and factors V, VIII, IX, X, XI and XII, and the normal range is 30–40 s. Prolonged aPTTs are associated with acquired or congenital bleeding disorders associated with coagulation factor deficiency, vitamin K deficiency, liver disease, DIC, von Willebrand disease, leukaemia, and haemophilia. The aPTT essentially measures the intrinsic clotting pathway and is particularly useful in monitoring heparin therapy.

Table 15.2 Screening test results in various bleeding disorders

Platelet count	PT	aPTT	Differential diagnosis
N	+	N	Factor VII deficiency (early liver disease, early vitamin K deficiency, early warfarin therapy) Dysfibrinogenemia Factor VII inhibitor Some cases of DIC
N	N	+	Factor VIII, IX, XI deficiency Inhibitors to factor VIII, IX, XI VWD Heparin Lupus inhibitor
N	+	+	Vitamin K deficiency Liver disease Warfarin Heparin Factor V, X deficiency
–	+	+	DIC Liver disease HIT
–	N	N	Increased platelet destruction Decreased platelet production Hypersplenism
+	N	N	Myeloproliferative disorders
N	N	N	Mild VWD Qualitative platelet defects Factor XIII deficiency

N = normal, – = decreased, + = increased

The prothrombin time (PT) is an assay designed to screen for defects in fibrinogen, prothrombin, and factors V, VII, and X and thus measures activities of the extrinsic pathway of coagulation. When any of these factors is deficient, then the PT is prolonged. A normal PT is 11.0–12.5 s. A PT greater than 20 s is indicative of coagulation deficit. The most common measure of PT is to divide the time of coagulation of a patient's blood by that of a known standard, and this value is referred to as the international normalized ratio (INR). The PT measures the vitamin K dependant clotting pathways (extrinsic pathway) and is therefore of particular use in measuring the effect of warfarin therapy (warfarin is a vitamin K antagonist).

Evaluation of further specific coagulation factors must be guided by these screening tests and should be discussed with the haematology team (Table 15.2).

15.5 Bleeding Disorders

Because of the complex nature of haemostasis, potential interference in the process can occur at many levels [15]. Platelet number or function can be insufficient to adequately support coagulation. Alternatively, abnormalities in the clotting factors may underlie an abnormality of haemostasis, either from an intrinsic defect in one of the factors or as the result of pharmacotherapy.

15.5.1 Platelet Disorders

A normal platelet count is 150–400 × 10^9/L. Thrombocytopenia can be congenital, due to impaired bone marrow production, i.e. aplastic anaemia, megaloblastic anaemia and bone marrow infiltration, or a result of increased platelet destruction/consumption. Examples include immune-related conditions like autoimmune thrombocytopenia (ITP), systemic lupus erythematosus and drugs and non-immune conditions such as disseminated intravascular coagulation (DIC), thrombotic thrombocytopenic purpura (TTP) and hypersplenism (splenic sequestration).

Bleeding disorders can also be due to abnormal platelet function in inherited conditions (Glanzmann's thrombasthenia, Bernard-Soulier syndrome and von Willebrand's disease) or acquired (e.g. uraemia and in myeloproliferative disorders). Antiplatelets medications such as aspirin and nonsteroidal anti-inflammatory drugs can often be continued perioperatively, but clopidogrel should be discontinued. Liasing with the cardiology team is essential in patients on dual antiplatelets therapy for recent coronary artery surgery.

15.5.2 Inherited Coagulation Disorders

The main bleeding disorders are genetically inherited. Haemophilia results from defects in secondary haemostasis. Haemophilia A is due to deficiency of factor VIII, and haemophilia B is due to deficiency of factor IX [16]. Deficiency in either of these proteins causes a very similar bleeding phenotype characterized by excess bruising and spontaneous bleeding into the joints, muscles, internal organs and brain. Factor VIII and factor IX are both X-linked genes. Thus haemophilia is primarily expressed in males, with haemophilia A present in about 1 in 5000 males and haemophilia B present in about 1 in 20,000 males. Depending on the mutation, haemophilia can be severe (<1% function), moderate (1–5%), or mild (5–20%). Haemophilia A and haemophilia B are treated mainly by infusion of recombinant factor VIII or factor IX, respectively.

Von Willebrand disease (VWD) is a bleeding disorder caused by deficiency or defect in von Willebrand factor (VWF). VWF is involved in platelet aggregation and is also a carrier for factor VIII. VWF is an autosomal gene, so the disease is present equally in men and women. The severity of the different types of VWD varies, and various therapies are available and preferred for different forms of the disease. Recommendations for factor replacement and duration of perioperative therapy vary according to disease severity and the magnitude of the surgical procedure.

The main drug used for treatment is desmopressin (DDAVP), which is a vasopressin analogue that stimulates release of VWF from endothelial cells and therefore temporarily increases the concentration of VWF in the blood. Type 3 VWD is more severe, and it is treated by infusion with pasteurized plasma-derived pure VWF/factor VIII concentrate. Both of these drugs can also be supplemented with the antifibrinolytic tranexamic acid.

15.5.3 Acquired Bleeding Disorders

These commonly include liver disease, trauma, hypothermia, vitamin K deficiency, DIC, and anticoagulant therapy. Disorders of vessels and supporting tissues may also account for bleeding disorders, and the weakening of the supportive tissues and blood vessel abnormalities as occurs in the ageing process or corticosteroid usage should not be overlooked.

15.5.3.1 Liver Disease

Majority of clotting factors are synthesized in the liver; therefore, severe liver disease is associated with coagulopathy. The most common coagulation abnormalities associated with liver dysfunction are thrombocytopenia and coagulation function manifested as prolongation of the PT.

Thrombocytopenia in patients with liver disease typically is related to hypersplenism, reduced production of thrombopoietin, and immune-mediated destruction of platelets. Platelet transfusions are the mainstay of therapy; however, the effect typically lasts only several hours. Decreased production or increased destruction of coagulation factors as well as a vitamin K deficiency can contribute to a prolonged PT and increased INR in patients with liver disease. Coagulopathy caused by liver disease is most often treated with FFP.

Since the liver is also involved in the clearance of activated clotting factors and fibrinolytic products, it may predispose to DIC.

15.5.3.2 Coagulopathy of Trauma and Hypothermia

Traditionally recognized causes of traumatic coagulopathy include acidosis, hypothermia, and dilution of coagulation factors. However, a significant proportion of trauma patients arrive at the emergency department coagulopathic, and this early coagulopathy is associated with a significant increase in mortality.

Hypothermia must be prevented as is also associated with anticoagulatory effects, which are more pronounced in the presence of acidosis. The effects may result from platelet dysfunction in mild hypothermia (below 35 °C) to decreased synthesis of clotting enzymes and plasminogen activator inhibitors when temperatures is <33 °C.

15.5.3.3 Disseminated Intravascular Coagulation

Disseminated intravascular coagulation (DIC) is characterized by systemic activation of blood coagulation [17], which results in generation and deposition of fibrin, leading to microvascular thrombi in various organs and contributing to multiple organ dysfunction syndrome (MODS).

DIC occurs because of aberrant activation of the clotting cascade, leading to fibrin deposition in small vessels, combined with activation of fibrinolytic mechanisms, leading to bleeding. DIC is usually a common final haemostatic disorder caused by other conditions such as sepsis, pancreatitis, liver disease, pregnancy complications, burns, or trauma. Because they are consumed by the ongoing prothrombotic and fibrinolytic processes, coagulation proteins and platelets can become depleted, leading to bleeding. Thus, in DIC, haemorrhage and thrombosis can occur simultaneously.

In acutely ill hospitalized patients, DIC usually presents with prolongation of the PT and aPTT along with decreased fibrinogen and platelets; systemic bleeding may or may not be present. Typically, bleeding manifests as ecchymoses, purpura and petechiae; it also occurs at surgical incisions or insertion sites of vascular access catheters. Mucosal and urinary bleeding are common.

Thrombocytopenia; prolongation of the PT, aPTT and thrombin time; and hypofibrinogenaemia are characteristic. Because DIC tends to be secondary to other disorders, addressing the underlying disorder is the mainstay of treatment. Therapy is otherwise supportive.

15.5.3.4 Patients on Anticoagulation Therapy

The perioperative management of patients receiving long-term oral anticoagulation therapy is an increasingly common problem. Firm evidence-based guidelines regarding which patients require perioperative 'bridging' anticoagulation are needed. Bridging anticoagulation involves discontinuation of oral anticoagulation before surgery and the use of IV or SC agents for several days before and (sometimes) after surgery. Most studies have shown that preoperative bridging is associated with an acceptably low postoperative bleeding rate [18]. It is essential to consider the estimated procedural bleeding and the thromboembolic risk of the patient in order to determine the timing of anticoagulant interruption and the need for bridging anticoagulation, which is dependant on the anticoagulation agent used and on the clinical indication.

Spontaneous bleeding can be a complication of anticoagulant therapy with either heparin, warfarin, low molecular weight heparins, or factor Xa inhibitors. Examples include haematuria, soft tissue bleeding, intracerebral bleeding, skin necrosis, and abdominal bleeding. Bleeding into the abdominal cavity is by far the most common complication of warfarin therapy and may be intraperitoneal, extraperitoneal, or retroperitoneal. Bleeding secondary to anticoagulation therapy is also not an uncommon cause of rectus sheath hematomas. In most of these cases, reversal of anticoagulation is the only treatment that is necessary. Lastly, it is important to remember that one of the first symptoms of an underlying tumour may be bleeding in a patient who is receiving anticoagulation therapy.

Surgical intervention may prove necessary in patients receiving anticoagulation therapy. When the aPTT is <1.3 times the control value in a patient receiving heparin or when the INR is <1.5 in a patient taking warfarin, reversal of anticoagulation therapy may not be necessary. However, meticulous surgical technique is mandatory, and the patient must be observed closely throughout the postoperative period [19]. There remain two major risk groups who will require conversion to IV unfractionated heparin in the perioperative period to maintain therapeutic anticoagulation in the absence of postoperative bleeding. These are patients with mechanical cardiac valve prostheses and those with a history of acute venous thromboembolism within the previous 4 weeks or during a current pregnancy. The heparin must be stopped 6 h before the operation and restart 12 h after operation, and oral warfarin should be reintroduced as soon as possible thereafter. Epidural anaesthesia is best avoided for those on therapeutic heparin. The newer direct oral anticoagulants (eg, direct thrombin inhibitor dabigatran, factor Xa inhibitors rivaroxiban, apixaban, edoxaban) have shorter half-lives, making them easier to discontinue and resume rapidly, but lack an approved drug-specific antidote, raising concenrns on management of bleeding in patients requiring urgent surgery.

For more rapid reversal of anticoagulation, vitamin K can be administered in patients having warfarin, while use of protamine sulphate is effective in patients receiving IV heparin. However, significant adverse reactions may be encountered when administering protamine, especially in patients with severe fish allergies. Symptoms include hypotension, flushing, bradycardia, nausea, and vomiting. Rapid reversal of anticoagulation can be accomplished with FFP in an emergent situation. Liaison with the haematology team is essential [20] and institutional guidelines are strongly recommended.

Parenteral administration of vitamin K also is indicated in elective surgical treatment of patients with biliary obstruction or malabsorption who may be vitamin K deficient. However, if low levels of factors II, VII, IX, and X (vitamin K-dependent factors) are a result of hepatocellular dysfunction, vitamin K administration is ineffective. For patients who were taking warfarin preoperatively and are at high risk for thrombosis, low molecular weight heparin should be administered, while the INR is decreasing and should be restarted at prophylactic dosages as soon as possible after surgery.

15.6 Thrombotic Disorders

The constitutive or acquired disorders of thrombosis are termed as thrombophilia and are presented in Table 15.3.

There are a number of factors that are associated with the hypercoagulable states. In addition to the genetic and hereditary disorders that predispose to thrombosis [21], several risk factors such as smoking, obesity, pregnancy, immobility, malignancy, surgery and females on oral contraceptives may also contribute to its development. Disorders of ATIII deficiency and reduced protein C and protein S are inherited in autosomal dominant fashion and are associated with increased risk of thrombosis [22]. Acquired protein C and protein S deficiency may be observed in vitamin K deficiency, warfarin therapy, pregnancy, liver cirrhosis, and sepsis. The risk of thromboembolism in the perioperative period is well recognized. Therefore,

Table 15.3 Hereditary and acquired bleeding and thrombotic disorders

Hereditary	Acquired
Bleeding disorders	
Haemophilia A, B, C	Consumptive coagulopathies
Factor V, VII, X, XII deficiency	DIC
Prothrombin deficiency	Liver disease
Afibrinogenaemia	Vitamin K deficiency
	Microangiopathic haemolytic anaemias
Thrombotic disorders	
Antithrombin III deficiency	Antiphospholipid antibody syndrome
Protein C deficiency	Increased levels of factors VIII, IX, XI, fibrinogen
Protein S deficiency	Homozygous homocystinuria
Factor V Leiden	
Prothrombin mutation	

patients with hereditary thrombophilia should be given thromboprophylaxis in consultation with the haematology team. Even in the absence of any known thrombophilia markers, surgical patients are at increased risk of venous thromboembolism as a result of their immobility and the postoperative inflammatory response [23]. All should be assessed for their individual risk in relation to the procedure planned and advised about the importance of leg exercise and early mobilization. Appropriate antiembolism hosiery should be fitted, and anticoagulant prophylaxis with subcutaneous low molecular weight heparin must be ensured [24], and 28 days postoperative treatment must be considered after major colorectal surgery [25].

15.7 Technical Considerations in Colorectal Surgery

Excessive bleeding during or after a surgical procedure may be the result of ineffective haemostasis, blood transfusion, undetected haemostatic defect, consumptive coagulopathy and/or fibrinolysis. Excessive bleeding from the operative field not associated with bleeding from other sites usually suggests inadequate mechanical haemostasis.

Preoperative anaemia is common in colorectal cancer patients [26] and must be corrected [27], as it is a recognised risk factor for postoperative complications. Minimally invasive surgery reduces surgical trauma [28] and reduces blood loss compared to laparotomy [29]. Nevertheless, application of laparoscopic surgery in the emergency setting has a steep learning curve [30] and must be reserved to highly trained colorectal surgeons to minimize conversions and morbidity [31].

New vessel sealing devices and topical haemostatic agents play an important role in common or complex general surgical procedures [32]. These are not a substitute for meticulous surgical technique. The advantages and disadvantages of each agent must be weighed in selecting the correct agent to control bleeding. In general, the minimum amount of each topical haemostatic agent should be used to minimize toxic effects and adverse reactions, interference with wound healing and procedural cost, and surgeons must be familiar with them [33].

Patients with inflammatory conditions such as diverticulitis, peritonitis and inflammatory bowel disease are at significant risk of intraoperative bleeding, due to oedematous tissue planes and a thickened bowel mesentery. Inappropriate and excessive traction must be avoided, as catastrophic bleedings may occur, for example from the spleen or the gastrocolic common trunk of Henle, during mobilisation of the splenic and hepatic flexure of the colon, respectively. Presacral venous bleeding is a technically challenging and potentially life-threatening complication of rectal surgery. Rapid control is important to prevent a fatal outcome. The first temporary manoeuvre is direct pressure at the point of bleeding together with aspiration of the accumulated blood. Conventional haemostatic methods often fail and may occasionally further shear the delicate veins, extend the area of active haemorrhage and significantly worsen the problem. Pelvic packing controls presacral bleeding effectively and may be lifesaving [34]. Alternative methods of packing without the need for reoperation have been also described [35]. Metallic thumbtacks [36] can be used to control presacral bleeding, omental or muscle fragment welding [37] and bone wax use are also very effective techniques. It is imperative to consider the stability of the patient when using potentially time-consuming techniques to control intraoperative haemorrhage. When a patient begins developing the lethal triad of acidosis, coagulopathy and hypothermia, the surgeon must always consider packing to rapidly control haemorrhage and prevent further deterioration [38]. Resuscitation with large volumes of crystalloids and blood products may exacerbate hemodilution, thrombocytopenia and abnormal coagulations, and surgeons must promptly proceed to damage control in cases of severe intraoperative bleeding unresponsive to conventional measures. Anastomotic bleeding is also a not uncommon complication in patients on anticoagulants treatment in the perioperative period and while minor haemorrhage can be treated conservatively under close observation, unstable patients require return to theatre where experienced endoscopic support should be available. If an ileocolic anastomosis is performed, a hand-sewn technique should be considered to minimise the risk of staple line bleeding [39]. Postoperative intra-abdominal haemorrhage often occurs as diffuse bleeding from raw surfaces and requires correction of underlying coagulopathy and abdominal packing if adequate haemostasis cannot be achieved [40].

15.8 Conclusions

Patients with inherited bleeding disorders represent a higher-risk population in the perioperative setting. Although surgery in this group of patients will continue to be challenging, careful perioperative planning, coordinated by an experienced haematology team, should ensure a successful outcome in most cases. Therapeutic anticoagulation preoperatively and postoperatively is becoming increasingly more common. The patient's risk of intraoperative and postoperative bleeding and the estimated thromboembolic risk should guide the need for reversal of anticoagulation therapy preoperatively and the timing of its reinstatement postoperatively.

References

1. Versteeg HH, Heemskerk JW, Levi M, Reitsma PH. New fundamentals in hemostasis. Physiol Rev. 2013;93(1):327–58.
2. Tubbs RS. Surgery is simple-it requires only anatomy and hemostasis. Clin Anat. 2015;28(7):821.
3. Bombeli T, Spahn DR. Updates in perioperative coagulation: physiology and management of thromboembolism and haemorrhage. Br J Anaesth. 2004;93:275–87.
4. Heemskerk JW, Bevers EM, Lindhout T. Platelet activation and blood coagulation. Thromb Haemost. 2002;88:186–93.
5. Monroe DM III, Hoffman M, Roberts HR. Molecular biology and biochemistry of the coagulation factors and pathways of hemostasis. In: Williams hematology. 8th ed. New York, NY: McGraw-Hill Professional Publishing; 2010. p. 614–6.
6. Clemetson KJ. Platelets and primary haemostasis. Thromb Res. 2012;129(3):220–4.

7. Hvas AM. Platelet function in thrombosis and hemostasis. Semin Thromb Hemost. 2016;42(3):183–4.
8. Johari V, Loke C. Brief overview of the coagulation cascade. Dis Mon. 2012;58(8):421–3.
9. Chapin JC, Hajjar KA. Fibrinolysis and the control of blood coagulation. Blood Rev. 2015;29(1):17–24.
10. Ranucci M. Detection of inherited and acquired hemostatic disorders in surgical patients. Can J Anaesth. 2016;63(9):1003–6.
11. Mensah PK, Gooding R. Surgery in patients with inherited bleeding disorders. Anaesthesia. 2015 Jan;70(Suppl 1):112–20, e39–40.
12. Escobar MA, Maahs J, Hellman E, et al. Multidisciplinary management of patients with haemophilia with inhibitors undergoing surgery in the United States: perspectives and best practices derived from experienced treatment centres. Haemophilia. 2012;18:971–81.
13. Zulfikar B, Koc B, Ak G, Dikici F, Karaman İ, Atalar AC, Bezgal F. Surgery in patients with von Willebrand disease. Blood Coagul Fibrinolysis. 2016;27(7):812–6.
14. Bonhomme F, Ajzenberg N, Schved JF, Molliex S, Samama CM, French Anaesthetic and Intensive Care Committee on Evaluation of Routine Preoperative Testing; French Society of Anaesthesia and Intensive Care. Pre-interventional haemostatic assessment: guidelines from the French Society of Anaesthesia and Intensive Care. Eur J Anaesthesiol. 2013;30(4):142–62.
15. Kruse-Jarres R, Singleton TC, Leissinger CA. Identification and basic management of bleeding disorders in adults. J Am Board Fam Med. 2014;27(4):549–64.
16. Santagostino E, Fasulo MR. Hemophilia a and hemophilia B: different types of diseases? Semin Thromb Hemost. 2013;39(7):697–701.
17. Toh CH, Alhamdi Y. Current consideration and management of disseminated intravascular coagulation. Hematology Am Soc Hematol Educ Program. 2013;2013:286–91.
18. Iqbal CW, Cima RR, Pemberton JH. Bleeding and thromboembolic outcomes for patients on oral anticoagulation undergoing elective colon and rectal abdominal operations. J Gastrointest Surg. 2011;15(11):2016–22.
19. Tebala GD, Natili A, Gallucci A, Brachini G, Khan AQ, Tebala D, Mingoli A. Emergency treatment of complicated colorectal cancer. Cancer Manag Res. 2018;10:827–38.
20. Chic Acevedo C, Velasco F, Herrera C. Reversal of rivaroxaban anticoagulation by nonactivated prothrombin complex concentrate in urgent surgery. Futur Cardiol. 2015;11(5):525–9.
21. Bertina R, Koelman B, Koster T, Rosendaal F, Dirven R, De Ronde H, et al. Mutation in blood coagulation factor V associated with resistance to activated protein C. Nature. 1994;369:64–7.
22. Greaves M. Antiphospholipid syndrome. J Clin Pathol. 1997;50:973–4.
23. White CK, Langholtz J, Burns ZT, Kruse S, Sallee K, Henry DH. Readmission rates due to venous thromboembolism in cancer patients after abdominopelvic surgery, a retrospective chart review. Support Care Cancer. 2015;23(4):993–9.
24. Krell RW, Scally CP, Wong SL, Abdelsattar ZM, Birkmeyer NJ, Fegan K, Todd J, Henke PK, Campbell DA, Hendren S. Variation in hospital thromboprophylaxis practices for abdominal cancer surgery. Ann Surg Oncol. 2016;23(5):1431–9.
25. Rasmussen MS, Jørgensen LN, Wille-Jørgensen P. Prolonged thromboprophylaxis with low molecular weight heparin for abdominal or pelvic surgery. Cochrane Database Syst Rev. 2009;(1):CD004318.
26. Banerjee AK, Celentano V, Khan J, Longcroft-Wheaton G, Quine A, Bhandari P. Practical gastrointestinal investigation of iron deficiency anaemia. Expert Rev Gastroenterol Hepatol. 2018;12(3):249–56.
27. Liu L, Liu L, Liang LC, Zhu ZQ, Wan X, Dai HB, Huang Q. Impact of preoperative anemia on perioperative outcomes in patients undergoing elective colorectal surgery. Gastroenterol Res Pract. 2018;2018:2417028.
28. Maggiori L, Khayat A, Treton X, et al. Laparoscopic approach for inflammatory bowel disease is a real alternative to open surgery: an experience with 574 consecutive patients. Ann Surg. 2014;260(2):305–10.
29. Sulu B, Aytac E, Stocchi L, Vogel JD, Kiran RP. The minimally invasive approach is associated with reduced perioperative thromboembolic and bleeding complications for patients receiving

preoperative chronic oral anticoagulant therapy who undergo colorectal surgery. Surg Endosc. 2013;27(4):1339–45.
30. Celentano V, Finch D, Forster L, Robinson JM, Griffith JP. Safety of supervised trainee-performed laparoscopic surgery for inflammatory bowel disease. Int J Color Dis. 2015;30(5):639–44.
31. Giglio MC, Celentano V, Tarquini R, Luglio G, De Palma GD, Bucci L. Conversion during laparoscopic colorectal resections: a complication or a drawback? A systematic review and meta-analysis of short-term outcomes. Int J Colorectal Dis. 2015;30(11):1445–55.
32. Anderson CD, Bowman LJ, Chapman WC. Topical use of recombinant human thrombin for operative hemostasis. Expert Opin Biol Ther. 2009;9(1):133–7.
33. Spotnitz WD, Burks S. Hemostats, sealants, and adhesives III: a new update as well as cost and regulatory considerations for components of the surgical toolbox. Transfusion. 2012;52(10):2243–55.
34. Zama N, Fazio VW, Jagelman DG, et al. Efficacy of pelvic packing in maintaining hemostasis after rectal excision for cancer. Dis Colon Rectum. 1988;31:923–8.
35. McCourtney JS, Hussain N, Mackenzie I. Balloon tamponade for control of massive presacral haemorrhage. Br J Surg. 1996;83:222.
36. Timmons MC, Kohler MF, Addison WA. Thumbtack use for control of presacral bleeding, with description of an instrument for thumbtack application. Obstet Gynecol. 1991;78:313–5.
37. Harrison JL, Hooks VH, Pearl RK, et al. Muscle fragment welding for control of massive presacral bleeding during rectal mobilization: a review of eight cases. Dis Colon Rectum. 2003;46:1115–7.
38. Celentano V, Ausobsky JR, Vowden P. Surgical management of presacral bleeding. Ann R Coll Surg Engl. 2014;96(4):261–5.
39. Golda T, Zerpa C, Kreisler E, Trenti L, Biondo S. Incidence and management of anastomotic bleeding after ileocolic anastomosis. Colorectal Disease. 2013;15(10):1301–8.
40. Asher Hirshberg. Reoperation for Bleeding in Trauma. Archives of Surgery. 1993; 128(10):1163.

Medical and Surgical Management of Colorectal Cancer Emergencies in Elderly Patients

16

Filippo Landi and Eloy Espin

Abbreviations

CC	Colon cancer
CRC	Colorectal cancer
ECR	Emergency colorectal resection
EP	Emergency presentation
GI	Gastrointestinal
mFI	Modified frailty index
MM	Morbidity and mortality
RC	Rectal cancer

F. Landi · E. Espin (✉)
Colorectal Surgery Unit, General Surgery Service, Hospital Universitari Vall d'Hebron, Universitat Autonoma de Barcelona (UAB), Barcelona, Spain
e-mail: eespin@vhebron.net

N. de'Angelis et al. (eds.), *Emergency Surgical Management of Colorectal Cancer*, Hot Topics in Acute Care Surgery and Trauma,
https://doi.org/10.1007/978-3-030-06225-5_16

16.1 Introduction

The incidence of colorectal cancer (CRC) increases sharply with age. Approximately two-thirds of cases occur in adults over 65 years and one-quarter in those aged 80 and older. Life expectancy has increased steadily over the past three decades in high-income countries, as the risk of dying between ages 60 and 80 years has been decreasing approximately 1.5% per year due to decrease in cardiovascular and cancer mortality [1]. Average life expectancy for an 80-year-old alive today is >8 years [2]. The age-specific incidence of CRC is expected to rise linearly with aging and should reach a maximum at about age 90 years [3]. Even if several artifacts could bias age-specific incidence, an estimated incidence of RC of 132–137 new cases per 100,000 people per year between 80 and 89 years of age has been described in an European population, and an incidence around 250/100,000 per year of CC at 85 years has been calculated in a US study [3, 4].

16.2 Emergency Presentation of CRC in the Elderly

16.2.1 Risk Factors

Although there exists considerable variation regarding screening recommendation for CRC among developed countries, almost all cancer societies agree in stop systematic tests by 75 years of age [5]. As a result, CRC screening rates decrease with aging, and the rate of CRC in the population over 80 is about one-third of the rate of 50–64 years old [3, 6]. The absence of physician's recommendation both with other social and clinical factors may increase the risk of emergency presentation (EP) for CRC in the elderly, including lack of specific relevant symptoms [6–8]. In a large nationwide Dutch study including 9913 patients, 22% of the oldest old (≥85 years) had an ECR, comparing with 12% in younger population [9]. A UK population study found that older patients had a threefold probability to EP for CRC comparing patients aged 90 with those aged 70; in this study, age was the strongest risk factor of EP both with dementia and deprived socioeconomic background [10]. The relevance of advanced age as the most important risk factor related to EP and nonelective resection for CRC was confirmed by others recent studies; additional identified factors for EP in older population were female gender, comorbidity (i.e., liver disease), physical frailty, social deprivation, and non-white ethnicity [2, 7, 8, 10–14].

16.2.2 Tumor Staging

CRC is a malignancy where outcomes are strongly related to the stage of disease on presentation. Moreover, the EP is associated with higher rates of locally advanced (T4) and node-positive disease, extramural vascular invasion, metastatic disease, reduced chance of curative surgery, and poorer survival compared with patients diagnosed electively across all ages, but this is particularly true within the senior population [2, 8, 11, 15–20]. In the elderly, the more limited access to healthcare and screening programs boosts the negative impact of nonelective diagnosis on clinical stage and prognosis [10, 12, 17, 21, 22]. In a large Canadian study including 41,356 newly diagnosed CRC patients, 39% of those presenting urgently (which 63% of them were over 70) had metastatic disease, compared to 17% of non-EP [12].

16.2.3 Obstruction

About 15% of all patients with CRC present with obstruction, and a majority of them are older than 75 years [23–25]. Obstruction is responsible for about 60% of EP of CRC [26]. Symptoms such as intermittent abdominal pain, distension, nausea, and vomiting are often secondary to partial obstruction; the latter symptoms are poorly evaluable in the elderly with dementia, in which a palpable mass may exist in right-sided colon cancer (CC) overgrowing to other organs. Peritoneal dissemination may present with small bowel obstruction or palpable mass. The risk of complete obstruction is greater in the sigmoid or splenic flexure segment, while rectal cancer (RC) is less disposed to complication than CC; complete obstruction requiring emergency colorectal resection (ECR) has a higher morbidity and worse survival than partial obstruction [23, 24]. While right-sided obstruction is treated more often with ECR in the elderly [27], colonic stent placement as a bridge to elective surgery is an alternative to ECR in patients with left-sided obstruction. However, even after a recent meta-analysis showed lower short-term morbidity and stoma formation rates, benefits of stenting are still uncertain [28]. Strong data on CRC stenting in the elderly are lacking [21]. Mizrahi and co-workers [29] reported outcomes of 132 patients with obstructive RC and left-sided or proximal CC treated with stent; patients were divided into three groups according to age: <70, 70–79, or ≥80 years. This study reported no differences in stent-related mortality and stoma creation; in contrast, patients >70 years received significantly less surgery after stenting and had higher mortality during the same admission (4% vs. 22% in <70 vs. ≥80 years).

16.2.4 Perforation

Acute perforation is the second most common reason of ECR for CRC, with an incidence between 3% and 25% [19, 24, 26, 30]. Free perforation may occur at the site of the tumor or in the distended proximal colon and lead rapidly to septic shock with mortality up to 35% [30]. Chronic perforation, more common in left-sided CRC, may extend into the retroperitoneum as an abscess (mimicking diverticulitis or appendicitis) or the urogenital tract, with fistula formation. Peritonitis and sepsis are the strongest risk factors for morbidity and mortality (MM) in elderly patients undergoing ECR [30–32].

16.2.5 Bleeding

Colonic hemorrhage is a less frequent EP than obstruction and perforation and is more common in right-sided CC in the elderly [33]. The incidence of lower gastrointestinal (GI) bleeding increases with age, and most CRC are responsible for occult or chronic bleeding presenting mainly as hematochezia. Rectal bleeding was present during the 12 months before EP in 3.6% for CC and 9.2% for RC in a recent British study [7]. The prevalence of anemia reaches 25% among geriatric populations, and a third of these cases are found to be owing to iron deficiency; CRC may be responsible for up to 20% of microcytic anemia in oldest old patient [34]. In the case of T4 carcinoma with local overgrowth, erosion of adjacent arteries may lead to acute bleeding. Severe lower GI bleeding is related to CRC in up to 30% of cases; ECR for bleeding is necessary in up to a quarter of patients who require urgent blood transfusion [35]. Arterial embolization is now considered a first-line therapy for massive hemorrhage, although is considered a bridge to urgent surgery owing to the high risk of bowel ischemia.

16.3 Preoperative Medical Management

Resuscitation measures must begin immediately in case of instability, including the correction of any imbalance before ECR. Because intravascular volume is usually depleted in case of sepsis or obstruction, intravenous crystalloid fluid rehydration is required in case of EP. From a cardiovascular standpoint, rates of diastolic dysfunction rise significantly with age, and the incidence of congestive heart failure raises concomitantly, factors that should be considered in the management in the elderly as well as the concomitant reduced pulmonary physiologic reserve and renal or endocrine comorbidities. Wide broad-spectrum antibiotics should be started as soon as possible in case of obstruction and perforation. In the case of a partial obstruction, patients can be initially managed conservatively allowing an elective surgical procedure. A nasogastric tube is urgently necessary in older patients with neurological comorbidities in order to avoid aspiration pneumonia. In the presence of acute lower GI bleeding, management includes treatment of coagulopathy, volume replacement, and transfusions before colonoscopy or CT scan investigates the source of hemorrhage.

16.4 Preoperative Aging-Specific Considerations

Advanced chronological age couldn't be considered a contraindication for CRC curative surgery [36–38]. Nevertheless, postoperative MM increased progressively with increasing age after emergency surgery, because of several factors [18, 39]. Physical frailty refers to an aggregate susceptibility to poor outcomes owing to age-related and disease-related deficits with decrease of physiological reserve giving rise to vulnerability separate from the normal aging process [40]. Preoperative frailty is a well-established risk factor that defines increased rates of postoperative MM, institutional discharge, and resource use of the older population after emergency abdominal surgery and ECR, particularly [32, 40]. Although it is a useful metric for risk stratification, frailty can be difficult to measure in patients before ECR, as some score including up to 70 factors. To improve its implementation into the clinical setting, the modified frailty index (mFI) based on 11 comorbidity and functional status variables has been proposed in the colorectal surgery domain [41, 42]. A recent study validating the mFI for ECR identified significantly increased odds of 30-day mortality (up to 46%) in elderly patients with concurrently increasing mFI score [32]. Sarcopenia, the age-related decline in skeletal muscle mass and function, has been proposed to represent the biological substrate of the physical impairment that characterizes frailty and may improve the accuracy of mFI in GI cancer surgery [43]. Sarcopenia was independently associated with increased in-hospital, 90-day, and 1-year mortality after emergency abdominal surgery in the elderly [44]. A complete nutritional evaluation, including serum albumin, prealbumin, and transferrin levels, should be carried out; severe malnutrition may be identified in over 70 patients with BMI < 17.

16.5 Surgical Management

16.5.1 Right-Sided Colon Cancer

Complicated right-sided CC is the most frequent indication for nonelective CRC resection in the elderly [26, 45, 46]. Surgery should aim to achieve a curative resection in the case of localized disease. If adjacent organs are involved, en bloc resection is indicated in those patients with better preoperative physical status and less comorbidity. In case of sepsis with hemodynamic instability, compromised immunity, advanced disease, malnutrition, and cardiopulmonary or renal insufficiency, a resection without primary anastomosis should be considered in older patient. The two-staged procedure consists in the resection of the affected segment, right-sided terminal ileocolostomy, and subsequent anastomosis 3–6 months after primary resection [23]. Even if the placement of an ileo- or colostomy after the resection was not found to be protective against mortality after nonelective CRC resection in octogenarians [46], anastomotic leak after right colectomy remains a strong predictor of mortality after emergency surgery in the elderly [26, 47, 48]. Laparoscopic and robotic approach have been barely described in selected octogenarians with complicated right-sided CC [33].

16.5.2 Left-Sided Colon Cancer

Left CC EP consists most often in complete obstruction in the elderly [30]. The operative treatment of complicated left-sided CC should be to radically resect the tumor at the initial operation according to tumor location and patient's anatomy.

Procrastinating the resection of the tumor to a staged surgery has been shown to have poorer short-term outcomes and survival. In the elderly left CC emergent clinical presentation consists most often in complete obstruction, physical impairment, malnutrition, or heavy comorbidity, though the presence of peritonitis, hemodynamic instability, or other preoperative predictors of mortality may be seen by some authors as a contraindication to primary resection with colocolic or colorectal anastomosis. One-, two-, and three-staged procedures have been described in the management of colorectal emergencies in frail elderly [23, 46]. In selected patients without free perforation, initial bowel decompression followed by subsequent resection or immediate resection with or without primary anastomosis may be performed according to the general characteristics of patients, preoperative conditions, tumor location, stage of disease, and surgeon experience. The two-staged procedure included resection of the affected segment, left-sided terminal colostomy, and succeeding anastomosis few months after primary resection, if possible. The three-staged procedure, which has been described in obstructive splenic flexure or descending CC, involves a transverse loop colostomy, planned resection with anastomosis as soon as patient's conditions and imbalances have been partially corrected (usually 1–3 weeks later), and transverse colostomy closure 2–3 months following resection. The staged procedure should be considered in selected extremely ill and frail patients with advanced age, in which a time-consuming and complex procedure might impair the life prognosis, as a long surgical time is a well-established risk factor of mortality in elderly patients after ECR [31].

16.5.3 Rectal Cancer

RC surgery is a major procedure in the elderly, underlined by the postoperative MM [37]. The occurrence of complications is associated with a higher postoperative mortality, which, in elderly patients, persists for at least 6 months, compared with a few weeks after surgery in younger patients [4]. Anastomotic leakage is highly related with MM in the elderly, as well as poor tolerance to medical complications [4, 30, 37]. In the EP setting, a radical procedure with oncologic mesorectal resection should be performed, whenever possible [4]. In the absence of sepsis, obstruction can be considered urgent, not emergent, if the ileocecal valve is incompetent and the cecum is not distended. The Hartmann procedure, associated with partial or total mesorectal excision with terminal colostomy, is considered the standard of care in older and frail patients with important comorbidity presenting with obstructed or bleeding RC who might not tolerate an anastomotic complication or in those with fecal peritonitis and systemic sepsis owing to tumor perforation. Nonetheless, the residual rectal stump may itself be the cause of increased postoperative MM as a short rectal stump is associated with a high risk of pelvic infection (almost 50% of the cases). In those cases an abdominoperineal resection is preferable to a low Hartmann's procedure. Colorectal anastomosis after anterior resection with partial mesorectal excision may be considered in selected patients with a complication of

RC other than perforation, with good nutritional status, and without renal, neurological, or cardiopulmonary comorbidities in the absence of fecal incontinence. In case of synchronous lesions or obstruction with competent ileocecal valve, cecum distension >12 cm, or frank perforation, a subtotal colectomy and terminal ileostomy might be necessary. This aggressive procedure should be reserved for carefully selected patients, since it has a sevenfold increase in postoperative mortality when performed in ASA class 3 octogenarians; with this frequent clinical presentation, the 30-day mortality may exceed 40% (Table 16.1). Subtotal colectomy is also a strong predictor of surgical reintervention and prolonged length of stay in those patients who survive [46].

16.5.4 Palliative Management

Palliative treatment is performed in up to 37% of elderly patients with EP of CRC [17, 21, 30]. Depending on the patient's conditions, age, physical status, and stage of disease, various approaches are used for palliative care (limited and local surgery, endoscopic stenting, interventional radiology, pelvic radiotherapy, and chemotherapy in selected cases) [25, 30]. Limited non-oncologic resection should only be attempted with palliative intent to treat life-threatening complications in case of elevated comorbidity or locally advanced or disseminated disease to prevent the risk of local complications from the primary tumor, such as stenosis, bleeding, and tumor infiltration of adjacent organs. If resection of the primary tumor is not indicated (i.e., locally advanced RC), bowel transit can be reestablished by bypass procedures or stoma creation.

16.6 Morbidity and Mortality

A summary of recent studies reporting short-term outcomes after ECR for CRC in the elderly is shown in Table 16.1.

16.6.1 Mortality

Mortality after ERC in the elderly is between 10% and 48%. Identified independent factors related to mortality are age ≥ 80 [17, 18, 26, 38, 47], age ≥ 70 [30, 31, 46], male sex [30], Charlson score ≥ 2 [17, 26], ECOG PS ≥ 2 [17], neurological comorbidity [47], ASA class ≥ 3 [18, 26, 30, 46, 47], systemic sepsis [30, 31], high mFI [32], advanced CRC stage [18, 32], tumor perforation [26, 30, 31], right and transverse colectomy [26], left colectomy or subtotal colectomy [46], intraoperative splenectomy and intraoperative surgical events [30], significant blood loss [30, 31], palliative outcome [18, 30], postoperative medical complications [30, 31], and anastomotic leakage [26, 47].

Table 16.1 Morbidity and mortality of emergency resection for CRC in the elderly

Author, country, year	N° of patients	Age, mean	Indication of surgery	Tumor site	Overall morbidity	30-day mortality	Palliative care	Risk factors
Mothes [17], Germany, 2017	33	>80	n/r	n/r	n/r	36%	15%	Age ≥ 80; Charlson ≥ 2; ECOG ≥ 2
Tabola [27], Italy, 2017	32	75.5	20 obstruction, 8 perforation, 4 bleeding	RC	28%	12.5%	n/r	–
De Simone [48], Italy, 2017	19	92.5	14 obstruction, 5 perforation	8 RC, 8 LC, 2 TC	37%	21%	1 patient	Right-sided cancer
Schlichtemeier [45], Australia, 2016	62	91	n/r	58% RC; 23 LC; 17% rectum	n/r	9.7%	n/r	–
Pirrera [38], Italy, 2016	78	84	n/r	72% colon; 28 rectum	n/r	15.3%	n/r	Age ≥ 80
Ming-Gao [21], China, 2014	85	84.7	75 obstruction, 10 perforation	39% RC; 61% LC/rectum	71.8%	30.6%	13%	–
Kolfschoten [46], The Netherlands, 2012	268	>80	n/r	41% RC; 17% LC/TC; 36% rectum/sigmoid; 6% others	1 RF: 27% 2 RF: 50% 3 RF: 77%	1 RF: 7% 2 RF: 21% 3 RF: 41%	n/r	Age ≥ 80, ASA ≥ 3; left or subtotal colectomy
Iversen [30], Denmark, 2008	2157	74	73.9% obstruction, 21.3% perforation	35.9% RC; 10.4% TC; left flexure 7.7%; 46% LC	24.4%, medical morbidity; 20.4% surgical morbidity	Overall: 22.1% 81–90 years: 35% ≥91 years: 48%	37%	Age ≥ 71; male sex ASA ≥ 3; perforation; palliative care; splenectomy; medical complications

n/r = not reported

RC right colon, *LC* left colon, *TC* transverse colon, *RF* risk factor, *ASA* American Society of Anesthesiologists, *ECOG* Eastern Cooperative Oncology Group performance status

16.6.2 Morbidity

Morbidity after ERC in the elderly is between 28% and 77%. Identified independent factors related to morbidity are age ≥ 80 and ASA class ≥ 3 [32, 46], high mFI, lung comorbidity, resection with anastomosis, systemic sepsis [31, 32], long operative time and renal insufficiency [31], right-sided CRC [38, 48], and left or subtotal colectomy [46].

16.7 Survival

The overall 1-year survival for patients over 80 undergoing CRC surgery was 86% vs. 70% after elective and ECR in a large population US study including 31,574 individuals; factors associated with decreased overall and CRC-specific survival included advanced age, EP, being widowed, having more hospitalizations within the prior year, use of home oxygen, frailty, and dementia [2]. Other studies found that ECR for CRC is independently associated with decreased overall and disease-free long-term survival compared to elective resection both in elderly and younger patients [8, 16, 17, 19, 21]. On the other hand, it should be considered that oldest old CRC patients undergoing an ECR experience high 30-day mortality. High excess 1-year mortality (up to 43% in the elderly) after an ECR procedure is typically due to the prolonged impact of the surgery itself [49], and when elderly patients survive the first year, they show the same cancer-related survival as younger patients [50]. However, there is a considerable variation in survival outcomes in the literature across different populations: an Australian study reported a 1- and 3-year overall survival after ECR in nonagenarians of 81% and 46.8%, respectively, with no significant differences with elective procedure [45]; conversely, an Asian study reported a survival of 43.5% vs. 75.5% at 1 year and 12.7% vs. 46.4% at 3 years comparing emergent and elective resections in octogenarians [21].

16.8 Conclusion

Complicated CRC is a predominant disease in elderly patients. Colorectal resection for CRC in the elderly is a procedure that is frequently performed emergently in the critically ill patient with important pre-existing comorbidity and reduced physiologic reserve. Oftentimes, in the setting of sepsis, obstruction, or bleeding, colectomy is a lifesaving treatment and is associated with important MM. Moreover, elderly CRC patients undergoing ECR have a greatly increased 1-year mortality risk, as well as worst mid- and long-term survival compared to elective. Nevertheless, age should not be a contraindication for radical surgery, and a curative resection should be performed whenever allowed by disease stage or patient physical status. Families and patients should be carefully informed of outcomes and involved in the decision-making process. Future research should focus on preoperative risk appraisal based on nutritional status and physical factors to identify more frail individuals. The earlier screening diagnosis of CRC in oldest old at risk of EP represents a potentially modifiable factor of decreasing high-risk ECR by conversion to an elective surgery. Future research should also investigate on older patients being considered for elective surgery to identify those patients at an increased risk of poor short-term outcomes who may be better managed with a palliative management in case of EP.

References

1. Cao B, Bray F, Beltran-Sanchez H, Ginsburg O, Soneji S, Soerjomataram I. Benchmarking life expectancy and cancer mortality: global comparison with cardiovascular disease 1981–2010. BMJ. 2017;357:j2765.
2. Neuman HB, O'Connor ES, Weiss J, Loconte NK, Greenblatt DY, Greenberg CC, et al. Surgical treatment of colon cancer in patients aged 80 years and older: analysis of 31,574 patients in the SEER-Medicare database. Cancer. 2013;119(3):639–47.
3. Soto-Ortiz L, Brody JP. Similarities in the age-specific incidence of colon and testicular cancers. PLoS One. 2013;8(6):e66694.
4. Rutten HJ, den Dulk M, Lemmens VE, van de Velde CJ, Marijnen CA. Controversies of total mesorectal excision for rectal cancer in elderly patients. Lancet Oncol. 2008;9(5):494–501.
5. Ebell MH, Thai TN, Royalty KJ. Cancer screening recommendations: an international comparison of high income countries. Public Health Rev. 2018;39:7.
6. Berkowitz Z, Hawkins NA, Peipins LA, White MC, Nadel MR. Beliefs, risk perceptions, and gaps in knowledge as barriers to colorectal cancer screening in older adults. J Am Geriatr Soc. 2008;56(2):307–14.
7. Renzi C, Lyratzopoulos G, Card T, Chu TP, Macleod U, Rachet B. Do colorectal cancer patients diagnosed as an emergency differ from non-emergency patients in their consultation patterns and symptoms? A longitudinal data-linkage study in England. Br J Cancer. 2016;115(7):866–75.
8. Comber H, Sharp L, de Camargo Cancela M, Haase T, Johnson H, Pratschke J. Causes and outcomes of emergency presentation of rectal cancer. Int J Cancer. 2016;139(5):1031–9.
9. Govaert JA, Govaert MJ, Fiocco M, van Dijk WA, Tollenaar RA, Wouters MW, et al. Hospital costs of colorectal cancer surgery for the oldest old: a Dutch population-based study. J Surg Oncol. 2016;114(8):1009–15.
10. Wallace D, Walker K, Kuryba A, Finan P, Scott N, van der Meulen J. Identifying patients at risk of emergency admission for colorectal cancer. Br J Cancer. 2014;111(3):577–80.
11. Askari A, Malietzis G, Nachiappan S, Antoniou A, Jenkins J, Kennedy R, et al. Defining characteristics of patients with colorectal cancer requiring emergency surgery. Int J Colorect Dis. 2015;30(10):1329–36.
12. Rabeneck L, Paszat LF, Li C. Risk factors for obstruction, perforation, or emergency admission at presentation in patients with colorectal cancer: a population-based study. Am J Gastroenterol. 2006;101(5):1098–103.
13. Geraghty J, Shawihdi M, Devonport E, Sarkar S, Pearson MG, Bodger K. Reduced risk of emergency admission for colorectal cancer associated with the introduction of bowel cancer screening across England: a retrospective national cohort study. Colorectal Dis. 2018;20(2):94–104.
14. Aquina CT, Becerra AZ, Xu Z, Boscoe FP, Schymura MJ, Noyes K, et al. Nonelective colon cancer resection: a continued public health concern. Surgery. 2017;161(6):1609–18.
15. Scott NA, Jeacock J, Kingston RD. Risk factors in patients presenting as an emergency with colorectal cancer. Br J Surg. 1995;82(3):321–3.
16. Xu Z, Becerra AZ, Aquina CT, Hensley BJ, Justiniano CF, Boodry C, et al. Emergent colectomy is independently associated with decreased long-term overall survival in colon cancer patients. J Gastrointest Surg. 2017;21(3):543–53.

17. Mothes H, Bauschke A, Schuele S, Eigendorff E, Altendorf-Hofmann A, Settmacher U. Surgery for colorectal cancer in elderly patients: how can we improve outcome? J Cancer Res Clin Oncol. 2017;143(9):1879–89.
18. Heriot AG, Tekkis PP, Smith JJ, Cohen CR, Montgomery A, Audisio RA, et al. Prediction of postoperative mortality in elderly patients with colorectal cancer. Dis Colon Rectum. 2006;49(6):816–24.
19. Amri R, Bordeianou LG, Sylla P, Berger DL. Colon cancer surgery following emergency presentation: effects on admission and stage-adjusted outcomes. Am J Surg. 2015;209(2):246–53.
20. Oliphant R, Mansouri D, Nicholson GA, McMillan DC, Horgan PG, Morrison DS, et al. Emergency presentation of node-negative colorectal cancer treated with curative surgery is associated with poorer short and longer-term survival. Int J Colorect Dis. 2014;29(5):591–8.
21. Ming-Gao G, Jian-Zhong D, Yu W, You-Ben F, Xin-Yu H. Colorectal cancer treatment in octogenarians: elective or emergency surgery? World J Surg Oncol. 2014;12:386.
22. Goldvaser H, Katz Shroitman N, Ben-Aharon I, Purim O, Kundel Y, Shepshelovich D, et al. Octogenarian patients with colorectal cancer: characterizing an emerging clinical entity. World J Gastroenterol. 2017;23(8):1387–96.
23. Cuffy M, Abir F, Audisio RA, Longo WE. Colorectal cancer presenting as surgical emergencies. Surg Oncol. 2004;13(2–3):149–57.
24. Baer C, Menon R, Bastawrous S, Bastawrous A. Emergency presentations of colorectal cancer. Surg Clin N Am. 2017;97(3):529–45.
25. Winner M, Mooney SJ, Hershman DL, Feingold DL, Allendorf JD, Wright JD, et al. Incidence and predictors of bowel obstruction in elderly patients with stage IV colon cancer: a population-based cohort study. JAMA Surg. 2013;148(8):715–22.
26. Bakker IS, Snijders HS, Grossmann I, Karsten TM, Havenga K, Wiggers T. High mortality rates after nonelective colon cancer resection: results of a national audit. Colorect Dis. 2016;18(6):612–21.
27. Tabola R, Mantese G, Cirocchi R, Gemini A, Grassi V, Boselli C, et al. Postoperative mortality and morbidity in older patients undergoing emergency right hemicolectomy for colon cancer. Aging Clin Exp Res. 2017;29(Suppl 1):121–6.
28. Arezzo A, Passera R, Lo Secco G, Verra M, Bonino MA, Targarona E, et al. Stent as bridge to surgery for left-sided malignant colonic obstruction reduces adverse events and stoma rate compared with emergency surgery: results of a systematic review and meta-analysis of randomized controlled trials. Gastrointest Endosc. 2017;86(3):416–26.
29. Mizrahi H, Geron N, Parker MC. The outcome of self-expanding metal stents in elderly patients. J Soc Laparoendosc Surg. 2014;18(3):e2014.00038.
30. Iversen LH, Bulow S, Christensen IJ, Laurberg S, Harling H, Danish Colorectal Cancer Group. Postoperative medical complications are the main cause of early death after emergency surgery for colonic cancer. Br J Surg. 2008;95(8):1012–9.
31. McGillicuddy EA, Schuster KM, Davis KA, Longo WE. Factors predicting morbidity and mortality in emergency colorectal procedures in elderly patients. Arch Surg. 2009;144(12):1157–62.
32. Congiusta DV, Palvannan P, Merchant AM. The impact of frailty on morbidity and mortality following open emergent colectomies. Biomed Res Int. 2017;2017:5126452.
33. Felli E, Brunetti F, Disabato M, Salloum C, Azoulay D, De'angelis N. Robotic right colectomy for hemorrhagic right colon cancer: a case report and review of the literature of minimally invasive urgent colectomy. World J Emerg Surg. 2014;9:32.
34. Clere-Jehl R, Schaeffer M, Vogel T, Kiesmann M, Pasquali JL, Andres E, et al. Upper and lower gastrointestinal endoscopies in patients over 85 years of age: risk-benefit evaluation of a longitudinal cohort. Medicine. 2017;96(44):e8439.
35. Edelman DA, Sugawa C. Lower gastrointestinal bleeding: a review. Surg Endosc. 2007;21(4):514–20.
36. Vallribera F, Landi F, Espin E, Sanchez JL, Jimenez LM, Marti M, et al. Laparoscopy-assisted versus open colectomy for treatment of colon cancer in the elderly: morbidity and mortality outcomes in 545 patients. Surg Endosc. 2014;28(12):3373–8.

37. Landi F, Vallribera F, Rivera JP, Bertoli P, Armengol M, Espin E. Morbidity after laparoscopic and open rectal cancer surgery: a comparative analysis of morbidity in octogenarians and younger patients. Colorect Dis. 2016;18(5):459–67.
38. Pirrera B, Vaccari S, Cuicchi D, Lecce F, De Raffele E, Via BD, et al. Impact of octogenarians on surgical outcome in colorectal cancer. Int J Surg. 2016;35:28–33.
39. Turrentine FE, Wang H, Simpson VB, Jones RS. Surgical risk factors, morbidity, and mortality in elderly patients. J Am Coll Surg. 2006;203(6):865–77.
40. McIsaac DI, Moloo H, Bryson GL, van Walraven C. The association of frailty with outcomes and resource use after emergency general surgery: a population-based cohort study. Anesth Analg. 2017;124(5):1653–61.
41. Obeid NM, Azuh O, Reddy S, Webb S, Reickert C, Velanovich V, et al. Predictors of critical care-related complications in colectomy patients using the National Surgical Quality Improvement Program: exploring frailty and aggressive laparoscopic approaches. J Trauma Acute Care Surg. 2012;72(4):878–83.
42. Vermillion SA, Hsu FC, Dorrell RD, Shen P, Clark CJ. Modified frailty index predicts postoperative outcomes in older gastrointestinal cancer patients. J Surg Oncol. 2017;115(8):997–1003.
43. Buettner S, Wagner D, Kim Y, Margonis GA, Makary MA, Wilson A, et al. Inclusion of sarcopenia outperforms the modified frailty index in predicting 1-year mortality among 1,326 patients undergoing gastrointestinal surgery for a malignant indication. J Am Coll Surg. 2016;222(4):397–407.
44. Rangel EL, Rios-Diaz AJ, Uyeda JW, Castillo-Angeles M, Cooper Z, Olufajo OA, et al. Sarcopenia increases risk of long-term mortality in elderly patients undergoing emergency abdominal surgery. J Trauma Acute Care Surg. 2017;83(6):1179–86.
45. Schlichtemeier S, Logaraj A, Gill AJ, Engel A. Colorectal cancer resection in the Australian nonagenarian patient. Colorectal Dis. 2017;19(3):243–50.
46. Kolfschoten NE, Wouters MW, Gooiker GA, Eddes EH, Kievit J, Tollenaar RA, et al. Nonelective colon cancer resections in elderly patients: results from the dutch surgical colorectal audit. Digest Surg. 2012;29(5):412–9.
47. Modini C, Romagnoli F, De Milito R, Romeo V, Petroni R, La Torre F, et al. Octogenarians: an increasing challenge for acute care and colorectal surgeons. An outcomes analysis of emergency colorectal surgery in the elderly. Colorectal Dis. 2012;14(6):312–8.
48. De Simone B, Coccolini F, Ansaloni L, Tarasconi A, Baiocchi G, Vettoretto N, et al. Complicated colorectal cancer in nonagenarian patients: is it better not to perform anastomosis in emergency? Turk J Trauma Emerg Surg. 2017;23(1):15–22.
49. Dekker JW, Gooiker GA, Bastiaannet E, van den Broek CB, van der Geest LG, van de Velde CJ, et al. Cause of death the first year after curative colorectal cancer surgery; a prolonged impact of the surgery in elderly colorectal cancer patients. Eur J Surg Oncol. 2014;40(11):1481–7.
50. Dekker JW, van den Broek CB, Bastiaannet E, van de Geest LG, Tollenaar RA, Liefers GJ. Importance of the first postoperative year in the prognosis of elderly colorectal cancer patients. Ann Surg Oncol. 2011;18(6):1533–9.

Colorectal Cancer Surgical Emergency in Transplanted Patients

17

Lelde Lauka, Giulio Vitali, Thierry Berney, and Nicola de'Angelis

17.1 Colorectal Cancer in Transplanted Patients

Solid organ transplantation (SOT) has become well-established medical procedure with increasing rates worldwide. In 2015 there were 126,670 organ transplantations that is 5.8% of increase over 2014; raise was observed in all solid organs except the pancreas [1]. It is well established that the population after SOT has a higher risk of developing various cancers, with non-Hodgkin lymphoma, Kaposi sarcoma, non-melanoma skin cancer, and lip cancer being among the most common malignancies in these patients [2–4].

Although the risk of developing colorectal cancer (CRC) after solid organ transplantation is smaller in comparison with malignancies mentioned above, various studies have reported a significantly increased risk. Incidence in these studies varies from no differences from general population up to standardized incidence ratio (SIR) 4.5 [5]. In a meta-analysis of malignancies in immunosuppressed patients, SIR after SOT was reported to be 1.69 with confidence interval 95% [2]. In the same meta-analysis for SIR for colorectal cancer in HIV/AIDS, immunosuppressed population was only 0.92; that suggests that lifelong immunosuppression is only one of the risk factors for developing a cancer. Incidence of different cancer type is strongly related also to the transplanted organ. Data collected from UK Transplant registry revealed SIR of 1.8 for CRC, with highest risk after liver transplantation (SIR 2.4), followed

L. Lauka · N. de'Angelis (✉)
Service of Digestive, Hepato-Pancreato-Biliary Surgery and Liver Transplantation, Unit of Minimally Invasive and Robotic Surgery, Henri Mondor Hospital, AP-HP, Créteil, France

University of Paris Est, UPEC, Créteil, France

G. Vitali · T. Berney
Service of Abdominal Surgery and Liver Transplantation, Geneva University Hospital and Medical School, Geneva, Switzerland

N. de'Angelis et al. (eds.), *Emergency Surgical Management of Colorectal Cancer*, Hot Topics in Acute Care Surgery and Trauma,
https://doi.org/10.1007/978-3-030-06225-5_17

by kidney (SIR 1.8) and heart and lung transplantation (SIR 1.1) [6]. Data from the US Transplant Cancer Match (TCM) study showed highest SIR for liver (1.34) and lung (2.34) recipients [5]. Difference in incidences can be explained by underlying conditions and indications for solid organ transplantation. One of the well-established indications for liver transplantation is primary sclerosing cholangitis (PSC). Up to 80% of PSC patients have inflammatory bowel disease (IBD); for IBD the cumulative risk of developing CRC reaches 34% after 25 years of the onset of the disease [7]. Moreover, the combination of PSC and IBD has been reported to have even higher risk in comparison with IBD alone [8]. In the US study, SIR reached 5.69 in the subgroup of SPC-IBD. Patients with cystic fibrosis (CF) have five- to tenfold higher risk of developing CRC; that explains very high SIR of 27 for patients after lung transplantation for CF [5, 9]. Also life habits like smoking and excessive alcohol consumption are related to diseases that lead to necessity of organ transplantation (lung and liver) and at the same time are risk factors for many cancer types [6].

It is important to notice that the risk of developing CRC is increasing with time after SOT and all patients should be screened for this malignancy with precaution. US study showed growing incidence according to the time after SOT reaching SIR of 2.68 after 12 years for proximal colon cancer; increase was observed also in distal colon cancer. Interestingly, the same study described SOT as a protective factor for rectal cancer with SIR 0.64; so far there is no other data available in a literature to reassure this outcome.

Overall, patients with CRC after SOT have more aggressive disease course and limited life expectancy in comparison with patients without transplantation in their medical history. Large study from the USA compared outcomes in patients with CRC from the Israel Penn International Transplant Tumor Registry and patients from the National Cancer Institute Surveillance Epidemiology and End Results database (NCI SEER). It showed significantly earlier CRC diagnosis at the age of 58 years in comparison with 70 years in NCI SEER database. Also, it revealed reduced 5-year survival for all cancer stages: overall, 44% vs. 62%, $p < 0.001$; Dukes A&B, 74% vs. 90%, $p < 0.001$; Dukes C, 20% vs. 66%, $p < 0.001$; and Dukes D, 0% vs. 9%, $p = 0.08$ [10]. Impaired outcomes can be partially explained by immunosuppression of posttransplant patients, delayed diagnosis and advanced disease, possible limited treatment options, and changed tumor biology, but there are no clear evidences that fully describe precise mechanisms of limited survival in this patient subgroup.

17.2 Perioperative Considerations for Transplanted Patients Undergoing Emergency Surgery

With ever-growing solid organ transplantation rates and long-term graft survivals, there is an increasing chance nowadays that any general surgeon will face a case of a surgical emergency in a patient after SOT. In that situation, it is crucial to recognize if the surgical problem is related or non-related to the graft. In the former case, patient should be immediately transferred to a transplant center while initiating a treatment. If the emergency is clearly not related to the graft, it is possible to

Table 17.1 Perioperative considerations for patients after SOT

Perioperative considerations of CRC emergencies in the transplant patient (*obstruction, perforation, bleeding*)	
Masked symptoms	Full spectrum of exams
Net state of immunosuppression	Prophylactic a/b (60 min before incision)
	Fast clinical decision-making
High risk of cardiovascular event	β-blockers administration
Graft rejection due to hypotension	Timely transfusion
Adrenal insufficiency	"Rescue dose" steroids (only if hypotension unresponsive to standard measures)
Impaired wound healing	Nonabsorbable materials
	Delayed removal of sutures or staples

manage the patient in nonspecialized center by a general surgeon. However, it is mandatory that a medical team takes into consideration particularities in this patient subgroup. Ideally, a consultation from the transplantation specialist or treating physician managing immunosuppression should be done before any surgical intervention. Generally, the treatment course and medical decisions in patients after SOT should follow standard medical approach depending on the underlying condition. However, there are several concerns in this subgroup (Table 17.1).

All these patients are chronically immunosuppressed because of lifelong immunosuppressive therapy. Current immunosuppressive regimens typically consist of two phases: induction phase and maintenance therapy. There are no uniform induction regimens, but most transplant centers use either high doses of conventional immunosuppressive agents or polyclonal or monoclonal antibodies directed against T-cell antigens (more common in heart, lung, and kidney transplantation). Maintenance immunosuppression generally consists of a drug combination therapy, involving corticosteroids, calcineurin inhibitors, antiproliferatives, and mTOR inhibitors. With the standardization of immunosuppressive protocols, a pattern of susceptibility has been described, which appeared to be dependent on the dose, duration, nature, and temporal sequence of immunosuppressive therapy [11].

Before considering specific immunosuppression-related perioperative features, it is of paramount to perform full spectrum of clinical, biological, and radiological examinations as immunocompromised patients can present in clinically different fashion with masked signs and symptoms. It often can lead to underestimation of disease severity and worsen the outcomes [12].

Chronic immunosuppression results in (1) persistently low immune defense and (2) carries various side effects from immunosuppressive drugs.

Due to decreased immune defense, patients are at a higher risk of developing malignancies that has been previously discussed in this chapter; however, in an emergency setting, if a patient presents with acute abdominal symptoms, it is important to screen for abdominal malignancy as a possible underlying cause.

Other consideration for impaired immune response is increased risk for infections. It is well known that patients after transplantations will have "net state of immunosuppression" that comprises all the factors that contribute to risk for infection with duration and sequence of immunosuppressive therapies being the major determinant [13]. Patients have characteristic infections depending on the time after transplantation: donor or recipient derived or associated with technical considerations in first 4 weeks, activation of latent infections and opportunistic infections in 1–6 months, and community acquired in the late phase. Accordingly, all patients after SOT must be considered as patients "at risk" for surgical infections at any stage after SOT and prophylactic antibiotics should be routinely administered preoperatively. As usual, broader spectrum coverage to include Gram-positive and Gram-negative bacteria is warranted for intraabdominal procedures, given within 60 min before incision, ideally at the time of anesthetic induction [14, 15].

It must be considered that immunosuppressive therapy effects tissue integrity and wound healing. In particular, the use of glucocorticoids, even at low doses, is associated with consequent enhanced friability of the skin, superficial blood vessels, and intestinal wall, making a cautious and delicate handling of the tissues cardinal to avoid postoperative wound-healing complications. Moreover, the use of nonabsorbable sutures as well as keeping skin staples in place two to three times longer than usual is recommended in transplanted patients [12].

Immunosuppression therapy has impact on literally all organ systems; therefore careful perioperative examination should be done with particular attention on the cardiovascular system and kidney function. Cardiovascular diseases are a major risk factor for mortality after SOT with 2.5-fold greater risk of cardiovascular death and threefold increased risk for ischemic event in comparison with general population [16]. Patients after kidney transplantation are at particularly increased risk for CVD with twofold greater incidence than general population. High incidence in this group can be explained by an end-stage renal disease and its association with ischemic heart disease; other risk factors for CVD, such as hypertension, hyperlipidemia, obesity physical inactivity, and diabetes, are highly prevalent in kidney recipients [12]. Most popular as immunosuppression regimenS usually CONTAIN mentioned drugs—corticosteroids, calcineurin inhibitors and mTOR inhibitors—are associated with developing or worsening preexisting hypertension, dyslipidemia, and diabetes that are well-known risk factors for CDV [16]; this refers to all patients after SOT as immunosuppression regimen usually containing mentioned drugs independently of transplanted organ type.

Perioperative use of β-blockers can reduce CDV event risk in patients undergoing noncardiac surgery. A large analysis of studies about the administration of β-adrenergic receptor antagonists in patients undergoing noncardiac surgery reported 57% risk reduction for all-cause deaths in high-risk group (emergency and vascular surgery) as well as decreased risk of CV death in the same group in comparison with intermediate-high- and intermediate-low-risk surgery group [17]. Therefore, β-blockers administration is also suggested in patients after SOT undergoing emergency surgery. Chronic kidney disease is other main concern in patients after SOT. Long-term use of calcineurin inhibitors is associated with renal dysfunction and has acute and chronic nephrotoxicity. Though it can be reversible after discontinuation of calcineurin inhibitors, their prolonged use can cause irreversible structural changes and development of chronic kidney disease. Renal failure after transplantation is associated with fourfold increased risk for mortality [18].

Because most transplanted patients are maintained on chronic corticosteroids as part of their immunosuppressive regimen, the possibility of adrenal insufficiency is often raised when these patients develop emergent problems requiring surgical intervention. However, adrenal insufficiency has become less and less common because the current doses of steroids used for the maintenance therapy have been markedly reduced compared with previous standards. As a consequence, the practice of administering a prophylactic supraphysiologic dose of corticosteroids perioperatively (the so-called stress dose) appears to be unnecessary in most of the cases [19].

To avoid complications caused by immunosuppression therapies, withdrawal or diminution of immunosuppressive drugs has been discussed during the acute stage of surgical emergency. On contrary, the potential risk for graft dysfunction and even rejection should be considered. Many of transplanted organs have diminished reserve; thus any surgical intervention or alteration in immunosuppression therapy can lead to impaired graft function [12]. There are no specific guidelines for therapy adaption for patients after SOT in emergency setting. In general, oral administration of immunosuppressive drugs in usual doses should be continued if possible. In cases when active substance absorption can be impaired, such as high gastrointestinal tract obstruction, ileus, or increased gastrointestinal motility, parenteral forms should be administered as majority of commonly used immunosuppression drugs are available in intravenous forms. Discontinuation of immunosuppression therapy could be necessary in life-threatening situation, when no effect can be achieved by usual measures. There is little evidence in the literature to support this strategy although some reports have described total withdrawal of immunosuppressive drugs in patients with sepsis. A case report of two patients after kidney transplant described discontinuation of any therapy with maintained stable renal function over 2–6 months [20]. More recent report documented 12 cases in heart transplant recipients with sever sepsis treated with sparing all immunosuppressants. Mortality rate was 50%, and acute rejection episode was observed in one case [21]. These studies are limited of showing the safety of sparing immunosuppressants as a therapeutic approach; therefore a decision for this strategy should be discussed for each case with experienced transplant specialist (Fig. 17.1). If possible, this approach should be avoided during the early stages (induction phase) after transplantation as it carries major risk of acute graft rejection.

17.3 Colorectal Cancer Emergencies in Transplanted Patients

Significant part of colorectal cancer patients has emergency presentation during the course of the disease; the acute condition can be an initial event that leads to the diagnosis of CRC, and it can also occur in later stages. The diagnosis of colon and rectal cancer through emergency presentation is reported to be 31.4% and 15.1% accordingly [22]. Around 17% of hospitalized colon cancer patients require emergency surgery in 72 h, and this number can be even higher if "emergency presentation" is defined by a surgeon [23]. In the same Swedish study, 30 days mortality after emergency surgery was reported to be 11% in comparison with 5% in the

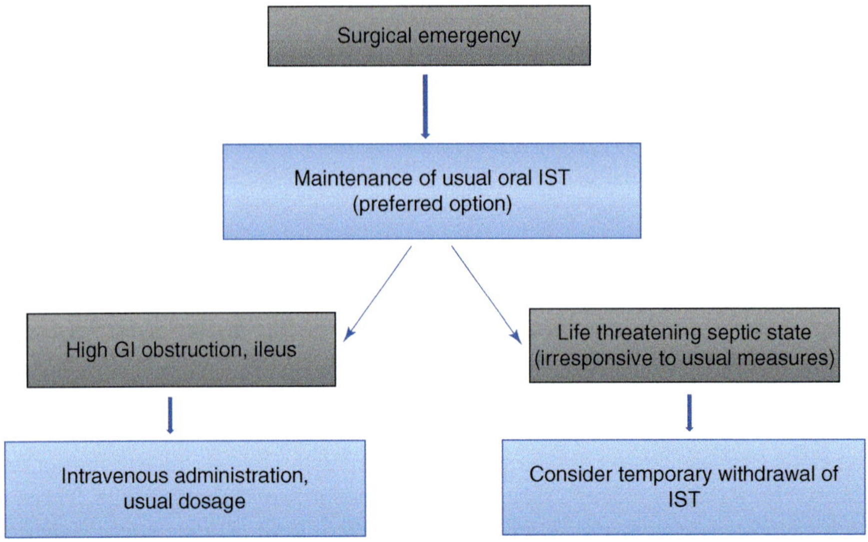

Fig. 17.1 Immunosuppression therapy adaptation in emergency setting. *GI* gastrointestinal, *IST* immunosuppression therapy

elective surgery group. Other studies have shown much higher perioperative mortality that can reach 34%. Also, higher postoperative complication rate is expected in emergency surgery group for CRC with up to 38.1% reported [24].

Emergency setting and, specially, emergency surgery are a prognostic factor for decreased long-term outcomes. In the Swedish study, patients requiring emergency surgery had 42% 2-year survival, while in elective surgery group, it was 62%. With up to 5-year follow-up, another study described median survival of 59 months in comparison with 82 months for elective surgery [25]. It has now become well accepted that the emergency surgery should follow oncological principles for improving long-term outcomes. It is described that good oncological surgical outcomes can be achieved also in the emergency setting; for colon cancer resection, R0 margins were reported to be achieved in 92% of cases and equal or more than 12 retrieved regional lymph nodes in 71% [26]; in other study for colorectal cancer resection, R0 margins were achieved in 90.5%, and more than 12 lymph nodes retrieved in 88.1% [27].

There is no comparative data available in a literature about CRC emergencies in the population after solid organ transplantation; nevertheless, it is expected that due to chronic immunosuppression caused conditions described earlier in this chapter, this subgroup has even more difficult management and worse prognosis in comparison with patients with no transplantation. In the literature, there exists one systemic review dedicated to emergency abdominal surgery after solid organ transplantation; however it does not include patients with emergencies CAUSED by malignant diseases [28]. As suggested by the same authors, surgery is often the preferable treatment since patients after SOT are not good candidates for medical treatment.

Emergency abdominal surgery in this population is associated with high risk of postoperative morbidity (32.7%) and mortality (17.5%) that highlights particularly challenging surgical management of transplanted patients [29].

There are three main surgical entities in an emergency setting related primary to colorectal cancer, that is, large bowel obstruction, perforation, and lower gastrointestinal bleeding [7]. This is true to both general population and population after solid organ transplantation, as there is no data available in the literature about possible differences in patients after transplantation.

17.3.1 Large Bowel Obstruction

Large bowel obstruction is the most common indication for emergency surgery in colorectal cancer making up to 77% of emergencies [26]. Colon cancer is also the most common cause of bowel obstruction in adult population [30]. The onset of the colon cancer can be vaguely symptomatic and is usually characterized by gradual worsening of symptoms like abdominal pain, distension, and obstipation [31]. These patients usually become urgent only when full obstruction has developed; that explains relatively high rates of primary presentation of colon cancer on emergency setting. The vague signs of colon cancer could be even more masked by immunosuppression therapy in patients after SOT that can lead to delayed referral to medical centers for treatment of obstruction. Rectal cancer with acute obstruction is usually associated with locally advanced disease resulting in difficult surgical management in emergency setting [30]. In a case of acute large bowel obstruction caused by colon cancer, there are several surgical treatment options and choice IS made in individual manner for each case. However, all emergency surgeries for colon cancer should follow goals proposed by the American Society of Colon and Rectal Surgeons: (1) avert the immediate negative impact of the complication (e.g., death, sepsis), (2) achieve the best possible tumor control, and (3) ensure timely recovery to permit the initiation of appropriate adjuvant or systemic treatment [32]. The oncological surgical principles of high ligation of blood vessels and safe margins should be upheld in a case of resection of the primary tumor in emergency settings for both colon and rectal cancer. In colon cancer with regional or distal metastases and locally advanced rectal cancer, perioperative systemic and/or local treatment is a standard of care. There are several reports in the literature where this principle has been applied also in patients after transplantation with immunosuppression therapy. In a case report of three patients with advanced rectal cancer after renal transplantation, two of them underwent abdominoperineal resection with total mesorectal excision and adjuvant chemotherapy with Xeloda. Follow-up in 8 months for first patient and 21 months of the second did not reveal the progression of the disease or signs of kidney rejection [33]. In the other report, patient who presented with locally advanced rectal cancer after kidney-pancreas transplantation received neoadjuvant treatment with radiotherapy and chemotherapy. However, chemotherapy of 5-FU and leucovorin was discontinued after the first cycle due to cardiac complications [34]. A case of systemic treatment for metastasis after colon cancer resection has been documented in a patient after kidney transplant; the patient received three courses of FOLFOX regimen with good tolerance and no disturbances in the graft function [35]. Although the data on neoadjuvant or adjuvant treatment for CRC in patients after SOT is anecdotal, this possibility should not be ruled out and considered when managing these patients also in the emergency setting.

In a case of large bowel obstruction, abdominal and pelvic CT scan is imaging modality of choice; using oral, rectal, and intravenous contrast, it can make an accurate diagnosis in up to 89% of cases [36]; moreover, it gives the necessary information for correct cancer staging and grafted organ anatomy. Colonoscopy is usually not feasible in patients presenting with acute obstruction and may be avoided if urgent surgery is necessary. It should be performed after the stabilization of the patient and diminution of obstruction symptom to localize the lesion and confirm the diagnosis with histological examination.

Proximal large bowel obstruction of colon cancer is usually associated with locally advanced tumor and late stages, as symptoms of full obstruction occur late due to larger diameter of the colon. Nonetheless, surgical decision for proximal tumors is simpler; in majority of cases oncologically safe resection with primary anastomosis can be performed; if there is a high risk for anastomotic leak, resection with ileostomy is an option still following oncological principles [30]. For distal tumors and large bowel obstruction, a surgeon has more possible approaches. Guidelines in the management of obstructing cancer of the left colon have been published by the World Society of Emergency Surgery and Peritoneum and Surgery Society. Hartman's procedure and primary segmental resection with anastomosis are both feasible options with former being preferred in patients with high surgical risk. Hartman's procedure is also recommended as superior to loop colostomy. Self-expanding metallic stents (SEMS) remain a nonsurgical option for palliation or bridge to surgery; placement of SEMS should be performed only by experienced endoscopist [37]. In the scope of obstructing cancer, primary resection with complete total mesorectal excision can be difficult as most of the cases in emergency surgery will reveal locally advanced cancer. Hartman's procedure avoids the risk of anastomosis-related complications that could be lethal in oncological patients on immunosuppression. Loop colostomy or ileostomy allows to make full work-up for correct staging and possible decision for neoadjuvant therapy [30].

17.3.2 Large Bowel Perforation

Large bowel perforation is the second most common cause for emergency surgery for CRC with an incidence up to 12%, and it is the most lethal complication of CRC with mortality rates associated with secondary peritonitis as high as 30–50% [30]. Knowing the high mortality after perforation and limited effect of medical treatment for patients with chronic immunosuppression, upfront surgery should be the treatment of choice.

In immunosuppressed transplanted patients, the signs and symptoms of perforation are often absent or non-specific. It has been reported that the interval from clinical onset to surgery was very large, ranging from 2 to 8 days in patients with gastrointestinal non-oncological perforations after SOT [28].

Abdominal and pelvic CT scan is imaging modality of choice for localizing the perforation site and extent of peritonitis with accuracy 95% [31].

Perforation most often occurs at the site of primary tumor but can also manifest proximal to the obstructing tumor due to increased pressure, distention, and ischemia of the colon wall. Free perforation into peritoneal cavity carries a very high mortality rate as patients rapidly can progress into septic shock and multisystem organ failure, in particularly those under lifelong immunosuppressive therapy after SOT; therefore, quick decision about surgical intervention should be taken. If the patient's general status allows surgery, it should be performed following oncological principles. Colon resection with peritoneal lavage is the only mean how to completely eliminate the source of intraabdominal infection. In majority of cases, resection is associated with colostomy or ileostomy. Contained perforation with a formation of intraabdominal abscesses is more characteristic for descending and sigmoid colon cancers, contrary of free perforations for colon cancers proximal to the splenic flexure [38]. Except the cases of metastatic disease when curative surgery is not anticipated and percutaneous drainage can be considered, Hartman's procedure is the treatment of choice.

A special subgroup of patients with CRC presenting with bowel perforation are patients with metastatic disease who are receiving bevacizumab as one of the treating modalities. It has been well described that one of the side effects caused by this monoclonal antibody is spontaneous bowel perforation; the incidence of bowel perforation in patients with mCRC attributed to the use of bevacizumab ranges from 1 to 4% [39]. As described before, the preferred choice of treatment is surgical intervention. Possible perforation site non-related to primary CRC in this subgroup of patients can be expected.

17.3.3 Bleeding

Colorectal bleeding has been reported in up to 50% of cases for patients with CRC and can present as an early symptom; however, mostly it is self-limited and does not alter the general status. Life-threatening bleeding from the tumor is rare. In cases of acute and life-threatening colorectal bleeding, emergency management for patients after SOT should follow the same principles as for immunocompetent patients.

It should be started with resuscitation and stabilization with crystalloids. Transfusion should be considered based on clinical findings and should be administered in the presence of continued active bleeding and signs of hypoperfusion, tachycardia, or hypotension after the administration of 2 l of crystalloid. Similar to elderly population, the threshold for transfusion should be lowered for patients after SOT to avoid graft complications caused by hypovolemic state. During the stabilization, assessment of underlying metabolic abnormalities and coagulopathies must be done. Lower endoscopy, angiography with embolization, and tagged red blood cell (RBC) scan are possible diagnostic and also treatment modalities. Surgery should be considered if less invasive approaches have failed to stabilize the patient; it is usually indicated in a continuous hemodynamic instability despite resuscitation with more than 6 units of blood products; inability to stop hemorrhage with endoscopic techniques or embolization; recurrent, uncontrollable bleeding after initial stabilization; recurrent hemorrhage associated with shock; and ongoing slow bleeding requiring more than 3 units of blood products per day [40]. Surgical resection should be oncologically safe with an intent to cure.

17.4 Conclusions

The treatment course and medical decisions in patients after SOT should follow standard medical practice depending on the surgical emergency; however, there are several considerations in the perioperative management in this population. At the time of admission in the emergency unit, all patients after SOT should receive full spectrum of exams as immunosuppressive state often masks symptoms and leads to delayed diagnosis. Patients after SOT have chronical immunosuppression that is associated with a high risk of infections; therefore broad-spectrum prophylactic antibiotics are warranted given within 60 min before skin incision. Skin closure materials after surgery should be kept two to three times longer than usual as an impaired wound healing is expected. Immunosuppressive therapy affects literally all organ systems with a particular impact on the cardiovascular system. Preoperative administration of β-blockers is recommended to decrease a risk of cardiovascular events.

Surgery is often the preferable approach since patients after SOT are not good candidates for medical treatment; moreover, due to impaired systemic response, decision about the intervention should to be taken without a holdup. When emergency surgery is performed, it should follow oncological principles with an intent to treat. Administration of the immunosuppressive therapy can be adapted; however, maintenance of usual dosage and oral administration route is the preferred choice, and it is a safe option in the majority of cases.

References

1. Carmona M, Alvarez M, Marco J, Mahíllo B. Organ donation and transplantation activities 2015 report. Global Observatory on Donation and Transplantation. September 2017. Available at: http://www.transplant-observatory.org.
2. Grulich AE, van Leeuwen MT, Falster MO, Vajdic CM. Incidence of cancers in people with HIV/ AIDS compared with immunosuppressed transplant recipients: a meta-analysis. Lancet. 2007;370(9581):59–67.
3. Engels EA, Pfeiffer RM, Fraumeni JF Jr, Kasiske BL, Israni AK, Snyder JJ, et al. Spectrum of cancer risk among US solid organ transplant recipients. JAMA. 2011;306(17):1891–901.
4. Chapman JR, Webster AC, Wong G. Cancer in the transplant recipient. Cold Spring Harb Perspect Med. 2013;3(7):a015677.
5. Safaeian M, Robbins HA, Berndt SI, Lynch CF, Fraumeni JF Jr, Engels EA. Risk of colorectal cancer after solid organ transplantation in the United States. Am J Transplant. 2016;16:960–7.

6. Collett D, Mumford L, Banner NR, Neuberger J, Watson C. Comparison of the incidence of malignancy in recipients of different types of organ: a UK Registry audit. Am J Transplant. 2010;10:1889–96.
7. Tsaitas C, Semertzidou A, Sinakos E. Update on inflammatory bowel disease in patients with primary sclerosing cholangitis. World J Hepatol. 2014;6(4):178–87.
8. Soetikno RM, Lin OS, Heidenreich PA, Young HS, Blackstone MO. Increased risk of colorectal neoplasia in patients with primary sclerosing cholangitis and ulcerative colitis: a meta-analysis. Gastrointest Endosc. 2002;56:48–54.
9. Hadjiliadis D, Khoruts A, Zauber AG, Hempstead SE, Maisonneuve P, Lowenfels AB. Cystic fibrosis colorectal cancer screening consensus recommendations. Gastroenterology. 2018;154(3):736–45.
10. Papaconstantinou HT, Sklow B, Hanaway MJ, et al. Characteristics and survival patterns of solid organ transplant patients developing de novo colon and rectal cancer. Dis Colon Rectum. 2004;47:1898–903.
11. Fishman JA, Issa NC. Infection in organ transplantation: risk factors and evolving patterns of infection. Infect Dis Clin N Am. 2010;24(2):273–83.
12. Gohh RY, Warren G. The preoperative evaluation of the transplanted patient for nontransplant surgery. Surg Clin North Am. 2006;86(5):1147–66.
13. Fishman JA, the AST Infectious Diseases Community of Practice. Introduction: infection in solid organ transplant recipients. Am J Transplant. 2009;9(Suppl 4):S3–6.
14. European Centre for Disease Prevention and Control. Systematic review and evidence-based guidance on perioperative antibiotic prophylaxis. Stockholm: ECDC; 2013.
15. Bratzler DW, et al. Clinical practice guidelines for antimicrobial prophylaxis in surgery. Am J Health Syst Pharm. 2013;70:195–283.
16. Girlanda R. Complications of post-transplant immunosuppression, Chapter 33. In: Regenerative medicine and tissue engeneering. Croatia: Intech; 2013.
17. Angeli F, Verdecchia P, Karthikeyan G, Mazzotta G, Gentile G, Reboldi G. β-Blockers reduce mortality in patients undergoing high-risk non-cardiac surgery. Am J Cardiovasc Drugs. 2010;10(4):247–59.
18. Ojo AO, Held PJ, Port FK. Chronic renal failure after transplantation of a nonrenal organ. N Engl J Med. 2003;349:931–8.
19. Kelly KN, Domajnko B. Perioperative stress-dose steroids. Clin Colon Rectal Surg. 2013;26(3):163–7.
20. Burke GW, Ciancio G, Cirocco R, Markou M, Coker D, Roth D, Nery J, Esquenazi V, Miller J. Association of interleukin-10 with rejection-sparing effect in septic kidney transplant recipients. Transplantation. 1996;61(7):1114–6.
21. Chou NK, et al. Sparing immunosuppression in heart transplant recipients with severe sepsis. Transplant Proc. 2006;38(7):2145–6.
22. Abel GA, Shelton J, Johnson S, et al. Cancer-specific variation in emergency presentation by sex, age and deprivation across 27 common and rarer cancers. Br J Cancer. 2015;112(Suppl 1):S129–36.
23. Gunnarsson H, Holm T, Ekholm A, Olsson LI. Emergency presentation of colon cancer is most frequent during summer. Colorectal Dis. 2011;13(6):663–8.
24. Kim J, Mittal R, Konyalian V, King J, Stamos MJ, Kumar RR. Outcome analysis of patients undergoing colorectal resection for emergent and elective indications. Am Surg. 2007;73(10):991–3.
25. Bass G, Flemin C, Conneely J, Martin Z, Mealy K. Emergency first presentation of colorectal cancer predicts significantly poorer outcomes: review of 356 consecutive Irish patients. Dis Colon Rectum. 2009;52(4):678–84.
26. Teixeira F, et al. Can we respect the principles of oncologic resection in an emergency surgery to treat colon cancer? World J Emerg Surg. 2015;10:5.
27. Weixler B, et al. Urgent surgery after emergency presentation for colorectal cancer has no impact on overall and disease-free survival: a propensity score analysis. BMC Cancer. 2016;16:208.

28. De'Angelis N, et al. Emergency abdominal surgery after solid organ transplantation: a systematic review. World J Emerg Surg. 2016;11(1):43.
29. De'Angelis N, Brunetti F, Azoulay D. Common surgical emergencies in transplanted patients. In: Di Saverio S, Catena F, Ansaloni L, Coccolini F, Velmahos G, editors. Acute care surgery handbook. Cham: Springer; 2017.
30. Baer C, Menon R, Bastawrous S, Bastawrous A. Emergency presentations of colorectal cancer. Surg Clin N Am. 2017;97:529–45.
31. Barnett A, Cedar A, Siddiqui F, Herzig D, Fowlkes E, Thomas CR Jr. Colorectal cancer emergencies. J Gastrointest Cancer. 2013 Jun;44(4):132–42.
32. Chang GJ, Kaiser AM, Mills S, Rafferty F, Buie WD. Practice parameters for the management of colon cancer. Dis Colon Rectum. 2012;55:831–43.
33. Liu HY, Liang XB, Li YP, Feng Y, Liu DB, Wang WD. Treatment of advanced rectal cancer after renal transplantation. World J Gastroenterol. 2011;17(15):2058–60.
34. Zittel TT, Mehl CFR, Reichmann U, Becker HD, Jehle EC. Treatment of advanced rectal cancer in a patient after combined pancreas–kidney transplantation. Langenbecks Arch Surg. 2004;389(1):6–10.
35. Fang W. Chemotherapy in patient with colon cancer after renal transplantation: a case report with literature review. Medicine (Baltimore). 2018;97(5):e9678.
36. Frago R, Ramirez E, Millan M, Kreisler E, del Valle E, Biondo S. Current management of acute malignant large bowel obstruction: a systematic review. Am J Surg. 2014;207(1):127–38.
37. Ansaloni L, et al. Guidelines in the management of obstructing cancer of the left colon: consensus conference of the World Society of Emergency Surgery (WSES) and Peritoneum and Surgery (PnS) Society. World J Emerg Surg. 2010;5:29.
38. Yeo ES. Perforated colorectal cancer: an important differential diagnosis in all presumed diverticular abscesses. Ann Acad Med Singap. 2011;40(8):375–8.
39. Abu-Hejleh T, Mezhir JJ, Goodheart MJ, Halfdanarson TR. Incidence and management of gastrointestinal perforation from bevacizumab in advanced cancers. Curr Oncol Rep. 2012;14(4):277–84.
40. Tavakkolizadeh A, Ashley S. Acute gastrointestinal hemorrhage. Sabiston textbook of surgery: the biological basis of modern surgical practice. Philadelphia: Elsevier; 2012.

18 Colorectal Cancer Surgical Emergencies in Patients with Inflammatory Bowel Disease

Niccolò Petrucciani, Nicola de'Angelis, Federica Gaiani, and Francesco Brunetti

18.1 Introduction

Inflammatory bowel diseases (IBDs) represent a well-known risk factor for the development of colorectal cancer. Screening programs are available for patients with IBDs to allow early detection of dysplastic and tumoral lesions and prompt treatments, in order to avoid potentially serious complications. However, non-observant patients or those with no previous diagnosis of IBD may present with complex clinical scenarios of complicated colorectal cancer on IBD, and may require emergency surgical treatment. The aim of this chapter is to discuss the incidence on colorectal cancer in IBDs patients, to examine the potential causes of emergency colorectal surgery in this setting, and to discuss treatment strategies in the light of the recent literature.

N. Petrucciani
Service of Digestive, Hepato-Pancreato-Biliary Surgery and Liver Transplantation, Henri Mondor Hospital, AP-HP, Creteil, France

University of Paris Est, UPEC, Creteil, France

N. de'Angelis · F. Brunetti (✉)
Service of Digestive, Hepato-Pancreato-Biliary Surgery and Liver Transplantation, Unit of Minimally Invasive and Robotic Surgery, Henri Mondor Hospital, AP-HP, Créteil, France

University of Paris Est, UPEC, Créteil, France
e-mail: francesco.brunetti@aphp.fr

F. Gaiani
Gastroenterology and Endoscopy Unit, University Hospital of Parma, University of Parma, Parma, Italy

N. de'Angelis et al. (eds.), *Emergency Surgical Management of Colorectal Cancer*, Hot Topics in Acute Care Surgery and Trauma,
https://doi.org/10.1007/978-3-030-06225-5_18

18.2 Colorectal Cancer and Inflammatory Bowel Diseases

Patients with IBDs have a higher risk of developing colorectal cancer (CRC) comparing to the general population [1]. IBDs are among the most important diseases increasing the risk of CRC, following familial adenomatous polyposis and hereditary nonpolyposis colorectal cancer syndrome [2].

18.2.1 Crohn's Disease and Colorectal Cancer

Concerning the risk of colorectal cancer in Crohn's disease, a meta-analysis of population-based data has pooled the results of six observational studies, reporting standardized incidence ratios for CRC ranging from 0.9 to 2.2. The pooled standardized incidence ratio for CRC in the meta-analysis was 1.9, significantly increased comparing to the general population. A pooled estimated standardized incidence ratio of 27.1 was found for the development of small bowel cancer [3].

Similar results were reported in the meta-analysis by Canavan et al., with a 2.5 (1.3–4.7) overall CRC relative risk in Crohn's disease, 4.5 (1.3–14.9) for patients with colonic disease, and 1.1 (0.8–1.5) in ileal disease [4]. A relative risk reduction over the past 30 years was reported. The relative risk of CRC following diagnosis of Crohn's disease was estimated at 2.9% (1.5–5.3%) at 10 years. Small bowel cancer relative risk in Crohn's disease was estimated at 33.2 (15.9–60.9), without reduction over the last 30 years [4].

Another meta-analysis published in 2011 by Laukotter et al. [5] included 20 clinical studies with a total of 40,547 patients. The incidence of colorectal cancer was 0.5/1000 person year duration (CI 0.3–0.6), with a risk increased by 2–3 comparing to age-matched standard population. Mean age at diagnosis of CRC was 51.5 years (20 years earlier than general population), with a mean duration of Crohn's disease of 18.3 years before diagnosis of CRC.

18.2.2 Ulcerative Colitis and Colorectal Cancer

In patients with ulcerative colitis (UC), a recent meta-analysis including eight population-based studies found that an average of 1.6% of patients with UC was diagnosed with CRC during the follow-up (mean follow-up duration = 14 years) [6]. A pooled standardized incidence ratio of 2.4 (95% CI, 2.1–2.7) was calculated. Among the risk factors for CRC, the male sex, the young age at UC diagnosis, and an extensive colitis were associated with increased standardized incidence ratio.

Other meta-analyses found contrasting results. Eaden et al. [7] raised concerns about the high risk of CRC associated to UC. They included 116 studies from several institutions in different geographic areas, analyzing the cumulative risk of CRC in UC patients. They found a cumulative risk of developing CRC that increases from 1.6% at 10 years to 8.3% at 20 years to 18.4% at 30 years after the diagnosis of UC [7].

An Australian study has reported a CRC cumulative incidence of 1% at 10 years, 3% at 20 years, and 7% at 30 years [8].

More recently, Castaño-Milla et al. [9] reported a meta-analysis of 81 studies including 181,923 patients. They reported a calculated incidence of CRC in patients with UC of 1.58 per 1000 patient years (CI 1.39–1.76). The extent of colitis and the decade of the disease were associated to a statistically significant increase of the risk of CRC. The incidence rate was higher (4.02/1000 py (95% CI = 2.74–5.31)) in studies that included only patients with extensive colitis, and 1.24/1000 py (95% CI = 1.01–1.47) in population-based studies. The incidence rate was 0.91/1000 py (95% CI = 0.61–1.2) in the first decade of disease, 4.07/1000 py (95% CI = 2.58–5.56) in the second, and 4.55/1000 py (95% CI = 2.64–6.46) in the third. Decreased incidence of CRC according to the time frame was also demonstrated, from 4.29/1000 py in the studies published in the 1950s to 1.21/1000 py in studies published in the last decade [9].

The results of this meta-analysis suggest a decrease in the risk of CRC in the last years, probably due to the implementation of surveillance strategies, the introduction of drugs that control inflammation more effectively, or the changing approach to maintenance therapy or colectomy.

Among the risk factors increasing the risk of CRC, also the extent of the colitis, the gender (relative risk higher in males), the severity of inflammation (histological activity of the disease), a family history of sporadic colorectal cancer, and coexistent primary sclerosing cholangitis are reported by the majority of authors, whereas the role of age at diagnosis is debated [10].

18.3 Prevention and Surveillance

Given the increased risk of CRC in IBD patients and that dysplastic changes in the colonic mucosa are associated with the possible development of CRC, endoscopic surveillance is recommended for prompt diagnosis and treatment. Endoscopic assessments are scheduled, along with revision of the patients' symptoms, medications, and laboratory test results and update of personal and family medical histories [11].

The Cochrane Collaboration analyzed the benefit of endoscopic surveillance in IBD, pooling the results of five observational studies (including 7199 patients) [12]. Three studies were pooled to assess the rate of cancer detected in the surveillance group compared to the non-surveillance group. The studies found a significantly higher rate of cancer detection in the non-surveillance group compared to the surveillance group. CRC was detected in 1.83% (53/2895) of patients in the surveillance group compared to 3.17% (135/4256) of patients in the non-surveillance group (OR 0.58, 95% CI 0.42–0.80; $p = 0.0009$). Four studies were pooled to assess the death rate associated with CRC in patients who underwent surveillance compared to patients who did not undergo surveillance. There was a significantly lower death rate associated with CRC in the surveillance group compared to the non-surveillance group. Eight percent (15/176) of patients in the surveillance group died from CRC compared to 22% (79/354) of patients in the non-surveillance group (OR 0.36, 95% CI 0.19–0.69, $p = 0.002$). Furthermore, a significantly higher rate of early stage CRC (Duke A & B) was detected in the surveillance group [12].

Surveillance programs permit in the majority of observant patients a precocious diagnosis, avoiding potential surgical complications of CRC in IBD. However, physicians should be aware of potential conditions due to CRC requiring emergency surgery in patients with IBD, including intestinal obstruction, lower gastrointestinal (GI) bleeding, or colonic perforation.

18.4 Indications for Emergency Surgery in CRC Associated to IBD

18.4.1 Crohn's Disease

Emergency surgery for Crohn's disease (CD) is required in approximately 6–16% of cases, regardless of the presence of an associated colorectal cancer (CRC) [13–16].

Among 972 patients with CD in the Sydney Inflammatory Bowel Disease cohort database, the overall risks of surgery within 5, 10, and 15 years of diagnosis were 31.7%, 43.3%, and 48.4%, with 6.7% of patients required emergency surgery within 5 years of diagnosis and 8.8% of patients required emergency surgery within 15 years [17]. The main indications for surgery were enteric stricture or obstruction, perianal disease, and intra-abdominal fistulas/abscess. Colorectal cancer was diagnosed in 11 patients (1.1%) in this cohort [17].

Colorectal cancer complicating CD and requiring emergency surgery is a rare condition, which however should not be neglected in order to avoid potentially serious consequences. It should be kept in mind that chronic colic strictures may be not easily accessible for biopsies (patients with long strictures with the proximal part not accessible for biopsies, which may hide a colic cancer) and may impede the endoscopic exploration of the proximal colon. Furthermore, imaging modalities such as CT or MR enterography have high accuracy (sensitivity 89% and specificity 99% for CT, sensitivity 89% and specificity 99% for MRI) for detection of strictures but are not able to differentiate fibrotic and inflammatory lesions from tumoral strictures [18].

18.4.2 Ulcerative Colitis

Emergency surgery for ulcerative colitis (UC) is required in case of several conditions: medical intractability of severe colitis, bleeding, perforation, obstruction, or megacolon. CRC on UC may be responsible of bleeding, perforation, or colonic obstruction, mainly if diagnosed at late stage in non-observant patients [19, 20].

Data of the American College of Surgeons National Surgical Quality Improvement Program database demonstrated that emergency colectomy represents approximately 6% of all colectomies for UC [21].

Comparison of patients undergoing elective versus emergency surgery for UC showed higher rate of pulmonary, cardiac, and renal comorbidities and more advanced age in patients undergoing emergency procedures. Open total abdominal without proctectomy with ileostomy was the most frequent procedure in the emergency setting. Postoperative complications, including surgical site infection, and respiratory, renal, cardiac, hematologic, and infectious complications, were more frequent in the emergency setting, such as reoperation and 30-day mortality (13% vs. 1% in elective procedures). No data were reported about CRC incidence in the two groups [21].

The main indication for emergency total colectomy in UC is toxic colitis, which occurs in about 10% of patients with UC [22]. Crohn's disease represents however 50% of cases of toxic colitis. Other causes of emergency surgery are intractable bleeding, which is often a sign of extensive colitis in UC (large areas of ulcerated mucosa), and perforation, which occurs approximately in 0–2% of patients with UC and is usually associated to toxic colitis. Strictures in UC are not common and should alert the physician toward a possible associated CRC. CRC may be occasionally a concomitant finding in case of toxic colitis or may be responsible of lower GI bleeding, perforation, or obstruction also in UC.

18.5 Causes of Emergency Colectomies for IBDs Complicated by CRC

The evaluation of patients with IBDs complicated by CRCs requiring emergency surgery is complex and requires a multidisciplinary approach [22]. Patients' evaluation includes assessment of severity of IBD, nutritional status, cancer staging, immunosuppressive drugs management, and previous history. Unfortunately, in emergency setting information may be incomplete, and the decision of emergency surgery and the strategy may be very difficult. Furthermore, not all centers and surgeons have specific expertise on IBD management or availability of a multidisciplinary team. Given the rarity of CRC on IBD presenting in emergency setting, large series are lacking, and the majority of recommendations are based on experts' opinions. A flowchart listing the objectives of the treatment in the emergency setting, the variables to be taken into account, and the possible treatment is proposed in Fig. 18.1.

Actually, the emergency treatment of complications of CRC on IBD has three main objectives: treatment of the emergency condition, which may impact short-term prognosis, treatment of CRC, and management of IBD.

After adequate patient stabilization, the first step of the management of patients presenting in emergency setting includes careful anamnesis and clinical

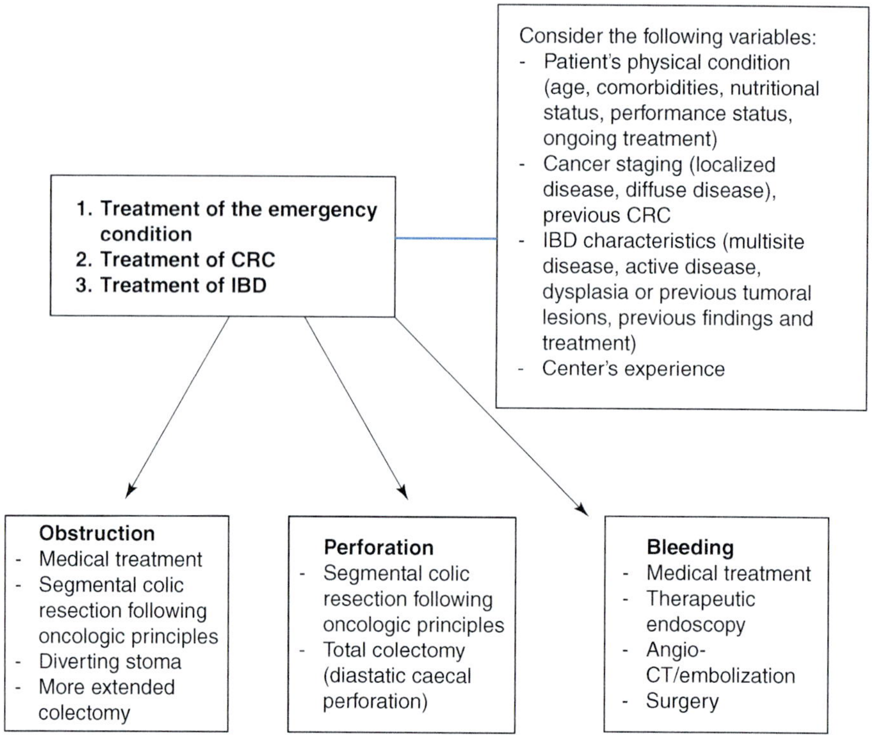

Fig. 18.1 Treatment of the surgical complications of CRC on IBD

examination. Blood tests are performed to detect inflammatory syndrome, anemia, electrolytes abnormalities, nutritional status, and hemostasis disorders. Tumor markers (CEA, CA 19.9) may be dosed if diagnosis of CRC is highly suspected. In the emergency setting, CT scan with contrast enhancement represents the most used imaging modality to identify possible complications of CRC on IBD requiring emergency surgery, including intestinal obstruction, perforation, or gastrointestinal (GI) bleeding. Endoscopic examinations may be contraindicated in emergency setting but may be performed in patients without suspected perforation or no risk of perforation or in a second time in patients responding to medical treatment.

Complete cancer staging should be performed whenever possible, including endoscopic examinations with biopsies, thoracic and abdominal CT scan, tumor markers dosage, eventually echoendoscopy, and pelvic or hepatic MRI. The IBD characteristics and history (type of IBD, extension of the disease, previous therapies) are also crucial to guide further treatments. Ideally, each patient should be discussed in a multidisciplinary meeting to define the best strategy, which is not always possible in the emergency setting.

The complications that may necessitate an emergency surgical treatment include bowel obstruction, colic perforation, or bleeding.

18.5.1 Colic Obstruction

Acute intestinal obstruction is more frequent in CD than in UC, and it is usually due to the presence of an inflamed or fibrotic intestinal segment, whereas the occurrence of cancer on the stenotic segment or the presence of an obstructing neoplasm at diagnosis is less frequent. Obstructive symptoms from colonic strictures occur in up to 17% of patients with CD, and the presence of carcinoma has been reported in approximately 7% of these cases. Advanced age, longer duration of the disease (3.3% if disease duration <20 years versus 11% if >20 years), and short strictures represent risk factors for malignant strictures [23]. In UC, the presence of stricture is highly suspect for CRC.

Symptoms of bowel obstruction include nausea, vomiting, distended abdomen, and the absence of gas or stool passage. Inflammatory syndrome and electrolyte disorders may be detected at blood tests. CT scan allows precise identification of the colic stenosis and of potential complications requiring emergency surgery (colic ischemia, colic perforation). In the absence of surgical complications, initial medical management consists in bowel rest, intravenous hydration, nasogastric decompression, and intravenous steroids or other anti-inflammatory drugs protocols in case of active inflammatory disease causing the obstruction. Response to medical treatment may allow tumor staging and accurate IBD evaluation. Multidisciplinary discussion is advisable to choose the best management.

The presence of an obstructive colorectal cancer on IBD represents an indication for surgery, with a variable degree of emergency. Several surgical options are possible, and the choice is made on a case-by-case basis, after careful evaluation of the variables listed in Fig. 18.1. In Figs. 18.2, 18.3, and 18.4, endoscopic aspect of an obstructing left-sided colic cancer in a patient affected by UC, not compliant to follow-up, is shown. Proximal colostomy can resolve the obstruction, prevent ischemia or perforation of the proximal colon, and allow complete exploration for tumor staging and IBD evaluation in the next days. Segmental colectomy, following oncologic principles, is a possible option, able to resolve the obstruction and treat the CRC, even in case of IBD. In emergency setting, often information about previous treatment and extension of the disease lack, and it is reasonable to avoid extensive resection, which may be not justified.

In case of symptomatic left-sided colonic obstruction in patients with an increased risk of postoperative mortality (age ≥70 years and/or ASA status ≥3), the possibility of endoscopic colonic stenting as a bridge to elective surgery should be evaluated [24].

In case of obstructive CRC, with associated colic ischemia or proximal colic perforation complicating the obstruction, more extensive colectomy until total colectomy is indicated, to remove the ischemic or perforated colon. Colectomy following the principles of oncologic colorectal surgery is recommended to obtain adequate tumor clearance and staging, regarding the colic segment affected by the tumor [25].

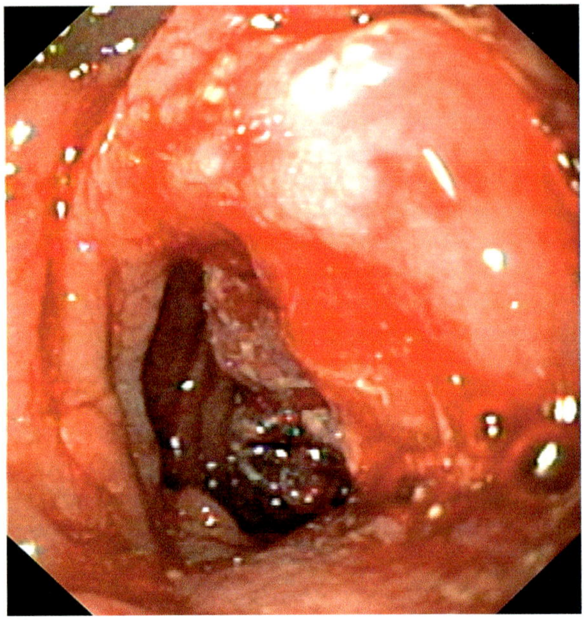

Fig. 18.2 Endoscopic aspect of an obstructing left-sided colic cancer in a patient affected by UC, not compliant to follow-up

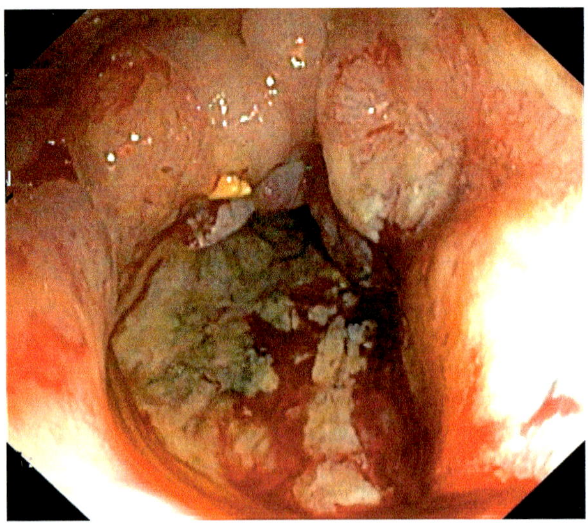

Fig. 18.3 Endoscopic aspect of an obstructing left-sided colic cancer in a patient affected by UC, not compliant to follow-up

18.5.2 Colonic Perforation

Free perforation of the small or large bowel represents a cause of emergency surgery in 1–16% of cases of CD [26, 27]. In UC, perforation is associated to toxic colitis or megacolon in the majority of cases and occurs in 0–2% of cases.

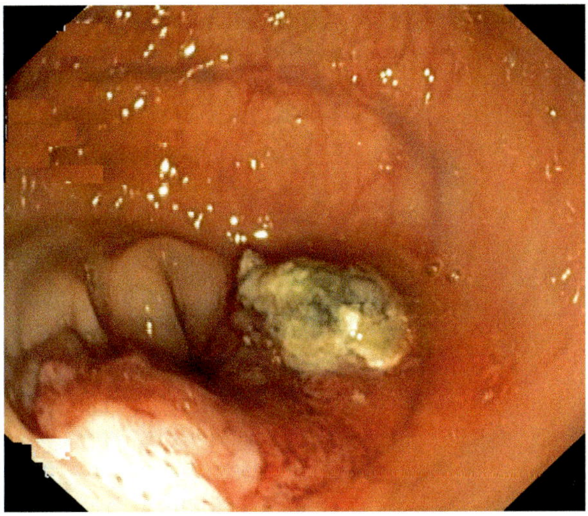

Fig. 18.4 Endoscopic aspect of an obstructing left-sided colic cancer in a patient affected by UC, not compliant to follow-up

The presence of an obstructive cancer with associated perforation or a perforated cancer is a rare but possible clinical condition in both diseases [28, 29].

Symptoms and signs are the same of colonic perforation for other etiologies, including abdominal pain, fever, and inflammatory biologic syndrome, CT scan showing pneumoperitoneum, abscess, or abdominal fluid. The treatment consists in colic resection following the principles of oncologic surgery, usually without intestinal continuity restoration due to a high risk of postoperative leakage [30]. In case of a cecal diastasic perforation complicating left-sided CRC, more extended colectomy is indicated to remove the perforated cecum.

18.5.3 Hemorrhage

Acute lower GI hemorrhage occurs in 0.9–6% of patients and represents rare complications of CD [31, 32]. Usually it is due to severe inflammation and blood vessels ulceration. In UC, bleeding is usually associated to extensive colitis. Initial management of hemorrhage in IBD patients includes resuscitation and patients' stabilization. CT angiography has sensitivity rates for acute GI bleeding up to 89% with specificity up to 92% and allows diagnosis of a concomitant CRC, which is a rare possibility. At CT, a contrast blush may be detected indicating the site of bleeding. Interventional radiology or endoscopy may be performed with diagnostic and therapeutic purpose. Surgical treatment is required only if the bleeding is life threatening, with persistent hemodynamic instability, and consists in segmental colic resection or more extended surgery depending on the site and origin of bleeding.

18.6 Emergency Surgical Treatment of CRC on IBD: Specific Considerations

The presence of CRC on IBD represents a particularly challenging scenario, even more if the patient requires an emergency management. Ideally, a complete oncologic evaluation should be performed, including a complete patients' evaluation (comorbidities, previous medical and surgical treatments, performance status, nutritional status), tumor markers' dosage, thoracoabdominal CT scan, and endoscopic evaluation with the aim to assess the characteristics of the tumor, to obtain diagnostic biopsies, and to explore the entire colon and ileon. Multidisciplinary evaluation including surgeons, gastroenterologists, and oncologists is recommended. Specific problems of colectomy for CRC on IBD include the extent of the resection, the timing of surgery, the strategy to treat the CRC, and the underlying disease in order to guarantee the better prognosis and quality of life after surgery.

Actually, the extent of the resection in case of CRC complicating CD is a matter of debate: surgical resection should follow the well-known principles of colorectal surgical oncology, including appropriate lymphadenectomy for colon cancer and total mesorectal excision for rectal cancer. Some authors support segmental bowel resection in case of CRC on CD, whereas others have advocated total colectomy with or without proctectomy, based on the possibility of developing metachronous large bowel malignancies, in 14–40% of patients [33–35].

Maser et al. reviewed data about 64 patients treated for CD and colon cancer who underwent segmental resection or subtotal colectomy [34]. Twenty-five of them had at least one metachronous cancer (39%) during follow-up, with a mean time to diagnosis of 6.8 years. Nineteen of the 47 patients (40%) who had a segmental resection for colon cancer developed metachronous cancer, and 6/17 patients (35%) with subtotal colectomy had metachronous cancer, with no significant difference ($p = 0.61$) between recurrence rates in patients with segmental resection versus subtotal colectomy.

Other authors advocate preservation of the rectum followed by endoscopic surveillance basing on a meta-analysis showing that the risk of rectal cancer is not increased [36].

In case of emergency surgery for colonic perforation or obstruction due to CRC on CD, segmental colectomy or subtotal colectomy, without restoration of the intestinal continuity, represents the most prudent option. Multidisciplinary evaluation including patients' characteristics, disease's features, and treatment history is recommended to choose the most adapted procedure case by case [37].

In general, a conservative approach should be chosen if possible in the emergency setting, when complete data about the IBD are lacking, to treat the emergency condition and the CRC (segmental colectomy following oncologic principles). In Crohn's disease, the presence of multi-segmental disease and of perineal disease need to be ruled out because they may change the surgical treatment in favor of more extended resection in the first case or contraindicate the realization of ileoanal pouch after proctocolectomy in the second case [38].

For UC in the emergency setting, total or subtotal colectomy with end ileostomy represents the most frequent and safe option in case of acute colitis. The goal of surgery in the acute setting is to remove the affected bowel, to restore the patient's global clinical conditions, and to preserve the possibility of reconstructive options. For the distal colic or rectal stump, Hartmann closure and creation of a mucous fistula both represent safe and effective options. Completion coloproctectomy and ileoanal anastomosis may be performed in a second time to remove the remaining disease and restore intestinal continuity, if diagnosis of UC is confirmed by histological examination [39]. Three steps procedure includes subtotal colectomy, followed by completion coloproctectomy, coloanal anastomosis, and lateral ileostomy (second step), followed by ileostomy closure after radiological control of the anastomosis (third step).

Total proctocolectomy has been almost abandoned in the setting of emergency surgery for UC for the higher risk of morbidity and mortality compared to total colectomy. Actually, an increased risk of postoperative hemorrhage, pelvic sepsis, pelvic nerve damage, and small bowel obstruction has been associated to total proctocolectomy [22].

In case of CRC complicating UC, if possible, a complete evaluation of patient's clinical conditions and of the IBD, as well as the CRC staging, should be performed. If no surgical complications (colic perforation or occlusion with ischemia) are present, a medical management may be started until complete evaluation and multidisciplinary discussion. For colic cancer discovered during acute colitis or in case of other complications requiring emergency surgery (colic perforation), emergency total colectomy with ileostomy represents a safe treatment option. Segmental colectomy is a possible option for CRC complicating UC in the emergency setting (e.g., obstructive CRC): this strategy has the advantages of a less demanding procedure, focused on the treatment of CRC and its complication, with less morbidity and faster recovery, which is particularly important in case additional oncologic treatments are needed. In these cases, decisions concerning the remaining colon may be delayed after patient recovery and postponed to CRC management. Colic resection should be performed following the oncologic principles of CRC surgery in the colic segment where the tumor is situated, to assure adequate lymphadenectomy and CRC clearance. For left-sided distal colic tumors, Hartmann closure of the rectal stump is the preferred option to have a clear distal margin. Diverting colostomy is also possible, for obstructive lesions, as a strategy allowing resolution of the obstruction, complete staging, and surgical treatment in the following days.

For patients with rectal cancer complicating UC and requiring emergency management, several considerations should be done: (1) optimal treatment of nonmetastatic rectal cancer includes complete local staging and rectal resection with total mesorectal excision, with preoperative neoadjuvant therapy in case of T3–4 or N+ tumors; (2) emergency proctectomy associated to total colectomy for acute UC has been associate to an increased risk of postoperative hemorrhage, pelvic sepsis, and pelvic nerve damage compared to not-emergency proctectomy [22]. In the light of these considerations, emergency proctectomy should be avoided, to limit morbidity and poor functional results (nerve damage) and to allow correct staging and management. If the rectal tumor causes obstruction, a diverting colostomy can relieve the obstruction and allows tumor and IBD staging and optimal treatment.

18.7 Role of Laparoscopy

Laparoscopic surgery has well-known advantages compared to open colorectal surgery, in reducing the postoperative morbidity and improving patients' recovery. In the setting of IBDs, laparoscopic surgery has been demonstrated to be safe and feasible and associated to lower rates of complications and length of stay compared to open surgery [40–42].

In the emergency setting, limited data have been published. However, laparoscopic surgery has been reported to be safe in experienced hands; even though generally laparoscopy has an increased operating time, it has demonstrated to allow a shorter hospital stay, while consequent morbidity has been shown to be similar or lower than open surgery in the different series [43].

The relevance of laparoscopic surgery is increasing also in the emergency surgical treatment of CRC [44, 45]. Recent data from the UK National Bowel Cancer Audit showed that the rate of laparoscopic surgery increased from 15.1% of cases to 30.2% in 2016 [44]. Predictive factors of the use of laparoscopy were ASA, T stage, N stage, age, socioeconomic status, hospital volume, and the presence of a dedicated colorectal emergency service. Laparoscopic patients had a shorter length of stay and lower 90-day mortality (8.1% vs. 13.0%) than patients undergoing open resection [44].

18.8 Prognosis

Several studies compared clinic-pathological characteristics of colorectal cancers arising on IBDs versus sporadic CRCs. Leowardi et al. [46] reported similar overall and disease-free survival for patients with CCR on UC versus those with sporadic cancers, even if the first group had more multifocal, high-grade, and mucinous carcinomas [46].

A Danish nationwide population-based study comparing 653 CRC on UC, 238 with CD with 107,024 CRC in patients without IBD showed younger age in IBD patients and an adjusted mortality at 5 years higher for patients with history of IBD comparing to those with sporadic CRC [47].

The analysis of the national Japanese database, including 169 CRCs associated to UC among a total population of 108,536 CRC patients, demonstrated that UC patients with CRC were younger and had more frequently multiple cancer lesions, superficial type lesions, and invasive type lesions and mucinous or signet ring cell carcinomas. Prognosis was poorer for stage III CRCs on UC compared to same stage sporadic CRCs, whereas no survival differences were found for stage I and II disease [48].

The recent meta-analysis by Reynolds et al. [49] included 20 studies with a total of 571,278 patients comparing data on outcome of CRC associated to IBD and sporadic CRC. Colorectal cancers associated with IBD were more frequently synchronous tumors (OR 4.403, 95% CI 2.320–8.359; $p < 0.001$), with poor differentiation (OR 1.875, 95% CI 1.425–2.466; $p < 0.001$); rate of rectal cancer was lower (OR 0.827, 95% CI 0.735–0.930; $p = 0.002$). No differences were retrieved in T stage, N stage, M status, sex, and 5-year survival.

18.9 Conclusions

Colorectal cancer surgical emergencies in patients with inflammatory bowel disease are rare, due to the diffusion of endoscopic screening programs for patients with IBDs. However, CRC may represent a potentially serious cause of emergency surgery in these patients in case of intestinal obstruction, perforation, or bleeding. Specific considerations should be kept in mind for the treatment of CRC on IBDs. The optimal management requires careful analysis of patient's characteristics and comorbidities, evaluation of both (IBD and CRC) diseases, and previous and actual pharmacological treatments, with the aim to choose the best treatment strategy. If possible, multidisciplinary discussion and experts' advice are recommended.

References

1. Huang LC, Merchea A. Dysplasia and cancer in inflammatory bowel disease. Surg Clin North Am. 2017;97:627–39.
2. Kim ER, Chang DK. Colorectal cancer in inflammatory bowel disease: the risk, pathogenesis, prevention and diagnosis. World J Gastroenterol. 2014;20:9872–81.
3. Jess T, Gamborg M, Matzen P, et al. Increased risk of intestinal cancer in Crohn's disease: a meta-analysis of population-based cohort studies. Am J Gastroenterol. 2005;100:2724–9.
4. Canavan C, Abrams KR, Mayberry J. Meta-analysis: colorectal and small bowel cancer risk in patients with Crohn's disease. Aliment Pharmacol Ther. 2006;23:1097–104.
5. Laukoetter MG, Mennigen R, Hannig CM, Osada N, Rijcken E, Vowinkel T, Krieglstein CF, Senninger N, Anthoni C, Bruewer M. Intestinal cancer risk in Crohn's disease: a meta-analysis. J Gastrointest Surg. 2011;15:576–83.
6. Jess T, Rungoe C, Peyrin-Biroulet L. Risk of colorectal cancer in patients with ulcerative colitis: a meta-analysis of population-based cohort studies. Clin Gastroenterol Hepatol. 2012;10:639–45.
7. Eaden JA, Abrams KR, Mayberry JF. The risk of colorectal cancer in ulcerative colitis: a meta-analysis. Gut. 2001;48:526–35.
8. Selinger CP, Andrews JM, Titman A, et al., Sydney IBD Cohort Study Group. Long-term follow-up reveals low incidence of colorectal cancer, but frequent need for resection, among Australian patients with inflammatory bowel disease. Clin Gastroenterol Hepatol. 2014;12:644–50.
9. Castaño-Milla C, Chaparro M, Gisbert JP. Systematic review with meta-analysis: the declining risk of colorectal cancer in ulcerative colitis. Aliment Pharmacol Ther. 2014;39:645–59.
10. Dyson JK, Rutter MD. Colorectal cancer in inflammatory bowel disease: what is the real magnitude of the risk? World J Gastroenterol. 2012;18:3839–48.

11. ECCO Guidelines. Inflammatory bowel disease. https://www.ecco-ibd.eu/publications/ecco-guidelines-science/published-ecco-guidelines.html. Accessed 25 Apr 2018.
12. Bye WA, Nguyen TM, Parker CE, Jairath V, East JE. Strategies for detecting colon cancer in patients with inflammatory bowel disease. Cochrane Database Syst Rev 2017;9:CD000279. doi: https://doi.org/10.1002/14651858.CD000279.pub4.
13. Annese V, Daperno M, Rutter MD, et al., European Crohn's and Colitis Organisation. European evidence-based consensus for endoscopy in inflammatory bowel disease. J Crohns Colitis. 2013;7:982–1018.
14. Magro F, Langner C, Driessen A, et al., European Society of Pathology [ESP]; European Crohn's and Colitis Organisation [ECCO]. European consensus on the histopathology of inflammatory bowel disease. J Crohns Colitis. 2013;7:827–51.
15. Smida M, Miloudi N, Hefaiedh R, Zaibi R. Emergency surgery for Crohn's disease. Tunis Med. 2016;94(3):210–5.
16. Kosmidis C, Anthimidis G. Emergency and elective surgery for small bowel Crohn's disease. Tech Coloproctol. 2011;15(Suppl 1):S1–4.
17. Toh JWT, Wang N, Young CJ, Rickard MJFX, Keshava A, Stewart P, Kariyawasam V, Leong R, the Sydney IBD Cohort Collaborators. Major abdominal and perianal surgery in Crohn's disease: long-term follow-up of Australian patients with Crohn's disease. Dis Colon Rectum. 2018;61:67–76.
18. Chan WPW, Mourad F, Leong RW. Crohn's disease associated strictures. J Gastroenterol Hepatol. 2018;33:998–1008.
19. Kinugasa T, Akagi Y. Status of colitis-associated cancer in ulcerative colitis. World J Gastrointest Oncol. 2016;8:351–7.
20. Yashiro M. Ulcerative colitis-associated colorectal cancer. World J Gastroenterol. 2014;20:16389–97.
21. Patel SS, Patel MS, Goldfarb M, et al. Elective versus emergency surgery for ulcerative colitis: a National Surgical Quality Improvement Program analysis. Am J Surg. 2013;205:333–7.
22. Berg DF, Bahadursingh AM, Kaminski DL, Longo WE. Acute surgical emergencies in inflammatory bowel disease. Am J Surg. 2002;184:45–51.
23. Yamazaki Y, Ribeiro MB, Sachar DB, Aufses AH, Greenstein AJ. Malignant strictures in Crohn's disease. Am J Gastroenterol. 1991;86:882–5.
24. van Hooft JE, van Halsema EE, Vanbiervliet G, et al. Self-expandable metal stents for obstructing colonic and extracolonic cancer: European Society of Gastrointestinal Endoscopy (ESGE) clinical guideline. Gastrointest Endosc. 2014;80:747–61.e1–75.
25. Winner M, Mooney SJ, Hershman DL, et al. Management and outcomes of bowel obstruction in patients with stage IV colon cancer: a population-based cohort study. Dis Colon Rectum. 2013;56:834–43.
26. Werbin N, Haddad R, Greenberg R, Karin E, Skornick Y. Free perforation in Crohn's disease. Isr Med Assoc J. 2003;5:175–7.
27. Roy MK, Delicata RJ, Carey PD. Crohn's disease presenting with acute colonic perforation. Postgrad Med J. 1997;73:645–6.
28. Fraschini A, Sella D, Gullotta R, et al. Free perforation due to colonic adenocarcinoma in Crohn's disease. Ital J Surg Sci. 1989;19:85–8.
29. Greenstein AJ, Gennuso R, Sachar DB, Aufses AH Jr. Free perforation due to cancer in Crohn's disease. Int J Colorectal Dis. 1987;2:201–2.
30. Ikeuchi H, Yamamura T. Free perforation in Crohn's disease: review of the Japanese literature. J Gastroenterol. 2002;37:1020–7.
31. Kim KJ, Han BJ, Yang SK, et al. Risk factors and outcome of acute severe lower gastrointestinal bleeding in Crohn's disease. Dig Liver Dis. 2012;44:723–8.
32. Driver CP, Anderson DN, Keenan RA. Massive intestinal bleeding in association with Crohn's disease. J R Coll Surg Edinb. 1996;41:152–4.
33. Kiran RP, Nisar PJ, Goldblum JR. Dysplasia associated with Crohn's colitis: segmental colectomy or more extended resection? Ann Surg. 2012;256:221–6.

34. Maser EA, Sachar DB, Kruse D, Harpaz N, Ullman T, Bauer JJ. High rates of metachronous colon cancer or dysplasia after segmental resection or subtotal colectomy in Crohn's colitis. Inflamm Bowel Dis. 2013;19:1827–32.
35. Strong S, Steele SR, Boutrous M, et al. Clinical practice guideline for the surgical management of Crohn's disease. Dis Colon Rectum. 2015;58:1021–36.
36. von Roon AC, Reese G, Teare J, Constantinides V, Darzi AW, Tekkis PP. The risk of cancer in patients with Crohn's disease. Dis Colon Rectum. 2007;50:839–55.
37. Bellolio F, Cohen Z, Macrae HM, et al. Outcomes following surgery for perforating Crohn's disease. Br J Surg. 2013;100:1344–8.
38. Martin ST, Vogel JD. Restorative procedures in colonic Crohn disease. Clin Colon Rectal Surg. 2013;26:100–5.
39. Ross H, Steele SR, Varma M, et al. Practice parameters for the surgical treatment of ulcerative colitis. Dis Colon Rectum. 2014;57:5–22.
40. Maggiori L, Khayat A, Treton X, Bouhnik Y, Vicaut E, Panis Y. Laparoscopic approach for inflammatory bowel disease is a real alternative to open surgery: an experience with 574 consecutive patients. Ann Surg. 2014;260:305–10.
41. Dasari BV, McKay D, Gardiner K, et al. Laparoscopic versus Open surgery for small bowel Crohn's disease. Cochrane Database Syst Rev. 2011;(1):CD006956.
42. Wu XJ, He XS, Zhou XY, Ke J, Lan P. The role of laparoscopic surgery for ulcerative colitis: systematic review with meta-analysis. Int J Colorectal Dis. 2010;25:949–57.
43. Chand M, Siddiqui MR, Gupta A, et al. Systematic review of emergent laparoscopic colorectal surgery for benign and malignant disease. World J Gastroenterol. 2014;20:16956–63.
44. Vallance AE, Keller DS, Hill J, et al. Role of emergency laparoscopic colectomy for colorectal cancer: a population-based study in England. Ann Surg. 2018. https://doi.org/10.1097/SLA.0000000000002752
45. Holder-Murray J, Marsicovetere P, Holubar SD. Minimally invasive surgery for inflammatory bowel disease. Inflamm Bowel Dis. 2015;21:1443–58.
46. Leowardi C, Schneider ML, Hinz U, et al. Prognosis of ulcerative colitis-associated colorectal carcinoma compared to sporadic colorectal carcinoma: a matched pair analysis. Ann Surg Oncol. 2016;23:870–6.
47. Ording AG, Horváth-Puhó E, Erichsen R, et al. Five-year mortality in colorectal cancer patients with ulcerative colitis or Crohn's disease: a nationwide population-based cohort study. Inflamm Bowel Dis. 2013;19:800–5.
48. Watanabe T, Konishi T, Kishimoto J, et al. Ulcerative colitis-associated colorectal cancer shows a poorer survival than sporadic colorectal cancer: a nationwide Japanese study. Inflamm Bowel Dis. 2011;17:802–8.
49. Reynolds IS, O'Toole A, Deasy J, McNamara DA, Burke JP. A meta-analysis of the clinicopathological characteristics and survival outcomes of inflammatory bowel disease associated colorectal cancer. Int J Colorectal Dis. 2017;32:443–51.

19 Emergency Surgical Management in Rectal Cancer Patients Following Radiotherapy

Hayim Gilshtein, Assaf Harbi, and Yoram Kluger

19.1 Introduction

Radiotherapy has become the mainstay of preoperative treatment in rectal cancer patients with locally advanced disease presenting as T3/T4 tumors with or without involved lymph nodes.

Radiotherapy is also practiced as an adjuvant setting and palliative care of non-resectable tumors. The widespread application of radiation brought into the awareness of the surgical community its ensuing toxic effects and potential complications both in the short and long run following treatment.

Herein we elaborate on the potential clinical situations that require the intervention of the surgeon.

19.2 Perforation

Rectal perforation as an adverse event of preoperative radiotherapy is an extremely rare event. Along with severe bleeding and obstruction, it usually occurs in the chronic phase and may manifest only months after therapy completion [1]. There are only few cases reported in the literature describing perforation as early complication during the course of the neoadjuvant therapy [2–5].

The mechanism of the radiotherapy-induced rectal perforations is believed to be secondary irreversible ischemia, fibrosis, and obliteration of small vessels which cause a massive inflammatory reaction and tissue necrosis [6].

There is a general agreement about the relation between the dose of radiation and radiation-induced gastrointestinal injuries. A total dose of 45–50 GY delivered to the

H. Gilshtein · A. Harbi · Y. Kluger (✉)
Department of General Surgery, Rambam Health Care Campus, Haifa, Israel
e-mail: y_kluger@rambam.health.gov.il

N. de'Angelis et al. (eds.), *Emergency Surgical Management of Colorectal Cancer*, Hot Topics in Acute Care Surgery and Trauma,
https://doi.org/10.1007/978-3-030-06225-5_19

pelvis generally causes very few early and late complications. However, treatment with escalated doses up to 70 GY increases significantly the risk of rectal perforations [1, 7].

Several potential risk factors for radiotherapy-induced rectal perforations were proposed: diverticular disease, collagen accumulation, and tumor ulceration.

The biological behavior of the tumor may have an impact on the occurrence of rectal perforations [2].

A pathological and immunohistochemical analysis demonstrated an association between tumor location, cell differentiation, and rectal perforation [8].

Short-course radiotherapy has been demonstrated to be less related with rectal perforations in comparison to long-course radiotherapy [9]; furthermore fractioned short-course radiotherapy (25 GY in five fractions) can reduce the incidence of rectal perforation [10].

It is obvious that both clinical presentation and management are depended on the site and magnitude of the perforation. Rectal perforations can manifest as an intraperitoneal perforation, extraperitoneal perforation, or as incomplete perforations. Perforations might occur into adjacent organs such as the urinary bladder, vagina, uterus, seminal vesicles, or the small bowel.

Management varies from observation with antibiotic treatment for incomplete and extraperitoneal perforations, drainage of organized fluid collections as demonstrated on CT, or surgical interventions.

In a setting of overt, intraperitoneal perforations, a diverting stoma is usually prudent. The resection of the tumor itself as a part of a Hartmann's procedure is advised for higher tumors in the hemodynamically stable patient and relatively straightforward dissection planes. Otherwise, especially in a setting of low-lying lesions, very rarely a more challenging operation as low anterior resection or abdominoperineal resections is undertaken. These surgeries must be under the supervision of an experienced colorectal surgeon.

The completion of the chemoradiotherapy course in the case it was ceased due to a perforation should be thoroughly discussed with the oncologists on an individual basis.

In some cases one need to consider a prophylactic diverting ostomy for impending perforation. There are some worrisome imaging features such as large tumor mass with an intraperitoneal component and an extension of the tumor through all intestinal layers with a contained perforation on presentation. The stoma of choice is usually a colostomy from the sigmoid or descending colon which can be undertaken laparoscopically. However, in large tumor masses with difficulty of mobilizing the colon, a diverting loop ileostomy is deemed appropriate.

19.3 Obstruction

Radiation proctitis is a disease with increasing prevalence.

The most frequent complication of high-dose pelvic irradiation is proctitis. There is a general consensus that the incidence of proctitis is directly proportional to the dose of radiation [11].

The incidence of postradiation proctitis is estimated to be 2–20% [12].

As mentioned before, doses lower than 45 GY are usually responsible for very few side effects, and doses above 75 GY are usually responsible for the side effects caused by a significant and long-standing injury to the tissues [7].

Radiation proctitis is usually divided into acute and chronic entities, considering the time of appearance of symptoms, and it has been accepted that 6 months is the period of distinction between the two forms of proctitis [13].

Large bowel obstruction is one of the most severe complications and usually appears in the chronic phase of the radiation proctitis [1].

The small bowel, mainly the ileum (enteritis), is the most frequently involved organ; however pelvic irradiation can cause rectum and sigma obstruction. The cause of the obstruction is edema and inflammation of the irradiated tissues [12] or occasionally due to tumor overgrowth during the radiation treatment.

The pathological features are usually nonspecific with inflammatory changes, fibrosis, obliterative vasculitis, edema, ischemic changes, and narrowing of the bowel wall [14].

The presentation of complete bowel obstruction is usually precipitated by a gradual onset of symptoms which include difficulty with bowel movements with laxative use, abdominal distention, persistent colicky abdominal pain, and dehydration with electrolyte abnormalities. Sometimes symptoms are sudden in onset and require an emergent attention [15].

The current availability of CT scan in the emergency departments, the high sensitivity (96%), and the high specificity (93%) mostly with the use of a triple-contrast protocol (oral-rectal and IV) made this technique the imaging modality of choice for the diagnosis of colonic obstruction [16].

Enema with a hydrosoluble contrast is also a valuable imaging technique, although it is now less commonly implemented in the everyday practice.

Colonoscopy is usually less pertinent in the emergency setting. When it is performed, mostly short colonoscopy can identify and localize the obstruction site as well as to perform biopsy to confirm the diagnosis. A simple rectoscopy is performed by the surgeon in prudent.

There are several options available to the surgeon facing the emergency of rectal obstruction, and there remains a wide controversy on the optimal management. It is important that the approach will be individually tailored for each patient with bearing in mind available resources and surgeon expertise.

19.3.1 Loop Colostomy

This surgical option can be facilitated in patients who cannot endure a resectional procedure, in those patients in which we prefer to proceed with the neoadjuvant chemoradiotherapy or in patients with locally advanced tumors that either preclude resection or make it too demanding.

19.3.2 Hartmann's Procedure

A fashioning of an end colostomy with resection of the obstructive site and closing the distal rectum is commonly performed procedure for distal obstruction. In the current literature, there are no differences in short- or long-term outcomes in these patients compared to patients undergoing only diverting colostomy [17].

19.3.3 Endoscopic Stent Insertion

Self-expandable metal stents are a non-operative option to treat a colonic obstruction. It is an alternative in those situations in which it is necessary to stabilize the patient or complete the oncologic staging and neoadjuvant therapy. Stent is more useful as a "bridge to surgery," and their placement is considered in the sigmoid colon or upper rectum [18]. More distant location of the stent is problematic due to both migration tendency and the patient intolerance.

19.4 Bleeding

Rectal bleeding is fairly common in the overall presentation of patients with rectal cancer, more so in the advanced stages of the disease.

In the majority of cases, the hemorrhage is self-limited, rarely requiring further workup or intervention. Radiation proctitis varies in its clinical presentation and is defined as acute or chronic, depending on the timing of symptom development [19].

The diagnosis of chronic proctitis is established when symptom last more than 3 months. Diarrhea, urgency, and abdominal pain are more common in the acute setting, while bleeding is mostly considered a later complication with accumulative risk and progression over time.

However, infrequently an acute presentation might occur. With the administration of radiotherapy, the tissue becomes friable, and the tendency toward bleeding is increased.

Several studies have demonstrated that complex and novel delivery methods of radiotherapy such as intensity-modulated radiation therapy (IMRT) might reduce the gastrointestinal side effect rate [20, 21]. The bleeding site of origin might be the tumor itself or its surrounding tissue. Most of the hemorrhagic episodes are self-limited with occasional need for blood products infusions. Rarely an active intervention is indicated.

The management approach is stepwise with medical therapy as the first line of treatment and endoscopic or surgical interventions usually reserved for failures or profound bleeding.

There are several medical therapies with reported effectiveness. Formalin instillation [22] and various enemas such as 5-ASA and antioxidants [23] are some of the described medications. When these fail and for more severe rectal bleeding, endoscopic procedures are warranted.

Endoscopic interventions consist of several optional modalities. Coagulation with electrocautery has reported success rates of 70–75%. Argon beam ablation has similar efficiency with a somewhat better safety profile [24]. Laser application is not commonly available with reported success of 66% in small series [25]. Radiofrequency ablation could be considered for chronic cases [26].

In patients suffering from massive rectal bleeding with preserved hemodynamics, computerized angiographic tomography followed by selective embolization of visible arterial blush was described [27]. However, the rich vascular supply of the rectum with additional angiogenesis caused by the tumor impedes these maneuvers in many instances.

Surgery is preserved for the most part for those patients who fail the previously described methods of action and those becoming hemodynamically unstable. The decision of what kind of surgical procedure to undertake is challenging. The surgical procedure performed can be also planned in a mounting manner. At first, in low-lying malignancies, local compression techniques with surgical pads or gauzes with addition of an antifibrinolytic agent such as tranexamic acid may be beneficial. If this proves unsuccessful, a more extensive surgery is needed. There have been reports of proximal diversion of feces via an ostomy with resultant bleeding control [28].

The anatomic access to the rectum is challenging, especially in the acute setting and irradiated tissues. In the operating theater, the surgeon might try to better visualize the area of bleeding with available retractors or sometimes transanal platforms such as transanal endoscopic microsurgery (TEM) or transanal minimally invasive surgery (TAMIS). With this achieved local pressure, packing, sewing, or application of various hemostatic materials such as Surgicel, Surgiflo, and others is advised. Local resections with flap reconstruction were considered in the past with unacceptable morbidity rates for refractory cases of chronic proctitis [29].

In the very uncommon cases of massive bleeding and failure of achieving hemostasis, a resection needs to be performed as the last resort. The choice of the surgical approach is dictated by the tumor location. For upper and middle rectal lesions, the abdominal approach is usually sufficient, while in the lower rectum, an addition of perineal dissection is needed. With completion of resection, an ostomy is created with refraining from a primary anastomosis in these extreme scenarios. Proctectomy and even pelvic exenteration though rarely described carry a high mortality and morbidity rates [30].

All the described surgical interventions need to be led by an experienced colorectal surgeon who is well familiar with the regional anatomy.

When facing with these patients and expert assistance or guidance is not available, transfer of the patient is prudent as long as the patients' hemodynamic status permits.

19.5 Conclusions

There is a relative paucity of data addressing the important issue of complications following radiotherapy in rectal cancer patients, in the acute setting with the need of emergent surgical attention.

Due to the ever-growing population that is undergoing radiotherapy, one needs to bear in mind its potential deleterious effects. Bleeding, perforation, and obstruction during or after completion of therapy might be life-threatening and requires a prompt intervention by the knowledgeable physician, a surgeon in particular. It is possible but yet to be further investigated and determined that novel methods of administering radiation such as IMRT might reduce the rate of complications and provide a safer course for the patients. The medical and surgical communities need to address this important issue in designing large good-quality studies in order to have evidence-based treatment algorithms.

References

1. Do NL, Nagle D, Poylin VY. Radiation proctitis: current strategies in management. Gastroenterol Res Pract. 2011;2011:917941.
2. Khan A, Suhaibani YA, Sharief AA. Rectal cancer perforation: a rare complication of neoadjuvant radiotherapy for rectal cancer. Internet J Oncol. 2009;7:1–2.
3. Lee J, Chen F, Steel M, Keck J, Mackay J. Perforated rectal cancer associated with neoadjuvant radiotherapy: report of four cases. Dis Colon Rectum. 2006;49:1629–32.
4. ElGendy K. Rectal perforation after neoadjuvant chemoradiotherapy for low-lying rectal cancer. BMJ Case Rep. 2015. https://doi.org/10.1136/bcr-2014-207105.
5. Takase N, et al. Local advanced rectal cancer perforation in the midst of preoperative chemoradiotherapy: a case report and literature review. World J Clin Cases. 2017;5(1):18–23.
6. Clarke RE, et al. Hyperbaric oxygen treatment of chronic refractory radiation proctitis: a randomized and controlled double-blind crossover trial with long-term follow-up. Int J Radiat Oncol Biol Phys. 2008;72(1):134–43.
7. Coia LR, Myerson RJ, Tepper JE. Late effects of radiation therapy on the gastrointestinal tract. Int J Radiat Oncol Biol Phys. 1995;31(5):1213–36.
8. Medina-Arana V, et al. Clinicopathological analysis of factors related to colorectal tumor perforation: influence of angiogenesis. Medicine (Baltimore). 2015;94(15):e703.
9. Bujko K, et al. Long-term results of a randomized trial comparing preoperative short-course radiotherapy with preoperative conventionally fractionated chemoradiation for rectal cancer. Br J Surg. 2006;93(10):1215–23.
10. Bujko K, Bujko M. Point: short-course radiation therapy preferable in the neoadjuvant treatment of rectal cancer. Semin Radiat Oncol. 2011;21(3):220–7. https://doi.org/10.1016/j.semradonc.2011.02.008. Review.
11. Di Staso M, et al. Late morbidity and oncological outcome after radical hypofractionated radiotherapy in men with prostate cancer. BJU Int. 2010;106(10):1458–62.
12. Tagkalidis PP, Tjandra JJ. Chronic radiation proctitis. ANZ J Surg. 2001;71(4):230–7.
13. Vanneste BG, et al. Chronic radiation proctitis: tricks to prevent and treat. Int J Colorectal Dis. 2015;30(10):1293–303.
14. Andreyev J. Gastrointestinal symptoms after pelvic radiotherapy: a new understanding to improve management of symptomatic patients. Lancet Oncol. 2007;8(11):1007–17.
15. Gordon PH. Malignant neoplasms of the colon. In: Gordon PH, Nivatvongs S, editors. Principles and practice of surgery for the colon, rectum and anus. 3rd ed. New York: Informa Healthcare; 2007. p. 534–5.
16. Frager D, et al. Prospective evaluation of colonic obstruction with computed tomography. Abdom Imaging. 1998;23(2):141–6.
17. Kronborg O. Acute obstruction from tumour in the left colon without spread. A randomized trial of emergency colostomy versus resection. Int J Colorectal Dis. 1995;10(1):1–5.

18. Baer C, et al. Emergency presentations of colorectal cancer. Surg Clin North Am. 2017;97(3):529–45.
19. Laterza L, Cecinato P, Guido A, Mussetto A, Fuccio L. Management of radiation-induced rectal bleeding. Curr Gastroenterol Rep. 2013;15:355.
20. Bazan JG, Hara W, Hsu A, Kunz PA, Ford J, Fisher GA, Welton ML, Shelton A, Kapp DS, Koong AC, Goodman KA, Chang DT. Intensity-modulated radiation therapy versus conventional radiation therapy for squamous cell carcinoma of the anal canal. Cancer. 2011;117:3342–51.
21. Staffurth J. A review of the clinical evidence for intensity-modulated radiotherapy. Clin Oncol (R Coll Radiol). 2010;22:643–57.
22. de Parades V, Etienney I, Bauer P, Bourguignon J, Meary N, Mory B, Sultan S, Taouk M, Thomas C, Atienza P. Formalin application in the treatment of chronic radiation-induced hemorrhagic proctitis—an effective but not risk-free procedure: a prospective study of 33 patients. Dis Colon Rectum. 2005;48:1535–41.
23. Feldmeier JJ, Jelen I, Davolt DA, Valente PT, Meltz ML, Alecu R. Hyperbaric oxygen as a prophylaxis for radiation-induced delayed enteropathy. Radiother Oncol. 1995;35:138–44.
24. Lenz L, Tafarel J, Correia L, Bonilha D, Santos M, Rodrigues R, Gomes G, Andrade G, Martins F, Monaghan M, Nakao F, Libera E, Ferrari AP, Rohr R. Comparative study of bipolar eletrocoagulation versus argon plasma coagulation for rectal bleeding due to chronic radiation coloproctopathy. Endoscopy. 2011;43:697–701.
25. Barbatzas C, Spencer GM, Thorpe SM, Sargeant LR, Bown SG. Nd:YAG laser treatment for bleeding from radiation proctitis. Endoscopy. 1996;28:497–500.
26. Rustagi T, Corbett FS, Mashimo H. Treatment of chronic radiation proctopathy with radiofrequency ablation (with video). Gastrointest Endosc. 2015;81:428–36.
27. Jacovides CL, Nadolski G, Allen SR, Martin ND, Holena DN, Reilly PM, Trerotola S, Braslow BM, Kaplan LJ, Pascual JL. Arteriography for lower gastrointestinal hemorrhage: role of preceding abdominal computed tomographic angiogram in diagnosis and localization. JAMA Surg. 2015;150(7):65.
28. Pricolo VE, Shellito PC. Surgery for radiation injury to the large intestine. Variables influencing outcome. Dis Colon Rectum. 1994;37:675–84.
29. Marks G, Mohiudden M. The surgical management of the radiation-injured intestine. Surg Clin North Am. 1983;63:81–96.
30. Turina M, Mulhall AM, Mahid SS, Yashar C, Galandiuk S. Frequency and surgical management of chronic complications related to pelvic radiation. Arch Surg. 2008;143:46–52.

Pathological Analyses of Colorectal Cancer

20

Gregoire Arnoux, Giulio Cesare Vitali, and Giacomo Puppa

20.1 Introduction

The pathological examination of colorectal cancer (CRC) specimens after surgery in an emergency setting follows the same rules as the elective one.

Essentially an accurate macroscopic analysis together with a careful microscopic examination allows both the assessment of the anatomic extent of disease (i.e., the tumor staging) and the identification of those non-anatomic, morphological factors affecting prognosis and further treatment [1, 2].

The long-term outcomes of colorectal cancers in an emergency setting are worse than their elective counterparts [3].

Thus the role of the pathologist is crucial to identify the factors accounting for such differences, in particular macroscopically the presence of perforation and occlusion and microscopically the anatomical staging factors and non-anatomical prognostic factors.

In this chapter all the staging and the morphological features, which characterize a CRC specimen resulting from an emergency procedure, are considered keeping as reference the more common resection performed electively.

G. Arnoux · G. Puppa (✉)
Service of Pathology, Geneva University Hospital and Medical School, Geneva, Switzerland
e-mail: giacomo.puppa@hcuge.ch

G. C. Vitali
Service of Abdominal Surgery and Liver Transplantation, Geneva University Hospital and Medical School, Geneva, Switzerland

N. de'Angelis et al. (eds.), *Emergency Surgical Management of Colorectal Cancer*, Hot Topics in Acute Care Surgery and Trauma,
https://doi.org/10.1007/978-3-030-06225-5_20

20.2 pT Category

In the current TNM eighth edition [4], the definitions of pT4a and pT4b are the same as in the seventh [5] where an inversion occurred in relation to the sixth edition. Therefore pT4a is applied when tumor invades through the visceral peritoneum, and pT4b is applied when the tumor directly invades or adheres to other adjacent organs or structures [6].

Compared with elective CRC cases, patients who had emergency surgery showed more deeply invading tumors with twice as much T4 occurrence [7, 8].

The median tumor size was significantly larger in the emergency surgery group compared with the screening colonoscopy group (5 cm vs. 3.0 cm, respectively) [9].

Moreover the emergency cases are more likely to have multiple tumors (OR = 2.816, $p = 0.001$), which is relevant [7].

20.3 Obstruction and Perforation

The left colon is more prone to obstruction, in particular the sigmoid. This is due to a greater tendency of annular lesions, a relatively narrow colonic luminal diameter (Fig. 20.1a, b), and a thicker stool consistency [3].

Because of the larger diameter of the cecum and ascending colon, right-sided obstructions are less common and thought to represent bulky tumors (Fig. 20.2a, b) of more advanced stage [3].

Perforations most commonly occur at the site of the primary tumor (Fig. 20.3a–c), due to a direct mechanism of local destruction [7] often associated to necrosis and friable tissue [3].

Depending on the location, these may progress to either free or contained perforations.

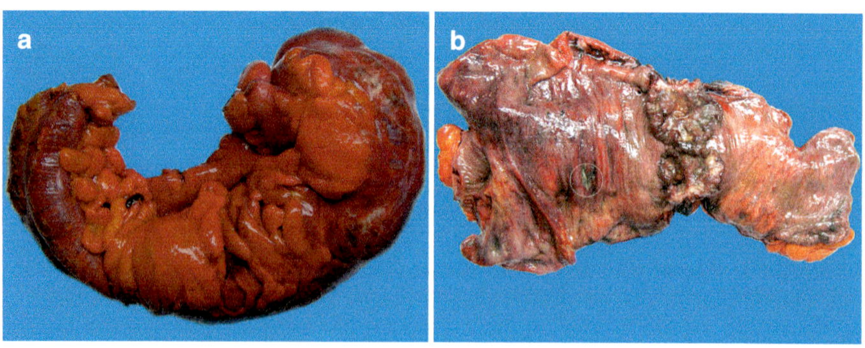

Fig. 20.1 (**a**) Left hemicolectomy with proximal dilatation (right half of the figure). (**b**) After opening an annular, centrally ulcerated neoplasm is evident accounting for the obstruction. The white circle indicates a focal ischemic necrosis

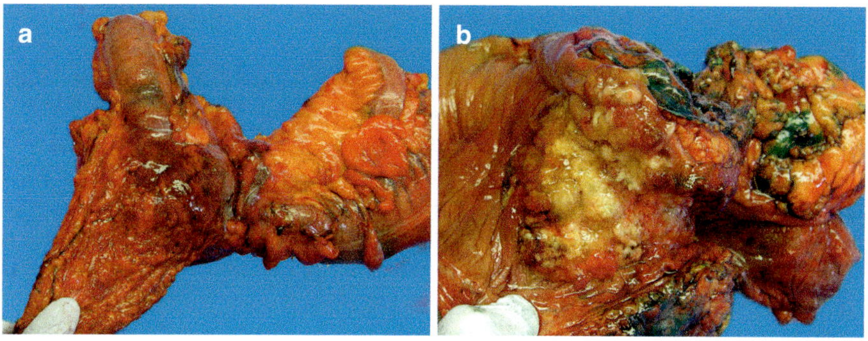

Fig. 20.2 (**a**) Right hemicolectomy extended to the colon transverse with a bulk at the flexure. (**b**) After opening a protruding tumoral mass is evident with some mucinous material evident at the surface corresponding at histology to a mucinous adenocarcinoma

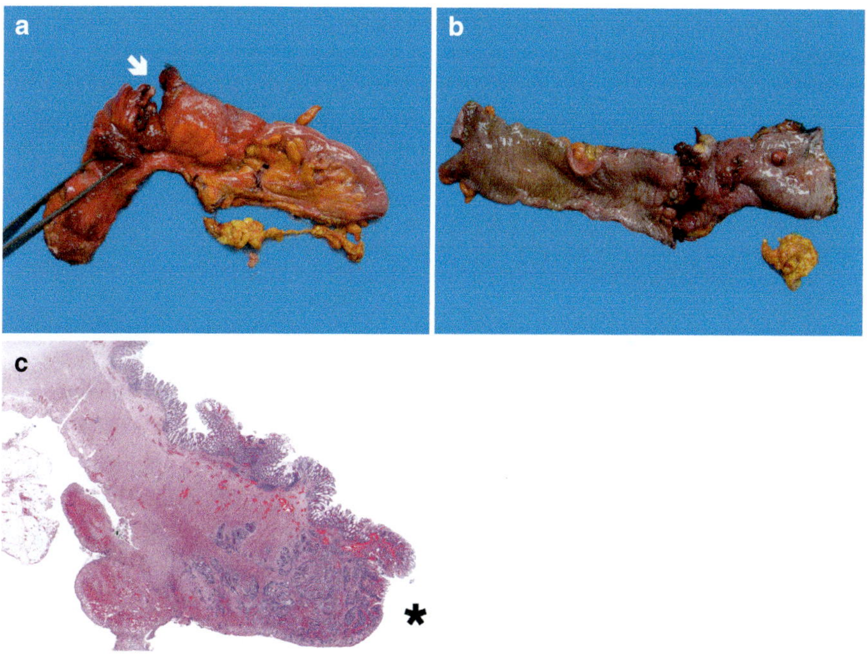

Fig. 20.3 (**a**) Left hemicolectomy showing a huge perforation (arrow) corresponding (**b**) to a circumferential neoplasm with intramural satellite metastases (right half of the specimen). (**c**) At histology at the perforation site (asterisk), there is evidence of an adenocarcinoma with full-thickness invasion and perforation of the wall

In about one-third of the cases of perforated colon, the perforation is located proximal to the cancer [7, 10].

Increasing pressure and distension from a complete distal obstruction follows the law of Laplace, which can ultimately result in ischemia of the proximal bowel (Fig. 20.1b, white circle) and perforations at remote proximal sites. The cecum is the most common site of this type of diastatic perforation [3]. A free perforation allows seeding into the peritoneal cavity resulting in poor survival [3].

Contained perforation corresponds to a peri-tumoral phlegmon or abscess (Fig. 20.4a–d), which is more common than free perforation in descending and sigmoid colon lesions [3].

Several tumor blocks from the suspect zone of perforation (Fig. 20.4a, b) should be taken (Fig. 20.4c) to assess if tumor cells are present at the peritoneum (making T4a category) or not (corresponding to T3 category, Fig. 20.4d).

In case of suspect of perforation or invasion of adjacent structures, a suture thread should be placed in the surgical theater in order to facilitate the pathologist to identify these zones (Fig. 20.4b) and allow a targeted sampling.

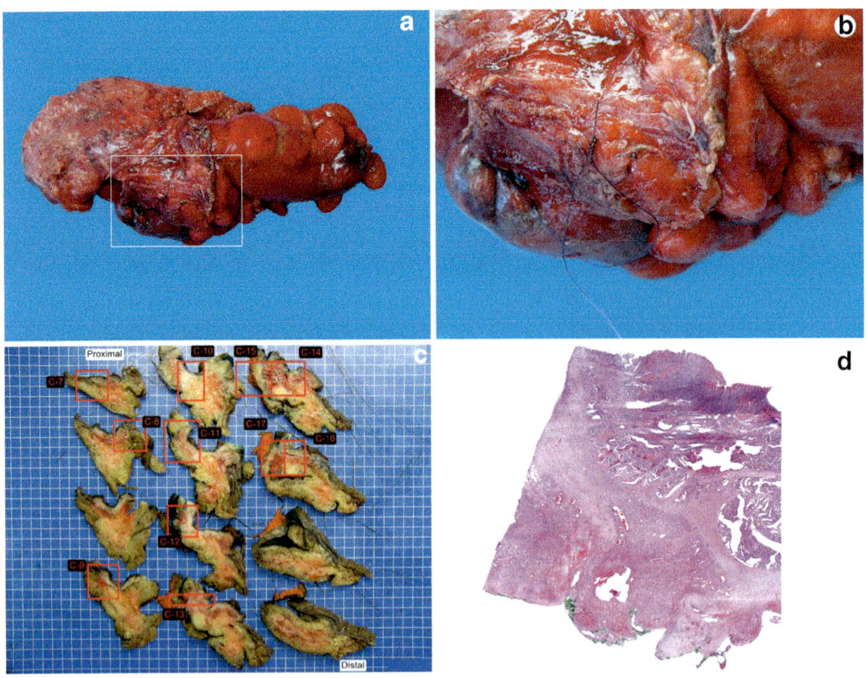

Fig. 20.4 (**a**) Left hemicolectomy for a lower sigmoid neoplasm. (**b**) Some suture thread was added to orientate the specimen indicating suspect for perforation and invasion of adjacent organs. (**c**) Several blocks are taken including the zone indicated by the suture as well where the tumor was closest to the serosa. (**d**) At histology there are peri-tumoral phlegmon and inflammatory peritoneal perforation, but the tumor is far away from the serosa thus making it category T3

20.4 pN Category

In the current and previous TNM editions, the only feature that has been taken into account for purposes of this category has been the number of metastatic regional lymph nodes [2, 4].

For practical purposes, it has been suggested that 12 lymph nodes should be considered as the minimum acceptable harvest, and this requirement was incorporated by the National Quality Forum as a quality surveillance indicator [2].

One study showed that an adequate lymph node yield (≥12) was reached in 70.6% of the elective group and 68.7% in the emergency group ($p = 0.004$) [11].

However this difference was small (1.9%), and accordingly another study showed almost an opposite trend 83% vs. 83.9% ($p = 0.79$), indicating that patients, undergoing emergency surgery, had no difference in the adequacy of nodal staging compared with their elective counterparts [11, 12].

When considering the proportion of metastatic regional lymph nodes, patients undergoing emergency surgery tend to have tumors with significatively more positive nodes (N1 and N2) compared with electively managed patients [7, 8].

20.5 M Category and R (Residual) Classification

In analogy to lymph node spreading, patients treated in an emergency setting have a higher proportion of advanced stages III and IV compared to elective group: this difference has been reported as significant in all the studies [3, 7–9, 11, 13, 14].

Differences in extent of disease at the time of diagnosis account for the results by Wong et al. showing that emergency patients were less likely to have a curative resection (60.2%) than elective patients (78.7%; $p < 0.0001$) [8].

Similar results presented by Pavlidis et al. demonstrated that macroscopic spread was not found in 57.8% of emergency cases and in 72% of elective cases ($p < 0.05$) [13].

Sites of metastases included the liver (18.2%), adjacent organ invasion (14%), and diffuse intra-abdominal dissemination (10%) [13].

Even following curative resection for CRC, the observed excess of both cancer-related and intercurrent deaths in patients who underwent surgery in emergency setting could be explained by occult hepatic metastases at the time of surgery [15].

Besides evident and/or occult metastatic disease, R1 resections are also more common among cases presenting as a surgical emergency (10% vs. 1%) [16].

20.6 Non-anatomic, Morphological Prognostic Factors

The prognostic heterogeneity of patients even in the same stage may be adjusted by adding prognostic factors, in particular in early disease (namely, stage II). In this event, if adverse prognostic indicators are present such as high tumor grade, vascular invasion, the involvement of peritoneal surface (pT4), and the acute presentation of intestinal wall perforation, the neoplasm is at high risk for recurrence, providing indications for adjuvant therapy [2].

Several studies about the perforation of colon cancer showed that these tumors would also be more likely to display lymphovascular [7, 16, 17] and/or perineural invasion [7] as well as poor differentiation [18].

Regarding mucinous differentiation, Ghazi et al. showed that there was no difference in mucin production. However, when the mucinous tumors of both groups were compared, those in the emergency group were more likely to have a signet ring cell component (OR = 3.267, $p = 0.001$) [7].

Bayar et al. also found an excess of signet ring carcinomas in the emergency group (2.2% vs. 0.9%) [18].

20.7 Conclusion

CRCs operated in an emergency setting display several differences when compared with elective cases, including a more advanced stage, a more aggressive histopathological profile, and a lower resectability.

They typically present as larger tumors, deeply infiltrating and protruding resulting in perforation and occlusion, the two common presentations in this setting.

All these factors account for the common concept that the long-term and oncologic outcomes for colorectal cancers presenting with emergency complications are worse than their elective counterparts [3].

As the type of surgery is not influenced by emergency setting (wide distance from margins and adequate lymphadenectomy: >12 are mandatory), the oncologic principles are upheld [3]. The pathology report for emergency cases should be accurate in order to document, at macroscopic and microscopic examination, all the tumor characteristics accounting for the different clinical presentations as well as the poorer outcome when compared to their elective counterparts.

References

1. Puppa G, Sonzogni A, Colombari R, et al. TNM staging system of colorectal carcinoma: a critical appraisal of challenging issues. Arch Pathol Lab Med. 2010;134:837–52.
2. Puppa G. TNM staging system of colorectal carcinoma: surgical pathology of the seventh edition. Diagn Histopathol. 2011;17:243–62.
3. Baer C, Menon R, Bastawrous S, et al. Emergency presentations of colorectal cancer. Surg Clin North Am. 2017;97:529–45.
4. Brierley J, Gospodarowicz MK, Wittekind C. TNM classification of malignant tumours. Hoboken, NJ: Wiley; 2017.
5. Sobin LH, Gospodarowicz MK, Wittekind C, editors. TNM classification of malignant tumors. New York: Wiley-Blackwell; 2009.
6. Puppa G, Caneva A, Colombari R, et al. For the sake of clarity about pT4 category of colorectal cancer. Arch Pathol Lab Med. 2009;133:340–1.
7. Ghazi S, Berg E, Lindblom A, et al. Clinicopathological analysis of colorectal cancer: a comparison between emergency and elective surgical cases. World J Surg Oncol. 2013;11:133.
8. Wong SK, Jalaludin BB, Morgan MJ, et al. Tumor pathology and long-term survival in emergency colorectal cancer. Dis Colon Rectum. 2008;51:223–30.

9. Moreno CC, Mittal PK, Sullivan PS, et al. Colorectal cancer initial diagnosis: screening colonoscopy, diagnostic colonoscopy, or emergent surgery, and tumor stage and size at initial presentation. Clin Colorectal Cancer. 2016;15:67–73.
10. Khan S, Pawlak SE, Eggenberger JC, et al. Acute colonic perforation associated with colorectal cancer. Am Surg. 2001;67:261–4.
11. Aquina CT, Becerra AZ, Xu Z, et al. Nonelective colon cancer resection: a continued public health concern. Surgery. 2017;161:1609–18.
12. Patel SV, Patel SV, Brackstone M. Emergency surgery for colorectal cancer does not result in nodal understaging compared with elective surgery. Can J Surg. 2014;57:349–53.
13. Pavlidis TE, Marakis G, Ballas K, et al. Does emergency surgery affect resectability of colorectal cancer? Acta Chir Belg. 2008;108:219–25.
14. Gunnarsson H, Jennische K, Forssell S, et al. Heterogeneity of colon cancer patients reported as emergencies. World J Surg. 2014;38:1819–26.
15. McArdle CS, Hole DJ. Emergency presentation of colorectal cancer is associated with poor 5-year survival. Br J Surg. 2004;91:605–9.
16. Bass G, Fleming C, Conneely J, et al. Emergency first presentation of colorectal cancer predicts significantly poorer outcomes: a review of 356 consecutive Irish patients. Dis Colon Rectum. 2009;52:678–84.
17. Metcalfe MS, Norwood MG, Miller AS, et al. Unreasonable expectations in emergency colorectal cancer surgery. Colorectal Dis. 2005;7:275–8.
18. Bayar B, Yilmaz KB, Akinci M, et al. An evaluation of treatment results of emergency versus elective surgery in colorectal cancer patients. Ulus Cerrahi Derg. 2016;32:11–7.

Postoperative Oncologic Management of Colorectal Cancer Emergencies

21

Emmanuelle Kempf, Isabelle Baumgaertner, and Christophe Tournigand

21.1 Introduction

Up to 30% of patients with colorectal cancer (CRC) present as surgical emergencies, such as intestinal obstruction or bowel perforation [1]. Both clinical complications might also occur while patients undergo chemotherapy for advanced CRC. The oncologic management of those patients following emergency surgery procedures remains a clinical challenge. The concerning issues include the postoperative complications themselves (see Chap. 12). This chapter will address the postoperative management of CRC emergencies, from the point of view of the oncologist. What are the best chemotherapy regimens for each kind of postoperative clinical presentation? How could we avoid a lasting interruption of active anticancer systemic treatment, so that surgical emergencies do not impair a patient's quality of life and overall survival (OS)? How could we choose the best chemotherapy regimen in order to achieve the optimal tumor response rate and therefore make CRC become resectable at the metastatic stage?

21.2 Surgical Emergencies as the Initial Clinical Presentation for CRC

Since the very end of the twentieth century, National Health Systems of developed countries have focused on the implementation of CRC screenings at a population level, based on the detection of blood in the individual feces. After a 30-year follow-up, randomized clinical trials show that this prevention measure might reduce by

E. Kempf · I. Baumgaertner · C. Tournigand (✉)
Department of Medical Oncology, Henri Mondor et Albert Chenevier Teaching Hospital, AP-HP, Créteil, France
e-mail: christophe.tournigand@aphp.fr

N. de'Angelis et al. (eds.), *Emergency Surgical Management of Colorectal Cancer*, Hot Topics in Acute Care Surgery and Trauma,
https://doi.org/10.1007/978-3-030-06225-5_21

32% and 22% the rate of disease-related mortality for annual and biennial testing, respectively [2]. However, across different countries, less than half of the targeted population seems to be keen on performing the free CRC screening test. Some reasons might explain such a poor adherence to the screening procedure, like an insufficient knowledge and/or communication from the general practitioners, people reluctance to perform a screening test based on stool sampling, and individuals' wish not to worry about cancer [3]. However, around every third of CRC case is currently diagnosed through an initial clinical complication requiring an emergency management [1].

Intestinal obstruction due to the intraluminal development of a CRC might be the first cancer-related symptom. Such acute clinical complication requires a surgical digestive derivation through the creation of an ileostomy. However, both medical and surgical managements might slightly differ according to the stage of tumor development. Fewer CRC cases present with a colon perforation, but this acute complication might predict poorer clinical outcomes than initial intestinal obstruction [4]. The acute prognosis of such mechanistic complication of the tumor development is mostly related to the presence of a septic peritonitis.

21.2.1 Localized Stage

In the case of a localized tumor stage, i.e., the absence of any distant metastasis, the carcinologic resection of the primary tumor might be performed during the same surgical procedure than the digestive derivation. Such tumor removal addresses three issues: the mechanistic complication, the tumor diagnosis, and the tumor curative treatment. The postoperative administration of adjuvant chemotherapy is recommended in such clinical presentations, as an initial intestinal obstruction is considered as a poor prognostic factor in stage II CRC [5, 6]. The FOLFOX regimen including the combination of leucovorin plus 5-fluorouracil and oxaliplatin administered every second week during 6 months has been the international standard since the MOSAIC study [7]. However, this therapeutic standard has been challenged by the recent IDEA collaboration published in *The Lancet Oncology* and the *Journal of Clinical Oncology* in 2018, respectively. Results of these international phase III randomized clinical trials claimed that a 3-month chemotherapy course might be a valid option for low-risk stage III CRC cases [8, 9]. Patients with tumor stage pT4, N1–N2, M0 or T1–T3, N2, M0 might be good candidates for such a shorter therapeutic procedure. This adjuvant treatment is expected to start after 4 weeks following the resection of the primary tumor. Two meta-analyses including more than 10,000 patients showed that any delay in the initiation of adjuvant chemotherapy was statistically associated with a worse overall survival [10, 11]. Yet, postoperative complications such as sepsis or general state impairment in elderly patients might delay the initiation of chemotherapy administration. An American observational study on 580 cases of resected localized CRCs concluded that postoperative complications were strong predictors of delays in the chemotherapy initiation (OR 2.4; 95% CI 1.6, 3.8) [12]. This issue is of special concern for the elderly undergoing urgent surgical procedures. An observational study from the SEER database performed on more than 30,000 patients showed that urgent surgical resections were associated with a poorer clinical outcome compared to elective tumor resections: 70% vs. 86% of 1-year OS rate, respectively [13]. In a real-life setting, patients aged 75 years and older are twice less likely to be provided with postoperative chemotherapy [14].

21.2.2 Advanced Stage

When the CRC development has reached distant organs, the clinical relevance of the initial resection of the primary tumor has been strongly debated according to the clinical presentation. In advanced CRC, bowel obstruction is a local complication of the tumor progression which is related to a poor prognosis. Therefore, the removal of the primary tumor should always be discussed in such clinical situation. A population-based study of the SEER database showed that the primary tumor removal in resectable stage IV CRC was associated with an absolute gain in overall survival rate of 60%, while it reduces the risk of a further digestive obstruction [15]. Randomized clinical trials are currently assessing the clinical relevance of such surgical procedure in the 20% of cases with unresectable metastasis [16]. Bowel obstruction in stage IV CRC is statistically associated with a proximal tumor site, a higher tumor grade or nodal status, a mucinous histological type, or an older CRC diagnosis [17]. For patients aged 65 years and over, surgical procedure has not shown any strong benefit compared to exclusive medical management [18]. Young patients diagnosed with unilobar liver metastasis, in the absence of any carcinomatosis, seem to be good candidates for radical surgery of both liver metastasis and primary tumor [19]. At the time of the initial presentation, creating an ileostomy might address the acute digestive obstruction, while a simple tumor sampling may confirm the tumor diagnosis. In case of potentially resectable metastasis, the primary tumor might be removed after a few chemotherapy cycles. Indeed, the urgent timing of CRC resection is likely to be associated with poorer short-term and long-term clinical outcomes compared to elective tumor removals [20]. Yet, a recent study showed that the poorer clinical outcomes of CRC patients undergoing urgent versus elective tumor resection were due to a bad selection of patients rather than to the urgent timing itself [21]. In the case of extensive metastatic disease, focusing on systemic treatments rather than on surgical procedures might improve clinical outcomes. In stage IV CRC patients undergoing laparotomy, up to 77% of patients experiencing postoperative complications were diagnosed with an extensive metastatic disease [19].

21.3 Surgical Emergency as a Complication for Patients with Advanced CRC Undergoing Chemotherapy

Bowel perforation is the main clinical complication requiring an emergency surgical procedure, once patients with advanced CRC have started a chemotherapy course. Such clinical event is likely to be due to the local tumor necrosis.

Anti-angiogenics are known to induce such complications in about 1% of the cases [22]. A meta-analysis performed on more than 12,000 patients included in randomized clinical trials showed that CRC tumors treated with bevacizumab were three times more likely to suffer a bowel perforation compared to cancers treated without bevacizumab [23]. In a very few cases, the colon perforation might be due to the progression of a chemotherapy-resistant tumor. The severity of the related infectious complications is the main prognostic factor of these clinical situations. On the one hand, the septic complications might directly impair the patient clinical outcomes. On the other hand, such infectious context might prevent anticancer active treatment from being administered again. Thus, the tumor might progress as long as the interruption of the chemotherapy administration lasts. Moreover, the general state of those patients, especially the elderly, might impair because of such septic complications, so that the further administration of chemotherapy cannot be initiated again. In this timeframe, some initial so-called potentially resectable advanced CRCs might become non-resectable at all.

21.4 How to Choose Among Chemotherapy Regimens in Order to Resect Advanced CRC?

After an emergency surgical procedure, the choice and the administration of the postoperative treatment are key prognostic factors. In case of potentially resectable metastasis, the main aim of such treatment is to achieve the best tumor shrinkage, assessed by the response rate (RR). The better the metastasis shrinkage, the easier the surgical procedure. Many chemotherapy regimens are available for the first line of treatment of advanced CRC. The tumor biology has been a key criterion for such a chemotherapy choice in the last decade. Since the discovery of the negative predictive value of *RAS* mutations in 2006 by Laurent-Puig et al., anti-EGFR monoclonal antibodies have been recommended solely for the treatment of *RAS*-wild advanced CRC in combination with standard chemotherapy [24]. In order to make stage IV CRC become resectable, the administration of anti-EGFR targeted therapies in *RAS*-wild tumors might be associated with a better RR and a deeper shrinkage compared to antiangiogenics [25, 26]. Other tumor characteristics might impact the choice of preoperative chemotherapy. A recent subanalysis of the CALGB/SWOG 80405 clinical trial showed that left-sided colon cancers might benefit more from anti-EGFR treatment than right-sided tumors [27]. *BRAF* mutation is likely to be exclusive from *RAS* mutation and accounts for 5% of advanced CRC cases [28]. This molecular abnormality is associated with a worse prognosis, an older age, a female sex, poorer differentiated, mucinous, MSI, and proximal tumors [29]. The combination of the FOLFOXIRI regimen with bevacizumab remains a valid option in those aggressive tumors [30, 31]. Also, clinicians must make sure that the patient's general state is good enough to undergo such triplet of chemotherapy. Grades 3 and 4 neurotoxicity, stomatitis, diarrhea, and neutropenia were significantly higher in the experimental arm. The development of immunotherapy is the current revolution within the oncology field. A phase 2 study showed that dMMR/MSI high molecular profile may carry a positive predictive value for checkpoint inhibitors such as nivolumab in the treatment of advanced CRCs. The disease control rate (DCR) reached 69% in yet-treated tumors with no available therapeutic options [32]. The combination of checkpoint inhibitors with ipilimumab might become the future option of the dMMR/MSI CRC population with a 80% DCR [33]. For the first time in its history, the Food and Drug Administration approved in 2017 checkpoint inhibitors for the treatment of tumors characterized by such molecular profile and previously treated, regardless of the histological tumor type. However, immunotherapy has not been accessible for CRC in European routine practice yet, and it remains a therapeutic option for yet-treated tumors. For other advanced CRC cases with *RAS* mutations and MSS profile, the standard of care for the first lines of treatment includes a chemotherapy doublet combined with antiangiogenics. Recently, a multicenter retrospective cohort showed that a slight modification of the FOLFIRI regimen combined with aflibercept, a VEGF trap, led to a dramatic improvement in terms of RR (FOLFIRI 3-aflibercept): the DCR reached 76.7% in irinotecan-naïve patients [34]. Splitting up the administration of irinotecan at days 1 and 3 of each chemotherapy cycle might have a promising future in advanced CRC with a project of further resectability.

21.5 Conclusion

Emergency surgical procedures remain a daily therapeutic option for the management of CRC. Such a postoperative context creates clinical issues which are likely to impair both quality of life and overall survival of the patient. The septic complications might delay the initiation of the chemotherapy administration, while the surgery-induced deterioration of patient general state might prevent any chemotherapy from ever starting. However, the adjuvant chemotherapy should begin within the first few weeks after the tumor resection at the localized stage. Its optimal duration has been challenged recently. At the metastatic stage, the emergency surgical procedure might address the mechanistic complication solely. The choice of the postoperative chemotherapy regimen is a key prognostic decision, which is based on the tumor biology and patient characteristics. The further resectability of such advanced cancers relies on an optimal tumor response rate and improves significantly the patient clinical outcomes.

References

1. Bass G, Fleming C, Conneely J, Martin Z, Mealy K. Emergency first presentation of colorectal cancer predicts significantly poorer outcomes: a review of 356 consecutive Irish patients. Dis Colon Rectum. 2009;52(4):678–84.
2. Shaukat A, Mongin SJ, Geisser MS, Lederle FA, Bond JH, Mandel JS, et al. Long-term mortality after screening for colorectal cancer. N Engl J Med. 2013;369(12):1106–14.
3. Vernon SW. Participation in colorectal cancer screening: a review. J Natl Cancer Inst. 1997;89(19):1406–22.

4. Chen T-M, Huang Y-T, Wang G-C. Outcome of colon cancer initially presenting as colon perforation and obstruction. World J Surg Oncol. 2017;15(1):164.
5. Kannarkatt J, Joseph J, Kurniali PC, Al-Janadi A, Hrinczenko B. Adjuvant chemotherapy for stage II colon cancer: a clinical dilemma. J Oncol Pract. 2017;13(4):233–41.
6. Schmoll HJ, Van Cutsem E, Stein A, Valentini V, Glimelius B, Haustermans K, et al. ESMO Consensus Guidelines for management of patients with colon and rectal cancer. a personalized approach to clinical decision making. Ann Oncol. 2012;23(10):2479–516.
7. Andre T, Boni C, Mounedji-Boudiaf L, Navarro M, Tabernero J, Hickish T, et al. Oxaliplatin, fluorouracil, and leucovorin as adjuvant treatment for colon cancer. N Engl J Med. 2004;350(23):2343–51.
8. Iveson TJ, Kerr RS, Saunders MP, Cassidy J, Hollander NH, Tabernero J, et al. 3 versus 6 months of adjuvant oxaliplatin-fluoropyrimidine combination therapy for colorectal cancer (SCOT): an international, randomised, phase 3, non-inferiority trial. Lancet Oncol. 2018;19(4):562–78.
9. Andre T, Vernerey D, Mineur L, Bennouna J, Desrame J, Faroux R, et al. Three versus 6 months of oxaliplatin-based adjuvant chemotherapy for patients with stage III colon cancer: disease-free survival results from a randomized, open-label, International Duration Evaluation of Adjuvant (IDEA) France, phase III trial. J Clin Oncol. 2018;36(15):1469–77.
10. Biagi JJ, Raphael MJ, Mackillop WJ, Kong W, King WD, Booth CM. Association between time to initiation of adjuvant chemotherapy and survival in colorectal cancer: a systematic review and meta-analysis. JAMA. 2011;305(22):2335–42.
11. Des Guetz G, Nicolas P, Perret G-Y, Morere J-F, Uzzan B. Does delaying adjuvant chemotherapy after curative surgery for colorectal cancer impair survival? A meta-analysis. Eur J Cancer. 2010;46(6):1049–55.
12. Wasserman DW, Boulos M, Hopman WM, Booth CM, Goodwin R, Biagi JJ. Reasons for delay in time to initiation of adjuvant chemotherapy for colon cancer. J Oncol Pract. 2015;11(1):e28–35.
13. Neuman HB, O'Connor ES, Weiss J, Loconte NK, Greenblatt DY, Greenberg CC, et al. Surgical treatment of colon cancer in patients aged 80 years and older: analysis of 31,574 patients in the SEER-Medicare database. Cancer. 2013;119(3):639–47.
14. Kahn KL, Adams JL, Weeks JC, Chrischilles EA, Schrag D, Ayanian JZ, et al. Adjuvant chemotherapy use and adverse events among older patients with stage III colon cancer. JAMA. 2010;303(11):1037–45.
15. Tarantino I, Warschkow R, Worni M, Cerny T, Ulrich A, Schmied BM, et al. Prognostic relevance of palliative primary tumor removal in 37,793 metastatic colorectal cancer patients: a population-based, propensity score-adjusted trend analysis. Ann Surg. 2015;262(1):112–20.
16. Kim CW, Baek J-H, Choi G-S, Yu CS, Kang SB, Park WC, et al. The role of primary tumor resection in colorectal cancer patients with asymptomatic, synchronous unresectable metastasis: study protocol for a randomized controlled trial. Trials. 2016;17:34.
17. Winner M, Mooney SJ, Hershman DL, Feingold DL, Allendorf JD, Wright JD, et al. Incidence and predictors of bowel obstruction in elderly patients with stage IV colon cancer: a population-based cohort study. JAMA Surg. 2013;148(8):715–22.
18. Winner M, Mooney SJ, Hershman DL, Feingold DL, Allendorf JD, Wright JD, et al. Management and outcomes of bowel obstruction in patients with stage IV colon cancer: a population-based cohort study. Dis Colon Rectum. 2013;56(7):834–43.
19. Rosen SA, Buell JF, Yoshida A, Kazsuba S, Hurst R, Michelassi F, et al. Initial presentation with stage IV colorectal cancer: how aggressive should we be? Arch Surg. 2000;135(5):530–5.
20. Baer C, Menon R, Bastawrous S, Bastawrous A. Emergency presentations of colorectal cancer. Surg Clin North Am. 2017;97(3):529–45.
21. Weixler B, Warschkow R, Ramser M, Droeser R, von Holzen U, Oertli D, et al. Urgent surgery after emergency presentation for colorectal cancer has no impact on overall and disease-free survival: a propensity score analysis. BMC Cancer. 2016;16:208.

22. Badgwell BD, Camp ER, Feig B, Wolff RA, Eng C, Ellis LM, et al. Management of bevacizumab-associated bowel perforation: a case series and review of the literature. Ann Oncol. 2008;19(3):577–82.
23. Hapani S, Chu D, Wu S. Risk of gastrointestinal perforation in patients with cancer treated with bevacizumab: a meta-analysis. Lancet Oncol. 2009;10(6):559–68.
24. Lievre A, Bachet J-B, Le Corre D, Boige V, Landi B, Emile J-F, et al. KRAS mutation status is predictive of response to cetuximab therapy in colorectal cancer. Cancer Res. 2006;66(8):3992–5.
25. Venook AP, Niedzwiecki D, Lenz H-J, Innocenti F, Fruth B, Meyerhardt JA, et al. Effect of first-line chemotherapy combined with cetuximab or bevacizumab on overall survival in patients with KRAS wild-type advanced or metastatic colorectal cancer: a randomized clinical trial. JAMA. 2017;317(23):2392–401.
26. Heinemann V, von Weikersthal LF, Decker T, Kiani A, Vehling-Kaiser U, Al-Batran S-E, et al. FOLFIRI plus cetuximab versus FOLFIRI plus bevacizumab as first-line treatment for patients with metastatic colorectal cancer (FIRE-3): a randomised, open-label, phase 3 trial. Lancet Oncol. 2014;15(10):1065–75.
27. Venook AP, Niedzwiecki D, Innocenti F, Fruth B, Greene C, O'Neil BH, et al. Impact of primary (1°) tumor location on overall survival (OS) and progression-free survival (PFS) in patients (pts) with metastatic colorectal cancer (mCRC): analysis of CALGB/SWOG 80405 (Alliance). J Clin Oncol [Internet]. American Society of Clinical Oncology; 2016;34(15_suppl):3504. Available from: http://ascopubs.org/doi/abs/10.1200/JCO.2016.34.15_suppl.3504.
28. Deshwar A, Margonis GA, Andreatos N, Barbon C, Wang J, Buettner S, et al. Double KRAS and BRAF mutations in surgically treated colorectal cancer liver metastases: an international, multi-institutional case series. Anticancer Res. 2018;38(5):2891–5.
29. Sanz-Garcia E, Argiles G, Elez E, Tabernero J. BRAF mutant colorectal cancer: prognosis, treatment, and new perspectives. Ann Oncol. 2017;28(11):2648–57.
30. Loupakis F, Cremolini C, Salvatore L, Masi G, Sensi E, Schirripa M, et al. FOLFOXIRI plus bevacizumab as first-line treatment in BRAF mutant metastatic colorectal cancer. Eur J Cancer. 2014;50(1):57–63.
31. Cremolini C, Loupakis F, Antoniotti C, Lupi C, Sensi E, Lonardi S, et al. FOLFOXIRI plus bevacizumab versus FOLFIRI plus bevacizumab as first-line treatment of patients with metastatic colorectal cancer: updated overall survival and molecular subgroup analyses of the open-label, phase 3 TRIBE study. Lancet Oncol. 2015;16(13):1306–15.
32. Overman MJ, McDermott R, Leach JL, Lonardi S, Lenz H-J, Morse MA, et al. Nivolumab in patients with metastatic DNA mismatch repair-deficient or microsatellite instability-high colorectal cancer (CheckMate 142): an open-label, multicentre, phase 2 study. Lancet Oncol. 2017;18(9):1182–91.
33. Overman MJ, Lonardi S, Wong KYM, Lenz H-J, Gelsomino F, Aglietta M, et al. Durable clinical benefit with nivolumab plus ipilimumab in DNA mismatch repair-deficient/microsatellite instability-high metastatic colorectal cancer. J Clin Oncol. 2018;36(8):773–9.
34. Carola C, Ghiringhelli F, Kim S, Andre T, Barlet J, Bengrine L, et al. FOLFIRI3-aflibercept as second- or later-line therapy in patients with metastatic colorectal cancer. J Clin Oncol [Internet]. American Society of Clinical Oncology; 2018;36(4_suppl):817. Available from: http://ascopubs.org/doi/abs/10.1200/JCO.2018.36.4_suppl.817.

Minimally Invasive Surgery for Colorectal Cancer in the Emergency Setting

22

Arianna Birindelli, Valeria Tonini, Justin Davies, Massimo Chiarugi, and Salomone Di Saverio

22.1 Introduction

Globally, colorectal cancer (CRC) is the third most commonly diagnosed cancer in males and the second in females, with 1.65 million new cases and almost 835,000 deaths in 2015 [1]. Its incidence is higher in developed countries most probably relating to dietary and environmental factors. About 30% of patients with CRC present as an emergency [2, 3]. Among these, large bowel obstruction is by far the most common presentation, accounting for about 80%, while the remaining 15% are perforated CRC and 5% are bleeding CRC [3].

According to the tumour site and symptoms, as well as the patient's haemodynamic stability and overall status (ASA score), the physicians' expertise and the level of healthcare facility, the management of CRC emergencies includes conservative measures, endoscopic stenting or haemostasis, angioembolisation or surgical treatment. Despite laparoscopy in elective CRC surgery is widely used and its advantages are much appreciated, its role in emergency colorectal setting is still debated, and no randomised controlled trials have been run on this topic yet. Although emergency laparoscopy has been proposed and is routinely used in some institutions, this is mainly for benign conditions, such as appendicitis, cholecystitis and diverticulitis, perforated peptic ulcer repair and assessment of abdominal trauma [4, 5]. The lack of diffusion of this technique in CRC emergencies is probably due

A. Birindelli · V. Tonini
Department of General Surgery, University of Bologna, S. Orsola Malpighi, Bologna, Italy

J. Davies · S. Di Saverio (✉)
Cambridge Colorectal Unit, Cambridge University Hospitals NHS Foundation Trust, Addenbrooke's Hospital, Cambridge, UK

M. Chiarugi
Department of Surgical, Medical, Molecular Pathology and Critical Care, Cisanello Hospital, University of Pisa Medical School, Pisa, Italy

N. de'Angelis et al. (eds.), *Emergency Surgical Management of Colorectal Cancer*, Hot Topics in Acute Care Surgery and Trauma,
https://doi.org/10.1007/978-3-030-06225-5_22

to the fact that the procedure may be more challenging due to the bowel distention, in case of obstruction, or abdominal contamination or inflammation, in case of perforation. In addition, in the absence of a highly skilled surgeon, these conditions may reduce the accuracy of the colonic resection in terms of oncologic criteria and lymph node harvesting. Furthermore, another limiting factor, in patients that are physiologically impaired, is the longer operative time usually required by laparoscopic procedures. This can also be a limiting factor to the common over-scheduling of emergency theatres.

In this chapter, we will describe the indications, patient selection, setting and equipment required, as well as the technical steps and useful tips to safely manage these conditions in a minimally invasive manner. Finally, we will review the available literature on laparoscopy in CRC emergencies.

22.2 Indications, Patient Selection, Setting and Surgical Technique in Colorectal Cancer Emergencies

First of all, in order to safely approach a minimally invasive procedure for colorectal cancer emergency, the patient should be haemodynamically stable, be able to tolerate a Trendelenburg position if needed and have no absolute contraindications to pneumoperitoneum. In case of haemodynamic instability, a fluid resuscitation can be attempted, and in case of good response, the patient can be approached laparoscopically. Secondly, the surgeon should have adequate surgical skills, in terms of being experienced in emergency, laparoscopic and colorectal surgery. Last but not least, adequate theatre time availability, collaborating theatre staff and good laparoscopic equipment are further fundamental requirements.

22.2.1 Obstructing Colorectal Cancer

Since the left colon is anatomically narrower than the right colon, cancers originating from this segment of the bowel commonly give obstructing symptoms at an earlier stage compared to right-sided tumours [6]. An exception is the tumour of the ileo-caecal valve that gives early small bowel obstruction symptoms [7].

According to the ESGE Guidelines, endoscopic stenting is indicated as the treatment of choice as bridge to elective surgery in elderly patients with obstructing left CRC who have an increased risk of postoperative mortality (age >70 years and/or ASA status ≥3) or in the setting of palliative care in case of metastatic disease [8]. Since controversies still exist regarding oncological safety and long-term outcomes of endoscopic colonic stenting in patients <70 years and/or ASA <3 presenting with obstructing left CRC [9, 10], in these patients the surgical resection is indicated [11]. Failed, contraindicated or unavailable endoscopic stenting is another indication to surgical treatment in obstructive CRC.

In the presence of the above-mentioned conditions, according to the location of the tumour, severity of obstruction and patient's status, a loop ileostomy (right-sided tumour) or colostomy (left-sided tumour), as well as an intestinal bypass, a right or left colectomy or a subtotal colectomy with or without primary anastomosis can be performed with a minimally invasive technique [7, 11, 12].

Preoperative CT scan with IV contrast can help getting an idea of the grade of obstruction as well as the competence or incompetence of the ileo-caecal valve. The patient's and trocars' positions are basically the same as for elective colonic procedures. However, we discourage the use of Verres needle in these patients because of the bowel distention. We recommend, instead, an umbilical open access technique or an optical blunt access at the Palmer's point. Bladeless trocars should be preferred in order to minimise risk of iatrogenic injuries due to gross visceral distension. In left obstructing CRC, due to the caecal distention, the operating trocars may need to be placed more medial than the standard position. Once the pneumoperitoneum is established, managing the distended bowel and gaining enough view and working space are the main challenge. This can be achieved by appropriate table tilting, the use of the 30° camera, retraction of the bowel with lap gauze and using atraumatic graspers. Distended and frail bowel loops should be handled with extreme care and shouldn't be directly grasped but bluntly mobilised or grasped from the mesentery [7, 11, 12].

Laparoscopic loop ileostomy is easily fashioned by gently grasping the terminal ileum at about 20 cm from the ileo-caecal valve, followed by the trephine abdominal wall incision down to the abdominal cavity and exteriorisation of the bowel checking the correct orientation. Although similar to loop ileostomy, laparoscopic loop colostomy can be slightly more complicated, especially if the tumour is proximal, because a grade of colonic medial mobilisation is required to exteriorise the bowel to the skin surface.

Colonic resections are obviously more challenging but feasible. For either right or left or subtotal colectomies, central vascular ligation and complete mesocolic excision should be aimed, to achieve adequate lymph node harvesting and the best oncologic prognosis. However, due to the bowel distention, the view can be severely impaired. In particular, when performing a laparoscopic sigmoidectomy for an obstructing CRC, instead of starting the procedure from the vascular ligation and mesocolic excision, a possible trick is to do the dissection downstream the obstruction, where the bowel is nicely collapsed and easier to approach, perform the distal bowel division with an endostapler at the level of the sacral promontory and only at this point, by pulling the bowel upwards, proceed with the mesocolic dissection and vascular ligation. If a proper mesocolic excision is not feasible, we recommend to convert the procedure to laparotomy.

Once the vascular ligation, mesocolic dissection and colonic mobilisation are completed, in case of resection without anastomosis, the distal bowel division can be performed intra-corporeally (with an endostapler), the diseased segment extracted through the stoma site and the proximal bowel edge divided extracorporeally at the time of the stoma fashioning (Fig. 22.1). We recommend to avoid primary anastomosis in patients with a bowel size discrepancy greater than 50% or with bowel poorly perfused.

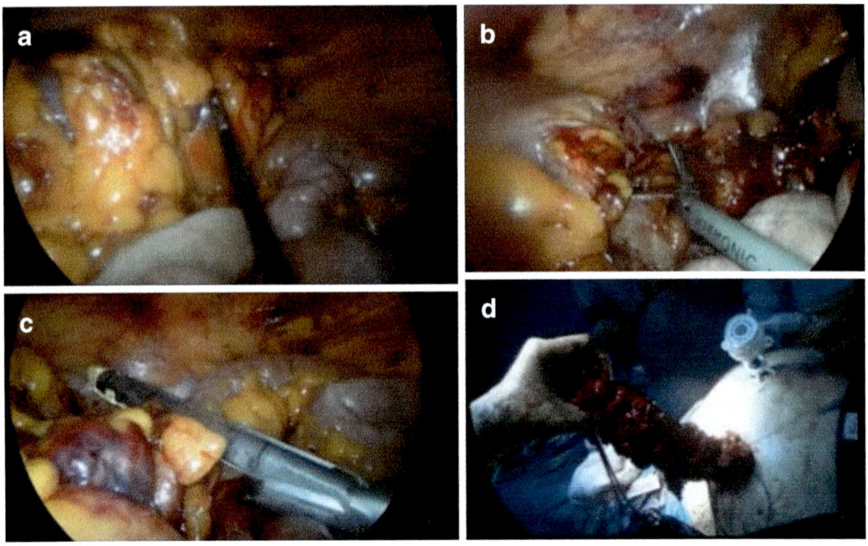

Fig. 22.1 Laparoscopic Hartmann's procedure for obstructing sigmoid cancer (**a**). IMV and IMA were intra-corporeally dissected, ligated and divided (**b**), as well as the stapled section of the rectum (**c**). Specimen was extracted through the colostomy site (**d**). (Operator Mr. Salomone Di Saverio MD FACS FRCS)

In the case of resection with anastomosis, after vascular ligation and complete mesocolic excision, the technique is different depending on the side. In left colectomy or sigmoidectomy, where the splenic flexure must be always fully mobilised, distal bowel division is performed intra-corporeally, the specimen is extracted through a mini-Pfannestiel incision and the proximal edge is separated extracorporeally at the skin level. Before inserting the anvil in the proximal stump, in order to avoid faecal spillage, this could be gently clamped with either the assistant fingers or a soft bowel clamp. After inserting and securing the anvil, the bowel is reinserted in the abdomen, and an intra-corporeal transanal colorectal anastomosis (Knight-Griffen) is fashioned [11] (Fig. 22.2). In right and subtotal colectomy, the whole procedure could ideally be performed intra-corporeally (proximal and distal bowel division and side-to-side stapled anastomosis) and the specimen extracted through a mini-Pfannestiel incision [12, 13]. However, considering the bowel distention and the impossibility of applying a laparoscopic bowel clamp in the proximal bowel stump, a targeted mini-laparotomy on top of the bowel stumps followed by an extra-corporeal anastomosis may be preferable to avoid massive enteric spillage at the time of enterotomy [7] (Fig. 22.3). A similar technique may be used to fashion an intestinal bypass in case of unresectable tumours. A distal small bowel loop can be laparoscopically identified and approached to the colon distal to the tumour. After slightly mobilising the latter, a targeted mini-laparotomy and an extracorporeal anastomosis can be performed. Another technical option in right colectomies is

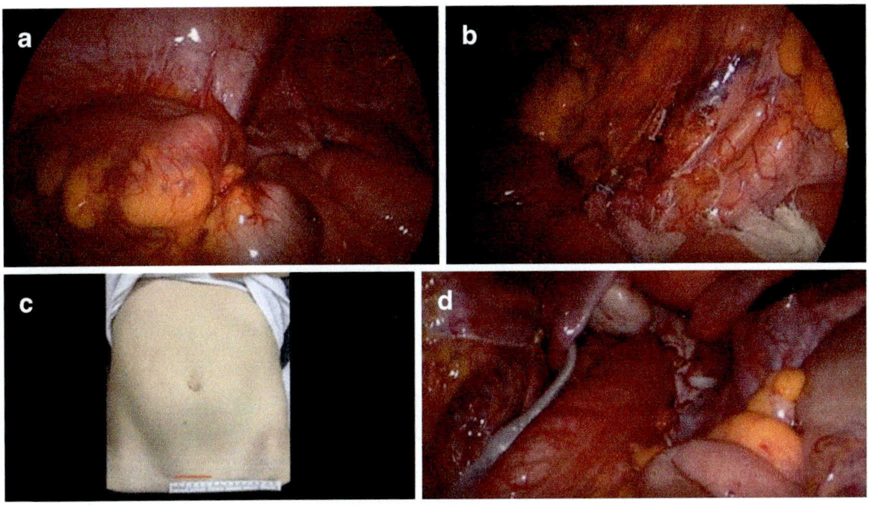

Fig. 22.2 Left colectomy for obstructing sigmoid cancer (**a**). IMV and IMA were intra-corporeally dissected, ligated and divided (**b**), as well as the stapled section of the rectum. Specimen was extracted through a mini-Pfannestiel incision (**c**), and an intra-corporeal transanal colorectal anastomosis was performed (**d**). (Operator Mr. Salomone Di Saverio MD FACS FRCS)

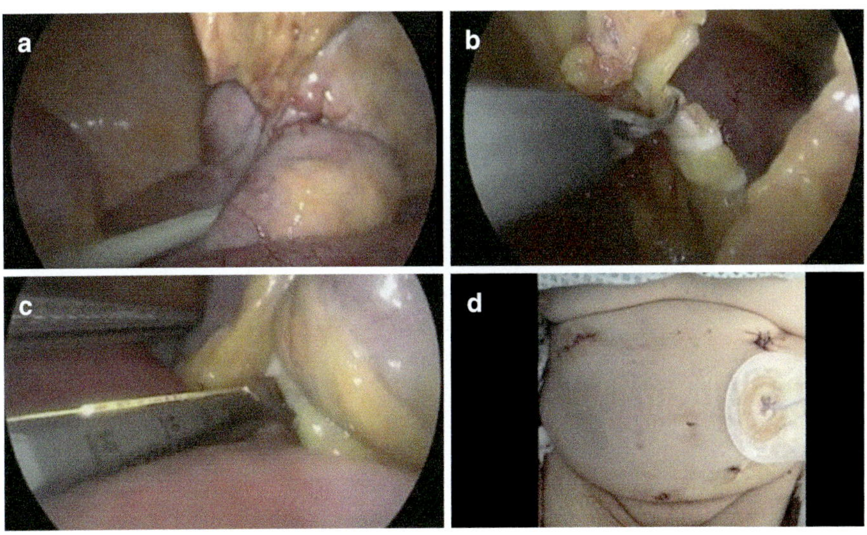

Fig. 22.3 Right colectomy for ileo-caecal valve obstructing cancer (**a**). Ileocolic vessel dissection, ligation and division were performed intra-corporeally (**b**), as well as the stapled section of the terminal ileum (**c**) and transverse colon. Specimen was extracted through a targeted mini-laparotomy in the RUQ, and through the same site, an extracorporeal handsewn side-to-side ileo-transverse anastomosis was performed (**d**). (Operator Mr. Salomone Di Saverio MD FACS FRCS)

performing both bowel division and anastomosis extracorporeally through a midline mini-laparotomy (*Barcelona* type), but this has increased short-term morbidity and increased length of hospital stay compared to intra-corporeal anastomosis [14].

Regardless the type of resection and anastomosis performed, as in elective procedures, this must be well perfused and without tension. At the end of any procedure, a careful laparoscopic check of haemostasis and correct orientation of the bowel are strongly recommended.

22.2.2 Perforated Colorectal Cancer

Perforated colorectal cancer is rare and usually associated with an advanced stage and a poor prognosis [15, 16]. Caecal perforation as a result of an obstructing CRC with competent ileo-caecal valve usually causes massive diffuse faecal peritonitis and septic shock that prevent the management by minimally invasive surgery. Otherwise provided haemodynamic stability and no absolute contraindications to pneumoperitoneum, perforated bowel cancer can be approached laparoscopically. In fact, either spontaneous or iatrogenic (as a colonoscopic complication) perforation that occurs at the site of the tumour is usually minor, detected by little pericolic bubbles at CT scan and causing localised peritonitis. Treatment of choice in these cases is the surgical resection following oncologic criteria.

The patient's and trocars' positions are basically the same as for elective colorectal resections. Bladeless trocars should be preferred in order to minimise risk of iatrogenic injuries in case of visceral distension and adhesions secondary to peritonitis. After an umbilical open access technique, pneumoperitoneum is established. In case of free peritoneal fluid, a pus swab should be taken in view of postoperative sepsis treatment, followed by a thorough cleansing of the abdominal cavity. Similar to what happens in perforated diverticulitis, since inflammation causes distortion of the anatomical planes, a gentle blunt dissection with suction tube is recommended to expose the perforation and avoid iatrogenic injuries [17]. Tilting of the bed and laparoscopic gauzes can be helpful in this step and throughout all the procedure to keep the small bowel out of the way and better expose the vessel roots. The other steps should be those of a standard radical colectomy following the surgical oncologic criteria. According to the surgeon's preference, the bowel division can be performed intra- or extracorporeally, while according to the patient's conditions, the surgeon can decide if an anastomosis (intra- or extracorporeal) or an end-stoma is performed (Fig. 22.4). If an anastomosis is fashioned, the specimen can be extracted through a mini-Pfannestiel incision, while in the case of an end-stoma, the specimen can be extracted through the stoma site.

22.2.3 Bleeding Colorectal Cancer

Colorectal cancer is an uncommon cause of acute lower GI bleeding. In the rare case of acutely bleeding CRC, angioembolisation or endoscopic haemostasis is the treatment of choice [18]. However, especially if the bleeding is venous and at a slow rate,

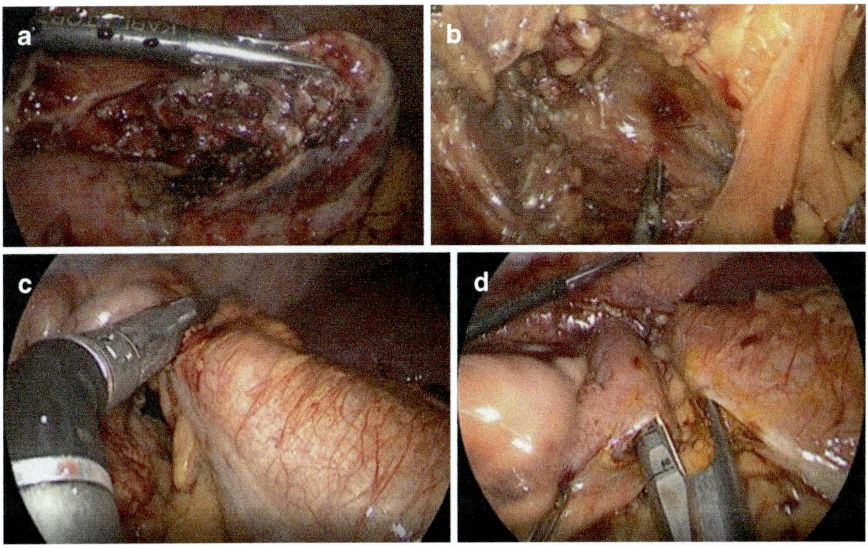

Fig. 22.4 Right colectomy for perforated right colon cancer (**a**). Ileocolic vessels were intra-corporeally dissected (**b**), ligated and divided, as well as the stapled section of the terminal ileum and transverse colon (**c**). An intra-corporeal staple side-to-side ileo-transverse anastomosis was fashioned (**d**), and the specimen was extracted through a mini-Pfannestiel incision. (Operator Mr. Salomone Di Saverio MD FACS FRCS)

the angioembolisation can fail to identify and treat the bleeding. Similarly, since the bowel is not prepared, the endoscopy can fail due to the poor visualisation of the bowel walls that can be completely covered by blood and stools. Therefore, in the case of a haemodynamically stable patient and failed, contraindicated or unavailable angio-embolisation or endoscopic haemostasis, a laparoscopic colon resection can be performed, with or without anastomosis according to patient's conditions. A very specific indication for laparoscopic colorectal resection is the colon ischaemia following an emergency angioembolisation for a bleeding CRC. The recommended surgical procedure in these patients is the colorectal resection following oncologic criteria. In case of active bleeding, it would be more appropriate to perform a medio-lateral approach with a vascular-first technique [19, 20]. The procedure is otherwise the same as an elective standard colectomy. The choice between end-stoma and anastomosis should be done according to patient's conditions and comorbidities. According to the surgeon's preference, the bowel division can be performed intra- or extracorporeally. If an anastomosis is fashioned, the specimen can be extracted through a mini-Pfannestiel incision, while in case of an end-stoma through the stoma site.

22.3 Discussion

Up to date, few papers have been published on the use of laparoscopy in emergency colorectal resection, most of them include both benign and malignant diseases and there are no RCT. Nevertheless, the results are mostly encouraging, with evidence of shorter length of stay and comparable morbidity and mortality between laparoscopic and open emergency colorectal resections. However, the fact that in many studies patients treated by laparoscopy tend to be younger, fitter and with earlier-stage diseases raises concerns of selection bias [21]. In the trial by Ng et al., including 43 patients with obstructing right CRC (14 laparoscopically assisted and 29 open), the two groups had comparable tumour stage, and minimally invasive surgery showed to be safe and feasible, significantly reduced the blood loss and allowed an earlier mobilisation [22].

In the observational propensity score-matched analysis of emergency CRC resections (36 laparoscopic vs. 72 open) performed by Odermatt et al., laparoscopy was associated with a significant higher lymph-node harvesting and shorter length of stay, with no difference in overall and recurrence-free 3-year survival between the two groups [23].

The recent systematic review and meta-analysis by Xu et al., including 11 studies on emergency colorectal resections for both benign and malignant conditions (286 laparoscopic vs. 466 open), showed how the minimally invasive technique is more time consuming but is associated with significant lower morbidity and shorter postoperative recovery (time to normal diet, bowel movements and length of stay). Comparable results between the two groups were found in terms of reoperation, mortality and lymph-node harvesting [24].

The British multicentre national prospective study is the largest and most recent published trial on minimally invasive surgery in emergency CRC resections (3435 laparoscopic vs. 12,081 open). Despite it is mainly used for young and fit patients with early right-sided CRC, laparoscopy has no higher readmission or reoperation rates and allows significantly shorter length of stay and a lower 90-day mortality [21].

22.4 Conclusions

Although laparoscopy is widely used in elective colorectal surgery, its acceptance in the emergency setting is still rare and considered unsafe. This is probably mainly due to the fact that in case of obstructing, perforated or bleeding tumour, the surgical field is impaired or the anatomical planes are unclear but also by the usual business of emergency theatres that don't allow long laparoscopic procedures. Even if no RCTs have ever been run yet, the scientific literature confirms the safety and feasibility of this technique that are associated with significant postoperative advantages. Undoubtedly, in order to safely perform these procedures, patients should be carefully selected, a highly skilled and experienced surgeon is required and adequate theatre time and setting as well as surgical equipment should be available.

References

1. Global Burden of Disease Cancer Collaboration, Fitzmaurice C, Allen C, et al. Global, regional, and national cancer incidence, mortality, years of life lost, years lived with disability, and disability-adjusted life-years for 32 cancer groups, 1990 to 2015: a systematic analysis for the Global Burden of Disease Study. JAMA Oncol. 2017;3:524.

2. Renzi C, Lyratzopoulos G, Card T, Chu TP, Macleod U, Rachet B. Do colorectal cancer patients diagnosed as an emergency differ from non-emergency patients in their consultation patterns and symptoms? A longitudinal data-linkage study in England. Br J Cancer. 2016;115(7):866–75. Epub 2016 Aug 18.
3. Jestin P, Nilsson J, Heurgren M, Påhlman L, Glimelius B, Gunnarsson U. Emergency surgery for colonic cancer in a defined population. Br J Surg. 2005;92(1):94–100.
4. Di Saverio S. Emergency laparoscopy: a new emerging discipline for treating abdominal emergencies attempting to minimize costs and invasiveness and maximize outcomes and patients' comfort. J Trauma Acute Care Surg. 2014;77(2):338–50.
5. Agresta F, Ansaloni L, Baiocchi GL, Bergamini C, Campanile FC, Carlucci M, Cocorullo G, Corradi A, Franzato B, Lupo M, Mandalà V, Mirabella A, Pernazza G, Piccoli M, Staudacher C, Vettoretto N, Zago M, Lettieri E, Levati A, Pietrini D, Scaglione M, De Masi S, De Placido G, Francucci M, Rasi M, Fingerhut A, Uranüs S, Garattini S. Laparoscopic approach to acute abdomen from the Consensus Development Conference of the Società Italiana di Chirurgia Endoscopica e nuove tecnologie (SICE), Associazione Chirurghi Ospedalieri Italiani (ACOI), Società Italiana di Chirurgia (SIC), Società Italiana di Chirurgia d'Urgenza e del Trauma (SICUT), Società Italiana di Chirurgia nell'Ospedalità Privata (SICOP), and the European Association for Endoscopic Surgery (EAES). Surg Endosc. 2012;26(8):2134–64. Epub 2012 Jun 27.
6. Faucheron JL, Paquette B, Trilling B, Heyd B, Koch S, Mantion G. Emergency surgery for obstructing colonic cancer: a comparison between right-sided and left-sided lesions. Eur J Trauma Emerg Surg. 2018;44:71–7.
7. Birindelli A, Segalini E, Kwan S, Biscardi A, Tonini V, Di Saverio S. Challenging emergency laparoscopic right colectomy for completely obstructing caecal carcinoma a video vignette. Colorectal Dis. 2017;19(5):504–6.
8. Self-expandable metal stents for obstructing colonic and extracolonic cancer. European Society of Gastrointestinal Endoscopy (ESGE) Clinical Guidelines. https://www.giejournal.org/article/S0016-5107%2814%2902197-X/pdf.
9. Sabbagh C, Browet F, Diouf M, Cosse C, Brehant O, Bartoli E, Mauvais F, Chauffert B, Dupas JL, Nguyen-Khac E, Regimbeau JM. Is stenting as "a bridge to surgery" an oncologically safe strategy for the management of acute, left-sided, malignant, colonic obstruction? A comparative study with a propensity score analysis. Ann Surg. 2013;258(1):107–15.
10. Maruthachalam K, Lash GE, Shenton BK, Horgan AF. Tumour cell dissemination following endoscopic stent insertion. Br J Surg. 2007;94(9):1151–4.
11. Di Saverio S, Birindelli A, Segalini E, Novello M, Larocca A, Ferrara F, Binda GA, Bassi M. "To stent or not to stent?": immediate emergency surgery with laparoscopic radical colectomy with CME and primary anastomosis is feasible for obstructing left coloncarcinoma. Surg Endosc. 2018;32(4):2151–5. Epub 2017 Aug 8.
12. Di Saverio S, Segalini E, Birindelli A, Mwangwemi C, Podda M. Laparoscopic extended right and transverse colectomy with completely intracorporeal ileodescending anastomosis for obstructing colon carcinoma a video vignette. Colorectal Dis. 2018;20(1):80–2.
13. Di Saverio S, Birindelli A, Mandrioli M, Podda M, Binda GA. Intracorporeal anastomoses in emergency laparoscopic colorectal surgery from a series of 59 cases: where and how to do it a technical note and video. Colorectal Dis. 2017;19(4):O103–7.
14. van Oostendorp S, Elfrink A, Borstlap W, Schoonmade L, Sietses C, Meijerink J, Tuynman J. Intracorporeal versus extracorporeal anastomosis in right hemicolectomy: a systematic review and meta-analysis. Surg Endosc. 2017;31(1):64–77. Epub 2016 Jun 10.
15. Zielinski MD, Merchea A, Heller SF, You YN. Emergency management of perforated colon cancers: how aggressive should we be? J Gastrointest Surg. 2011;15:2232–8.
16. Ogawa M, Watanabe M, Eto K, Omachi T, Kosuge M, Hanyu K, Noaki L, Fujita T, Yanaga K. Clinicopathological features of perforated colorectal cancer. Anticancer Res. 2009;29(5):1681–4.
17. Di Saverio S, Vennix S, Birindelli A, Weber D, Lombardi R, Mandrioli M, Tarasconi A, Bemelman WA. Pushing the envelope: laparoscopy and primary anastomosis are technically feasible in stable patients with Hinchey IV perforated acute diverticulitis and gross faeculent peritonitis. Surg Endosc. 2016;30(12):5656–64.

18. ASGE Standards of Practice Committee. The role of endoscopy in the patient with lower GI bleeding. Gastrointest Endosc. 2014;79(6). https://www.asge.org/docs/default-source/education/practice_guidelines/doc-2014_the-role-of-endoscopy-in-the-patient-with-lower-gi-bleeding.pdf?sfvrsn=8.
19. Poon JT, Law WL, Fan JK, Lo OS. Impact of the standardized medial-to-lateral approach on outcome of laparoscopic colorectal resection. World J Surg. 2009;33(10):2177–82.
20. Honaker M, Scouten S, Sacksner J, Ziegler M, Wasvary H. A medial to lateral approach offers a superior lymph node harvest for laparoscopic right colectomy. Int J Colorectal Dis. 2016;31(3):631–4. Epub 2016 Jan 22.
21. Vallance AE, Keller DS, Hill J, Braun M, Kuryba A, van der Meulen J, Walker K, Chand M. Role of emergency laparoscopic colectomy for colorectal cancer. A population-based study in England. Ann Surg. 2018. https://doi.org/10.1097/SLA.0000000000002752
22. Ng S, Lee J, Yiu R, Li J, Leung W, Leung K. Emergency laparoscopic-assisted versus open right hemicolectomy for obstructing right-sided colonic carcinoma: a comparative study of short-term clinical outcomes. World J Surg. 2008;32:454–8.
23. Odermatt M, Miskovic D, Siddiqi N, Khan J, Parvaiz A. Short- and long-term outcomes after laparoscopic versus open emergency resection for colon cancer: an observational propensity score-matched study. World J Surg. 2013;37:2458–67.
24. Xu S, Jia Z, Zhu Y, Zhang R, Wang P. Emergent laparoscopic colectomy is an effective alternative to open resection for benign and malignant diseases: a meta-analysis. Indian J Surg. 2017;79(2):116–23.

23 Indications for Open Abdomen in Colorectal Cancer Emergency

Gennaro Perrone and Fausto Catena

23.1 Introduction

Temporary abdominal closure (TAC) or open abdominal (OA) techniques have been described for the first time over 120 years ago by McCosh [1].

The OA procedure is defined as intentionally leaving the non-approximate abdominal fascia edges (laparotomy). From that moment, this technique has been used more and more frequently. However this clinical approach to a critically ill patient at that time was unusual and while again referred to by Ogilvie in the mid-1940s only recently became popular in patients undergoing damage control surgery (DCS) [2]. The "old" paradigm of closing the abdomen at "any cost" has been definitively overcome by the evidence of literature. Obviously this technique must be performed by expert surgeons, especially because it provides precise timing for the closure of the abdomen and the eventual restoration of intestinal continuity.

Despite the OA being applied in many situations where it is necessary to prevent or treat intra-abdominal hypertension (IAP) and possibly abdominal compartment syndrome (ACS), until a few years ago there were no univocal works regarding epidemiology, the various techniques of execution of the procedure and the deferred closure due to the heterogeneity of the same studies and the large cohorts of the patients treated with the same procedures. In this chapter, the various wall closing techniques and the packaging of the procedure in the first instance will not be dealt with. The World Society of Emergency Surgery (WSES) and the Panamerican Trauma Society (PTS) promoted the International Register of Open Abdomen (IROA) [3]. The register has had the merit not only of bringing together all the cases involved but also of comparing them and finding a common front for the improvement of the procedures in order to bring order to such a chaos. In fact, it served as a stimulus for the execution of targeted studies and guidance for newbies.

G. Perrone · F. Catena (✉)
Emergency Surgery Department, Parma University Hospital, Parma, Italy

N. de'Angelis et al. (eds.), *Emergency Surgical Management of Colorectal Cancer*, Hot Topics in Acute Care Surgery and Trauma,
https://doi.org/10.1007/978-3-030-06225-5_23

23.2 Why OA in Colorectal Cancer?

The use of OA associated with the DCS is directed towards two objectives that are controlling the bleeding and contamination of the peritoneal cavity, leaving the abdomen open to decompress or facilitate the subsequent planned re-laparotomy.

Among the causes that most require the use of this technique, we have above all the peritonitis and the traumas that represent about 70% of the cases. Pancreatitis, haemorrhages, intestinal infarcts and increased intra-abdominal pressure after surgery are other possible causes that require OA [4].

Colorectal cancer, in certain cases, can benefit from OA as a primary treatment. This cause falls within 4% of various causes that the IROA identifies as possible cases from OA. However, approximately 20% of patients with colorectal carcinoma are initially seen with stage IV disease, and their 5-year survival is dismal [5].

Obstruction was an important indicator of prognosis, independent of Dukes' stage. Bowel perforation is associated with poor prognosis in disease-free survival. Rectal bleeding had a positive impact on survival. Thus, obstruction, perforation, and rectal bleeding (but not location) are found to be prognostic factors in patients with Dukes' B2 or C colon cancer [6].

The perioperative mortality rate for perforated colorectal cancer at the site of the cancer was 9% and for obstructive colorectal cancer, 5%. Perioperative mortality was much greater for perforations of the colon and rectum occurring proximal to the cancer (31%). Survival was worse for patients with obstruction (33%) or perforation proximal to the cancer (33%). The site of perforation did not appear to impact the 5-year survival, although the numbers are relatively small [7].

Neoplastic colonic stenosis mainly affects the left colon. This event can occur slowly and subtly while the explosion of the symptomatology is dramatic. The patient shows all the classic signs of low intestinal obstruction. In case of continence of the caecal valve, an abnormal colonic distension occurs which can in many cases, after failure of endoscopic decompression, lead to emergency surgery. When the treatment is not timely, upstream perforation can occur, especially at the caecal level where the distension creates points of parietal weakness. Loop colostomy is a historical component of the therapeutic scheme staged for intestinal occlusion by left colon cancer. Initially, as a first step, the obstruction is managed by decompressive colostomy. The second step takes place a few weeks later when the tumour is resected and the colostomy is closed. Alternatively, the colostomy can be closed in a third step based on the patient's clinical picture [8].

Usually in situations of this type, after careful evaluation of the surgeon and the resuscitator, OA can be a valid therapeutic option. The reasons for this choice are linked to a cleaning of the peritoneal cavity which leads to a reclamation of the peritonitis and to a revaluation of the vascular tropism of the intestinal stumps (Photos 23.1–23.3). Advantages of a choice of this type are linked to the execution of an anastomosis in a stable anaesthesiological phase and with the inflammatory focus under control. When valve is incontinent, generalized intestinal distension, severe bowel wall oedema and inflammation can be present. Such situations of

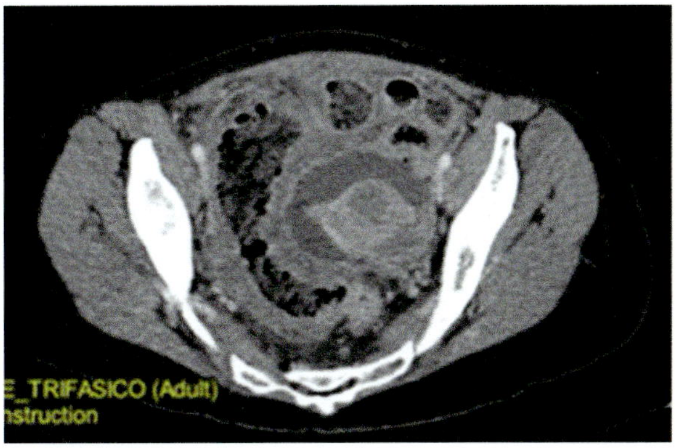

Photo 23.1 Abscess

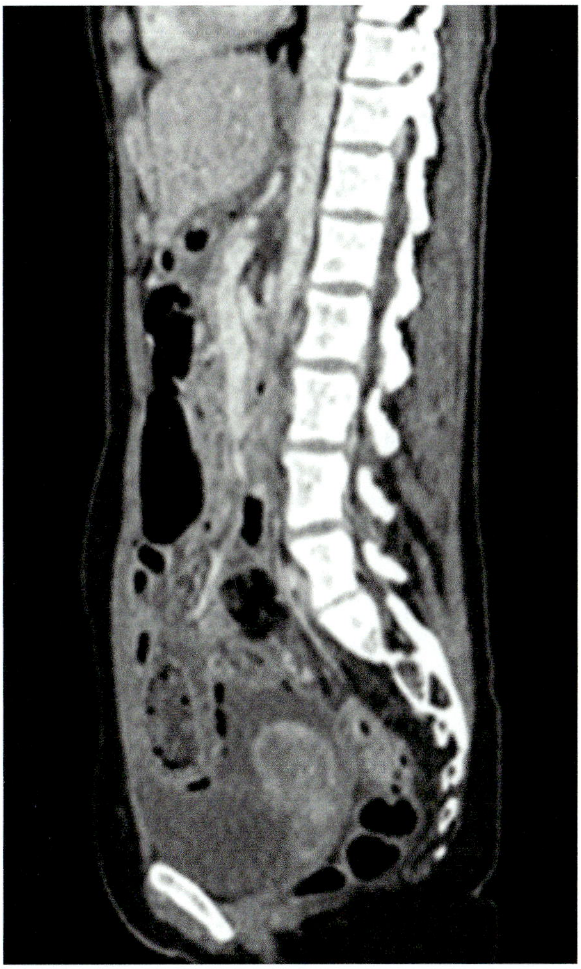

Photo 23.2 Colorectal cancer

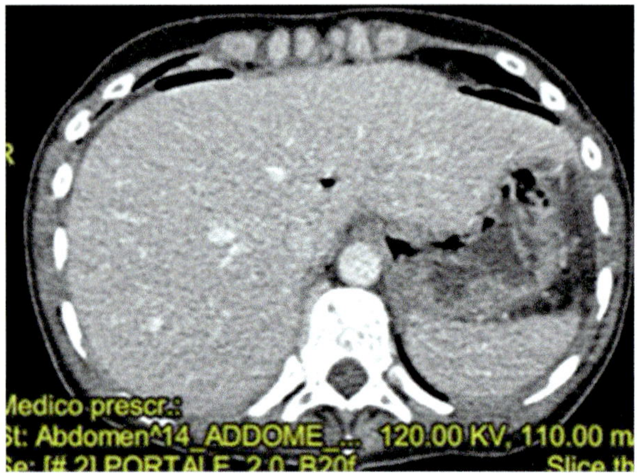

Photo 23.3 Free perihepatic liquid

intestinal distension can lead in rare cases to an increase in intra-abdominal pressure (IAP) which can result in abdominal compartment syndrome.

When obstructive colitis becomes fulminant, it is known as "acute necrotizing colitis". In these conditions, all the more reason, since there is no scientific evidence about the causes, the intestinal revaluation after a few days allows us to re-evaluate the visceral vasculature to establish a more adequate surgical strategy [9].

Patients who arrive with a critical situation and who need a DCS, whatever their aetiology, are candidates for OA. This procedure in patients with colon cancer does not have any prognostic improvement in the neoplastic pathology but only serves to give the possibility of immediate survival. The neoplastic cause will be faced in conditions of clinical stability of the patient in compliance with the DCS. Obviously in cases where colic resection is possible in case of perforation, it is strongly recommended in the first instance to eliminate the underlying cause of sepsis [10].

References

1. McCosh AJ. The treatment of general septic peritonitis. Ann Surg. 1897;25(6):687–97.
2. Ogilvie WH. The late complications of abdominal war wounds. Lancet. 1940;2:253–6. https://doi.org/10.1016/S0140-6736(01)08769-4.
3. Coccolini F, Catena F, Montori G, Ceresoli M, Manfredi R, Nita GE, Moore EE, Biffl W, Ivatury R, Whelan J, et al. IROA: the International Register of Open Abdomen: an international effort to better understand the open abdomen: call for participants. World J Emerg Surg. 2015;10:37. Epub 2015 Aug 16.
4. Coccolini F, Montori G, Ceresoli M, Catena F, Ivatury R, Sugrue M, Sartelli M, Fugazzola P, Corbella D, Salvetti F, Negoi I, Zese M, Occhionorelli S, Maccatrozzo S, Shlyapnikov S, Galatioto C, Chiarugi M, Demetrashvili Z, Dondossola D, Yovtchev Y, Ioannidis O, Novelli G, Nacoti M, Khor D, Inaba K, Demetriades D, Kaussen T, Jusoh AC, Ghannam W, Sakakushev B, Guetta O, Dogjani A, Costa S, Singh S, Damaskos D, Isik A, Yuan K-C, Trotta F, Rausei S, Martinez-Perez A, Bellanova G, Fonseca VC, Hernández F, Marinis A, Fernandes W, Quiodettis M, Bala M, Vereczkei A, Curado RL, Fraga GP, Pereira BM, Gachabayov M, Chagerben GP, Arellano ML, Ozyazici S, Costa G, Tezcaner T,

Ansaloni L. IROA: International Register of Open Abdomen, preliminary results. World J Emerg Surg. 2017;12:10.

5. Young A, Rea D. ABC of colorectal cancer: treatment of advanced disease. BMJ. 2000;321(7271):1278–81.
6. Steinberg SM, Barkin JS, Kaplan RS, Stablein DM. Prognostic indicators of colon tumors. The Gastrointestinal Tumor Study Group experience. Cancer. 1986;57(9):1866–70.
7. Chen HS, Sheen-Chen SM. Obstruction and perforation in colorectal adenocarcinoma: an analysis of prognosis and current trends. Surgery. 2000;127(4):370–6.
8. Ansaloni L, Andersson RE, Bazzoli F, Catena F, Cennamo V, Di Saverio S, Fuccio L, Jeekel H, Leppäniemi A, Moore E, Pinna AD, Pisano M, Repici A, Sugarbaker PH, Tuech JJ. Guidelines in the management of obstructing cancer of the left colon: consensus conference of the World Society of Emergency Surgery (WSES) and Peritoneum and Surgery (PnS) society. World J Emerg Surg. 2010;5:29. https://doi.org/10.1186/1749-7922-5-29.
9. Matsunaga H, Shida D, Kamesaki M, Hamabe Y. Acute necrotizing colitis due to sigmoid colon cancer. World J Surg Oncol. 2014;12:19.
10. Beckman M, Paul J, Neideen T, Weigelt JA. Role of the open abdomen in critically ill patients. Crit Care Clin. 2016;32(2):255–64. https://doi.org/10.1016/j.ccc.2015.12.003.

Difficult Decisions in Colorectal Cancer in Emergency Settings

24

Gianluca Pellino, António S. Soares, and Matteo Frasson

24.1 Introduction

Colorectal cancer is an extremely common disease (see Chap. 2). This means that the range of possible presentations can be dramatically varied posing significant problems for the treating clinician, be it a surgeon or not. In this chapter we will approach difficult decisions in the management of critically ill patients and pregnant patients with colorectal cancer. Given the necessity of optimal communication with the patient, a short section on communication about serious illness is included in the end of the chapter.

24.2 Concomitant Colorectal Cancer in Critically Ill Patients

If a patient with colorectal cancer (CRC) become critically ill, it is fundamental to answer two questions: (1) should the patient be admitted to the intensive care unit (ICU) and if so (2) to what extent should intensive care measures be provided [1]?

Gianluca Pellino and António S. Soares contributed equally to this chapter.

G. Pellino
Unit of Colorectal Surgery, University Hospital "La Fe", Valencia, Spain

Department of Advanced Medical and Surgical Sciences,
Università della Campania "Luigi Vanvitelli", Naples, Italy

A. S. Soares
Department of Surgery and Interventional Sciences, University College London Hospitals, NHS Trusts, GENIE Centre, University College London, London, UK
e-mail: antonio.soares.17@ucl.ac.uk

M. Frasson (✉)
Unit of Colorectal Surgery, University Hospital "La Fe", Valencia, Spain

N. de'Angelis et al. (eds.), *Emergency Surgical Management of Colorectal Cancer*, Hot Topics in Acute Care Surgery and Trauma,
https://doi.org/10.1007/978-3-030-06225-5_24

It is important to consider not only the short-term prognosis of ICU and hospital discharge and 30-day mortality, but also consideration should be given to the long-term outcome and quality of life of the patient. These questions are highly complex, and therefore the need for a multidisciplinary approach should be emphasized. This section will cover epidemiology of CRC patients requiring ICU admission, criteria and timing of ICU admission, end of life in ICU and gaps in current literature. Management of specific complications have been addressed in previous chapters and therefore will not be approached in this chapter.

24.2.1 Epidemiology and Outcomes

Surgical patients can be admitted to ICU after elective surgery, after urgent/emergent surgery and for medical reasons. Variability in the definition of these patient groups in the literature makes comparisons across studies difficult. The admission of patients to ICU after elective cancer surgery has been described in the Dutch National Intensive Care Evaluation registry in admissions from 2007 to 2012, including 28,973 patients (9% of total ICU admissions) [2]. Patients submitted to surgery for gastrointestinal cancer had the highest ICU and hospital mortality, specifically in the case of CRC (OR 1.41, $p < 0.05$) on multivariate analysis. Median ICU admission length after elective surgery was 0.9 days and mechanical ventilation and vasopressor use were the most prevalent supportive measures in place. A different cohort study followed patients for 2 years after the diagnosis of cancer in the west region of Scotland, including 2561 cases of colorectal CRC [3]; 16.5% of these patients required ICU admission. Non-planned admission was associated with lower mortality if patients were admitted for surgical causes as opposed to medical admissions (38.2% versus 52.6%, respectively). In a longitudinal cohort study of 39,734 cancer patients in England, Wales and Northern Ireland between 1997 and 2013, 33.8% of which had CRC, unplanned admission after either elective (OR 0.27) or urgent (OR 0.57) surgery was significantly related to decreased mortality compared with medical admissions in patients with cancer [4]. In a European cohort study, patients with solid tumours represented 12.8% of admissions from a total of 3147 patients admitted to ICU [5]. Patients with cancer had a significantly higher mortality if they presented with at least three organ failures—75% vs. 45% in patients admitted with no cancer.

A prospective cohort study assessed the longer-term survival and quality of life of cancer patients admitted to ICU in two units in Brazil [6]; 792 patients were included, of which 35.1% had digestive tract cancer, and were assessed over 18 months after admission. Half of patients were admitted after elective surgery. In surgical patients, survival at 12 months was significantly higher after elective admissions (60%) than after urgent admissions (25%). Quality of life after elective admission, assessed through EQ-5D-3L and its utility dimension, improved at the end of follow-up (baseline 0.57 vs. 0.68). Care should be taken in examining these results due to the immortal time bias.

24.2.2 Admission to ICU

Critical illness can occur at every stage of CRC natural history, from diagnosis to terminal disease. It is important to bear in mind that the lack of physiological reserve can have a profound impact on the way colorectal cancer can be approached. A working group has provided recommendations on the criteria and goals of ICU admissions for cancer patients [7] while also noting that these should not replace the individual clinical judgement as the correct assessment of an individual patient's prognosis is far from perfect. Interestingly, the existence of a daily meeting between an oncologist and an intensivist has shown to be associated with decreased mortality in cancer patients admitted to ICU, as well as improved use of resources [8]. There is no mention to the role of a daily meeting between surgeons and intensivists in the same paper.

Admission criteria: curative admission without primary limitations can be recommended for the following group of patients [9] (Table 24.1).

The cut-off for substantial lifespan is arbitrary but has been considered as 1 year for some authors [1].

Other clinical situations: patients do not always fall in these categories [1]. For these patients, who may have the option of life-prolonging therapies, a time-limited ICU trial may be proposed. All the available therapeutic options are employed, and a readjustment of treatment goals takes place after a defined period. This should be no less than 3 days but ideally should be at least 5 days. This allows for an assessment of the patient's response to treatment [9]. The proposal of the ICU trial is based on the work by Lecuyer et al. [10]. In this trial, organ failure scores at the day 6 of ICU admission were better predictors of survival than the scores on admission or 3 days after admission. The best duration for a time-limited trial can also be biased by clinical judgement. This question has been assessed by a simulation-based approach by Shrime et al. [11] which concluded that for solid cancers a duration of 1–4 days may be sufficient as survival was similar compared with unlimited duration of admission. This clinical situation should be an exception and therefore a minority of cases. After admission for a trial, the clinical team should bear in mind the risk of disproportionate care and try to mitigate it. Patients with no further life-prolonging cancer treatment, with a predicted lifespan <1 year, on anticancer treatment or with a poor performance status in the months before critical illness should generally not be admitted to ICU [1]. Patients can however be admitted exceptionally if the poor performance status is due to cancer and there is a possibility of antineoplastic treatment. Patients on clinical trials can also fall within this group. Furthermore, prophylactic ICU admissions can occur if there is a strong possibility of clinical deterioration. In the postoperative period, this can be justified for some patients. While this is not consensual, there can be admissions for palliative reasons [1]. This situation should be preceded by a careful consideration of the goals of treatment which should be defined in advance.

Table 24.1 Cancer patient groups with indication for ICU admission without primary limitations [9]

Curative therapeutic options available
Cure is not likely but expected lifespan is substantial
Remission of malignancy

24.2.3 Timing of Admission

Early ICU admission leads to improved outcomes. This has been shown in the case of respiratory failure [10, 12] and severe sepsis or septic shock [12, 13]. Such studies are limited with regard to the applicability to colorectal cancer patients due to the heterogeneous groups of patients included but remain nonetheless a useful framework. This approach has been recommended by expert consensus [1, 9]. Organ dysfunction should be assessed daily in patients admitted to wards.

24.2.4 End of Life in ICU

While not applied specifically to CRC patients, specific literature has been dedicated to the topic of dying in ICU. An honest discussion should be held with the patient, or a surrogate should take place as soon as possible and ideally before the appearance of critical illness [14, 15]. These are associated with better quality of life, reduced use of nonbeneficial medical care near death, enhanced goal-consistent care, positive family outcomes and reduced costs [16]. In a cohort of patients with metastatic lung or colorectal cancer, a discussion about end-of-life decisions has shown that early discussion (before last 30 days of life) was associated with less aggressive care and increased use of hospice services [17]. Specific recommendations on the withdrawal of care can be found elsewhere [18].

24.2.5 Gaps in Research

There is currently a paucity of data on the overall management of patients with cancer in ICU and specifically cases of colorectal cancer. Marked heterogeneity on the case mix of patients (with regard to disease, disease stage, reason for ICU admission and discharge, patient comorbidities) has hindered comparisons between centres and the synthesis of evidence [7]. Haematological disease is very frequently considered when assessing outcomes of patients with cancer, which may bias results in patients with solid tumours. Larger cohorts of patients admitted to ICU with colorectal cancer should be published, with longitudinal follow-up of survival, disease-free survival and quality of life assessments.

24.3 Colorectal Cancer Diagnosed During Pregnancy: Challenging Treatment Priorities in Emergency Settings

Even if rare, colorectal cancer (CRC) in pregnant women represent a treatment challenge and warrant discussion when dealing with difficult decisions in colorectal surgery in emergency settings.

Several cases of CRC in pregnancy have been reported in the literature; however no agreed guidelines exist on how to deal with these patients. The first unequivocal case was reported in 1842 by Cruveilhier, which described a rectal cancer found during the autopsy of a lady who died days after giving birth to a stillborn baby [19]. According to a recent systematic review of the literature which only included patients diagnosed with CRC during pregnancy (hence removing those who were diagnosed after childbirth), 119 patients have been described between 1947 and 2016 [20]. The pooled incidence risk was as high as 0.002%. There has been an increased trend over time, with papers from the 1950s reporting incidence between 1/100,000 and 1/50,000 [21, 22] versus approximately 1/13,000 deliveries in more recent publications (0.008%) [23]. The age at diagnosis seems to have been decreasing over time [20].

Up to 11% of pregnant patients with CRC might have an emergency presentation, including acute small bowel obstruction and perforation, whereas up to 14% might have constipation which would need subsequent hospitalization and bowel rest [20], overall accounting for one patient out of four requiring emergency surgery. CRC is equally distributed in colon and rectum in pregnant women (53% and 44%, with the remaining having multiple locations) [20], although authors have hypothesized an inverse proportion as compared with the general population of patients with CRC, meaning higher rates of colon cancers in pregnancy [23]; however, this is not the case when CRC diagnosed at delivery are not included [20]. Most patients with CRC diagnosed during pregnancy do not have any risk factors, but more than 3/4 of the patients already had pregnancies [20]. The wide majority of patients are diagnosed during II and III trimester, and they already have distant disease at diagnosis, found in almost 50% of patients [20].

Managing pregnant patients with CRC raises major ethical issues due to the difficulties in establishing priorities. Delayed diagnosis further complicates such a delicate management. Unfortunately, common CRC markers (e.g. carcinoembryonic agent) seem to be less accurate in pregnancy than in general population [24]. However, bleeding is the most common symptom in reported cases, occurring in almost half of patients, probably being overlooked because of misdiagnosed haemorrhoidal disease, a common finding in pregnant women.

There is no agreed treatment algorithm in CRC in pregnancy in emergency settings, but following a stepwise approach could help emergency surgeons in dealing with challenging choices. Approach should be based on cancer site, stage, age of gestation and mother/family will [20].

In patients with resectable disease at diagnosis, if the foetus is viable, a caesarian section/delivery could be considered. When the foetus maturation is yet to be completed, an option could be performing a colostomy in rectal cancer and delay treatment; this should be then guided by mother's will to continue pregnancy. If this is the case, intensive follow-up would be advisable, considering elective resection and facilitation of delivery when possible, delaying stoma closure at a later stage. Should the mother decide not to continue the pregnancy, then conventional treatment options should be evaluated following abortion. In patients with colon cancer and nonviable foetus, either colon stenting or resection with stoma could be considered in obstructing tumours, potentially reserving the latter if stenting fails. Studies have suggested that colon cancer stenting can be a useful bridge to surgery but also to delivery in pregnant patients [25, 26]. Successful stenting would allow elective resection at a later stage, but this should be carefully weighed against the risk of tumour perforation or micro-perforation. Subsequent consequences on the newborn cannot be anticipated. It should also be considered that colon stenting could not be possible because of tumour features and location. Following resolution of the emergent presentation, subsequent treatment should again rely on mother's will.

It has been showed that it is relatively safe for the foetus to continue a pregnancy with CRC, as metastases to the placenta and invasion to the foetus are anecdotal events [27]. Instead, the ideal approach to ovaries and tubes during surgery for CRC in pregnancy is still controversial. Authors failed to show a survival benefit with removal of ovaries at the time of surgery [28], but studies suggested that the risk of metastases to the ovaries is more than 15% higher in pregnant women with CRC [29, 30]. Options include removing ovaries at a later stage, after the delivery, to avoid miscarriage if pregnancy is continued, removing only one ovary, and sampling ovaries intraoperatively to detect tumour growth [20].

Unfortunately, most of CRC during pregnancy are diagnosed at a later stage, and diagnostic modalities to assess distant disease are to be advocated after considering the potential benefits and harms associated with them. Intuitively, MRI should be the ideal tool in pregnant women, in order to reduce exposure to radiation [31]. MRI is the ideal tool to assess local disease in rectal cancer, but its accuracy in detecting distant disease and in staging colon cancer is questionable as compared with CT scan. Lastly, in emergency settings, MRI scan is of limited value because of timing, costs and availability. FDG-PET scan is an important imaging modality in CRC, and its role in ruling out distant disease in primary and recurrent cancers is widely accepted [32, 33]. However, even if the quality of the test could be reduced, low-dose PET scans (18.5 MBq) have been safely performed in pregnant women, bearing in mind that the foetus is more sensitive to radiation at earlier gestational age [34]. PET/MRI has been proposed as an useful tool in oncologic patients, capable of reducing the amount of radiation even if preserving the advantages of a simultaneous morphological and functional study [35]. However, this test has high costs, and most units do not have access to it. Newer imaging modalities and techniques could contribute much to enhancing the quality of care of these patients, eventually improving the outcomes of treatment. Imaging biomarkers and algorithm-based technologies are being studied and could possibly find application in pregnant women in whom the suspicion of CRC is raised.

Irrespective of the imaging assessment of CRC in pregnancy, it is rather disappointing to note that, as above reported, the most common presenting symptom is rectal bleeding. Almost always, a careful history taking and early specialist assessment by a colorectal surgeon could have been able to detect cancer earlier. With regard to this clinical picture (rectal bleeding), when strongly indicated, lower gastrointestinal tract endoscopy can be safely performed in experienced hands even in pregnant women, with cautious manoeuvers [36].

In the event of unresectable distant disease in patients with colon cancer, stenting remains an option, as well as a stoma; delivery or caesarian section should be considered with viable foetus. Under the same circumstances, patients with rectal cancer could benefit from a colostomy, advocating a caesarian section when possible. Vaginal delivery should be discouraged in patients with rectal cancer in pregnancy, because of the possible risks of obstruction to delivery and compression to the mass [21]. Women who have weight loss, unjustified anaemia and fatigue should also be carefully interviewed and assessed.

Timing to start adjuvant or neoadjuvant treatment in pregnant women is debated, and foetus exposure to antineoplastic agents has been investigated only in limited series. Radiotherapy is proscribed unless the mother decides to have abortion or a caesarian section is feasible, according to gestational age. Among cytotoxic agents, 5-fluorouracil seems to have an acceptable safety profile, even if newborns may be smaller and suffer from other long-term effects (e.g. hypothyroidism) [37, 38]. One of the largest series on in utero exposure to chemotherapy included more than 230 patients with breast or ovarian cancer who received taxanes during pregnancy and found that newborns did not have an increased risk of anomalies or growth retardation with a follow-up extending beyond 10 years from birth [39]. Case series have suggested the safety of oxaliplatin treatment as well, either alone or combined with leucovorin and 5-fluorouracil [40, 41].

Survival after surgery for CRC in pregnancy is disturbingly poor as compared with CRC occurring in general population, both because of a trend towards advanced stage at diagnosis and because of intrinsic, biological features of aggressiveness showed by the former. It is likely that hormones and growth factors contribute to a complex carcinogenetic effect [42–44], triggering incipient lesions or promoting rapidly growing tumours, with mechanisms which are yet to be understood. In the context of individual-surgeon variations of outcomes and preferences in CRC, the decision-making is even more challenging in these patients [45, 46]. No guidelines can replace common sense or identify treatment priorities when dealing with two patients at the same time, and treatment must be individualized [47]. Under this light, women with CRC diagnosed during pregnancy needing emergency surgery should be involved in any decision, as long as the condition allows for it. A multidisciplinary team approach is warranted, and—even if it might not always be possible in the acute phase of urgent presentation—individual/single specialty approaches are to be discouraged. Patients and their family should be offered a balanced and sincere view of the possible treatment options and provided with realistic hope.

24.4 Communication

Communication assumes a vital importance with regard to difficult decisions in the management of CRC. Therefore, it is essential to have adequate training in communication and an optimized framework of reference [16]. The discussion of prognosis may be hindered by the perception of the clinician that this will cause harm to the patient. When prognosis is discussed, clinicians tend to be overly optimistic as demonstrated in the systematic review of 1563 individual prediction-survival dyads by Glare et al. [48]. They documented that prediction was correct within 1 week in 25% of patients but incorrect by more than 4 weeks in 27% of cases. When addressing serious illness care planning, the following topics have been proposed to be discussed with the patient [16]: the patient's understanding of prognosis, the decision-making and information preferences, a prognostic disclosure, the patient's goals and fears, acceptable function, trade-offs and family involvement. A checklist has been formulated to facilitate these conversations.

24.5 Conclusions

The optimal management of critically ill or pregnant patients with CRC is still not consensual, and there is no high-level evidence to guide it. Further research should be pursued in this field to improve outcomes, ideally through collaborative efforts. Communication between surgeon and patient remains a cornerstone of good care.

References

1. Schellongowski P, Sperr WR, Wohlfarth P, et al. Critically ill patients with cancer: chances and limitations of intensive care medicine—a narrative review. ESMO Open. 2016;1:e000018. https://doi.org/10.1136/esmoopen-2015-000018.
2. Bos MMEM, Bakhshi-Raiez F, Dekker JWT, et al. Outcomes of Intensive Care Unit admissions after elective cancer surgery. Eur J Surg Oncol. 2013;39:584–92. https://doi.org/10.1016/j.ejso.2013.02.014.
3. Puxty K, McLoone P, Quasim T, et al. Risk of critical illness among patients with solid cancers. JAMA Oncol. 2015;1:1078. https://doi.org/10.1001/jamaoncol.2015.2855.
4. Ostermann M, Ferrando-Vivas P, Gore C, et al. Characteristics and outcome of cancer patients admitted to the ICU in England, Wales, and Northern Ireland and national trends between 1997 and 2013. Crit Care Med. 2017;45:1668–76. https://doi.org/10.1097/CCM.0000000000002589.
5. Taccone F, Artigas AA, Sprung CL, et al. Characteristics and outcomes of cancer patients in European ICUs. Crit Care. 2009;13:R15. https://doi.org/10.1186/cc7713.
6. Normilio-Silva K, De Figueiredo AC, Pedroso-De-Lima AC, et al. Long-term survival, quality of life, and quality-adjusted survival in critically ill patients with cancer. Crit Care Med. 2016;44:1327–37. https://doi.org/10.1097/CCM.0000000000001648.
7. Azoulay E, Soares M, Darmon M, et al. Intensive care of the cancer patient: recent achievements and remaining challenges. Ann Intensive Care. 2011;1:5. https://doi.org/10.1186/2110-5820-1-5.
8. Soares M, Bozza FA, Azevedo LCP, et al. Effects of organizational characteristics on outcomes and resource use in patients with cancer admitted to intensive care units. J Clin Oncol. 2016;34:3315–24. https://doi.org/10.1200/JCO.2016.66.9549.
9. Kiehl MG, Beutel G, Böll B, et al. Consensus statement for cancer patients requiring intensive care support. Ann Hematol. 2018;97:1271–82. https://doi.org/10.1007/s00277-018-3312-y.
10. Lecuyer L, Chevret S, Thiery G, et al. The ICU trial: a new admission policy for cancer patients requiring mechanical ventilation. Crit Care Med. 2007;35:808–14. https://doi.org/10.1097/01.CCM.0000256846.27192.7A.
11. Shrime MG, Ferket BS, Scott DJ, et al. Time-limited trials of intensive care for critically ill patients with cancer how long is long enough? JAMA Oncol. 2016;2:76–83. https://doi.org/10.1001/jamaoncol.2015.3336.
12. Lee D-S, Suh GY, Ryu J-A, et al. Effect of early intervention on long-term outcomes of critically ill cancer patients admitted to ICUs. Crit Care Med. 2015;43:1439–48. https://doi.org/10.1097/CCM.0000000000000989.

13. Torres VB, Azevedo LC, Silva UV, et al. Sepsis-associated outcomes in critically ill patients with malignancies. Ann Am Thorac Soc. 2015. https://doi.org/10.1513/AnnalsATS.201501-046OC.
14. Cook D, Rocker G. Dying with dignity in the intensive care unit. N Engl J Med. 2014;370:2506–14. https://doi.org/10.1056/NEJMra1208795.
15. Kostakou E, Rovina N, Kyriakopoulou M, et al. Critically ill cancer patient in intensive care unit: issues that arise. J Crit Care. 2014;29:817–22. https://doi.org/10.1016/J.JCRC.2014.04.007.
16. Bernacki RE, Block SD. Communication about serious illness care goals: a review and synthesis of best practices. JAMA Intern Med. 2014;174:1994–2003. https://doi.org/10.1001/jamainternmed.2014.5271.
17. Mack JW, Cronin A, Keating NL, et al. Associations between end-of-life discussion characteristics and care received near death: a prospective cohort study. J Clin Oncol. 2012;30:4387–95. https://doi.org/10.1200/JCO.2012.43.6055.
18. Downar J, Delaney JW, Hawryluck L, Kenny L. Guidelines for the withdrawal of life-sustaining measures. Intensive Care Med. 2016;42:1003–17. https://doi.org/10.1007/s00134-016-4330-7.
19. Cruveilhier J. Anatomie pathologique du corps humain, ou descriptions, avec figures lithographiées et coloriées, des diverses altérations morbides dont le corps humain; 1835.
20. Pellino G, Simillis C, Kontovounisios C, et al. Colorectal cancer diagnosed during pregnancy. Eur J Gastroenterol Hepatol. 2017;29:743–53. https://doi.org/10.1097/MEG.0000000000000863.
21. McLean DW, Arminski TC, Bradley GT. Management of primary carcinoma of the rectum diagnosed during pregnancy. Am J Surg. 1955;90:816–25.
22. Moran BJ, Yano H, Al Zahir N, Farquharson M. Conflicting priorities in surgical intervention for cancer in pregnancy. Lancet Oncol. 2007;8:536–44. https://doi.org/10.1016/S1470-2045(07)70171-7.
23. Bernstein MA, Madoff RD, Caushaj PF. Colon and rectal cancer in pregnancy. Dis Colon Rectum. 1993;36:172–8.
24. Mechery J, Ikhena SE. Cancer of the descending colon during pregnancy. J Obstet Gynaecol (Lahore). 2007;27:311–2. https://doi.org/10.1080/01443610701241159.
25. Alonso-Lázaro N, Bustamante-Balén M, Pous-Serrano S, et al. Insertion of self-expanding metal stent for treatment of malignant obstruction in a pregnant woman. Rev Esp Enferm Dig. 2014;106:216–9.
26. Healey AJ, Bansi D, Dhanjal MK, et al. Colorectal stenting: a bridge to both Caesarean section and elective resection in malignant large-bowel obstruction in pregnancy: a multidisciplinary first. Colorectal Dis. 2011;13:e248–9. https://doi.org/10.1111/j.1463-1318.2010.02429.x.
27. Potter JF, Schoeneman M. Metastasis of maternal cancer to the placenta and fetus. Cancer. 1970;25:380–8.
28. Pitluk H, Poticha SM. Carcinoma of the colon and rectum in patients less than 40 years of age. Surg Gynecol Obstet. 1983;157:335–7.
29. Tsukamoto N, Uchino H, Matsukuma K, Kamura T. Carcinoma of the colon presenting as bilateral ovarian tumors during pregnancy. Gynecol Oncol. 1986;24:386–91.
30. Mason MH, Kovalcik PJ. Ovarian metastases from colon carcinoma. J Surg Oncol. 1981;17:33–8.
31. Sayar H, Lhomme C, Verschraegen CF. Malignant adnexal masses in pregnancy. Obstet Gynecol Clin N Am. 2005;32:569–93. https://doi.org/10.1016/j.ogc.2005.08.003.
32. Shim J-R, Lee SD, Han S-S, et al. Prognostic significance of 18F-FDG PET/CT in patients with colorectal cancer liver metastases after hepatectomy. Eur J Surg Oncol. 2018;44:670–6. https://doi.org/10.1016/j.ejso.2018.01.243.
33. Selvaggi F, Fucini C, Pellino G, et al. Outcome and prognostic factors of local recurrent rectal cancer: a pooled analysis of 150 patients. Tech Coloproctol. 2015;19:135–44. https://doi.org/10.1007/s10151-014-1241-x.
34. Loevinger R, Budinger TF (Thomas F, Watson EE, Society of Nuclear Medicine (1953-)). Medical Internal Radiation Dose Committee. MIRD primer for absorbed dose calculations. Rev. ed. New York, NY: Society of Nuclear Medicine; 1991.

35. Catalano OA, Coutinho AM, Sahani DV, et al. Colorectal cancer staging: comparison of whole-body PET/CT and PET/MR. Abdom Radiol (New York). 2017;42:1141–51. https://doi.org/10.1007/s00261-016-0985-3.
36. de Lima A, Zelinkova Z, van der Woude CJ. A prospective study of the safety of lower gastrointestinal endoscopy during pregnancy in patients with inflammatory bowel disease. J Crohns Colitis. 2015;9:519–24. https://doi.org/10.1093/ecco-jcc/jjv079.
37. Woods JB, Martin JN, Ingram FH, et al. Pregnancy complicated by carcinoma of the colon above the rectum. Am J Perinatol. 1992;9:102–10. https://doi.org/10.1055/s-2007-994680.
38. Nesbitt JC, Moise KJ, Sawyers JL. Colorectal carcinoma in pregnancy. Arch Surg. 1985;120:636–40.
39. Cardonick E, Bhat A, Gilmandyar D, Somer R. Maternal and fetal outcomes of taxane chemotherapy in breast and ovarian cancer during pregnancy: case series and review of the literature. Ann Oncol. 2012;23:3016–23. https://doi.org/10.1093/annonc/mds170.
40. Jeppesen JB, Østerlind K. Successful twin pregnancy outcome after in utero exposure to FOLFOX for metastatic colon cancer: a case report and review of the literature. Clin Colorectal Cancer. 2011;10:348–52. https://doi.org/10.1016/j.clcc.2011.06.003.
41. Gensheimer M, Jones CA, Graves CR, et al. Administration of oxaliplatin to a pregnant woman with rectal cancer. Cancer Chemother Pharmacol. 2009;63:371–3. https://doi.org/10.1007/s00280-008-0731-9.
42. Slattery ML, Samowitz WS, Holden JA. Estrogen and progesterone receptors in colon tumors. Am J Clin Pathol. 2000;113:364–8. https://doi.org/10.1309/5MHB-K6XX-QV50-PCJQ.
43. Sica V, Contieri E, Nola E, et al. Estrogen and progesterone binding proteins in human colorectal cancer. A preliminary characterization of estradiol receptor. Tumori. 1981;67:307–14.
44. Arem H, Park Y, Felix AS, et al. Reproductive and hormonal factors and mortality among women with colorectal cancer in the NIH-AARP Diet and Health Study. Br J Cancer. 2015;113:562–8. https://doi.org/10.1038/bjc.2015.224.
45. Augestad KM, Lindsetmo R-O, Stulberg J, et al. International preoperative rectal cancer management: staging, neoadjuvant treatment, and impact of multidisciplinary teams. World J Surg. 2010;34:2689–700. https://doi.org/10.1007/s00268-010-0738-3.
46. García-Granero E, Navarro F, Cerdán Santacruz C, et al. Individual surgeon is an independent risk factor for leak after double-stapled colorectal anastomosis: an institutional analysis of 800 patients. Surgery. 2017;162:1006–16. https://doi.org/10.1016/j.surg.2017.05.023.
47. Pellino G, Warren O, Mills S, et al. Comparison of Western and Asian guidelines concerning the management of colon cancer. Dis Colon Rectum. 2018;61:250–9. https://doi.org/10.1097/DCR.0000000000001012.
48. Glare P, Virik K, Jones M, et al. A systematic review of physicians' survival predictions in terminally ill cancer patients. BMJ. 2003;327:195–8. https://doi.org/10.1136/bmj.327.7408.195.

Future Perspectives in Colorectal Cancer Treatments

25

Mahir Gachabayov and Roberto Bergamaschi

25.1 Introduction

It may have been around two centuries ago that the concepts of tumor excision (transanal for rectal cancer) as well as bowel resection (via laparotomy for colon cancer) surfaced in Germany [1] and France [2], respectively. For decades, surgery has been led by expert opinions legitimizing rituals characterized by corrective (rather than preventive) actions aiming at avoiding recurrence (rather than occurrence) of adverse events. Even when evidence-based medicine became widely accepted, the random-order study design [3] had limited impact on innovation, which by far has to be attributed to individual surgeons [4–6]. In fact, one of the most disappointing grants of the National Institute of Health was assigned to randomizing open colectomy to a laparoscopic-facilitated colectomy, where nothing except the mobilization of the colon was performed laparoscopically. In the COST trial, most surgeons were learning laparoscopy during the study, and the only part of the operation actually randomized was the order with which the colon mobilization and the laparotomy were carried out [7]. The opposite should be said for the Swedish Rectal Cancer Trial, which must be acknowledged as a true random-order effort to improving the cancer-specific outcomes of rectal cancer patients [8]. Rightfully so, the inherent limitations as well as safety hazards of chemotherapy have become widely known contributing to alternative therapies [9]. An attempt is made herein to give the reader a succinct insight of the immediate and near future perspectives in

Disclaimers: Conflict of interest—None; Previously copyrighted material—None; Funding—None.

M. Gachabayov · R. Bergamaschi (✉)
Section of Colorectal Surgery, Department of Surgery, Westchester Medical Center, New York Medical College, Valhalla, NY, USA

N. de'Angelis et al. (eds.), *Emergency Surgical Management of Colorectal Cancer*, Hot Topics in Acute Care Surgery and Trauma,
https://doi.org/10.1007/978-3-030-06225-5_25

colorectal cancer treatments. This chapter does not intend to offer a comprehensive review of the topic; rather, it highlights some controversial issues and then outlines the role of future perspectives in value-based care.

25.2 Currently Unfolding Innovations

25.2.1 Indocyanine Green Fluorescence Imaging to Minimize Anastomotic Leak Rates

Assessing the blood supply of the bowel during surgery can be a difficult task even for experienced surgeons. Laser-assisted indocyanine green (ICG) fluorescent dye angiography can provide intraoperative visual assessment of blood flow to the bowel wall and surrounding tissues, allowing for modification to the surgical plan, which often is in the patients' best interest. We have used ICG angiography for small bowel ischemia and left colorectal resections and collected data prospectively in a single center during a 1-year period. ICG angiography played a major role in the intraoperative decision-making of several patients. In case of acute small intestine ischemia, resection was not warranted unless absolute perfusion units were below 19 (relative 21%). When evaluating blood supply to the left colon prior to anastomosing in the context of a Hartmann's reversal, resection is recommended with absolute units lower than 18 (relative 31%) even if the bowel appears macroscopically perfused [10].

25.2.2 Could D3 Extended Mesenterectomy Improve Accuracy of N Staging for Adjuvant Chemotherapy?

Although we have come a long way since 1732, when George Arnaud de Ronsil performed the first right colectomy [11], we are still performing D2 node dissection in the Western world. Despite sharing a common goal, high tie, complete mesenteric excision (CME), and D3 extended mesenterectomy may not be synonymous [12]. While a high tie clearly alludes to a central vascular ligation, it does not necessarily entail removal of all mesenteric adipose tissue with lymph nodes surrounding the vessel origins. On the other hand, CME represents a combination of such a high tie with meticulous dissection along embryological planes, the benefit of which is generally accepted but not proven. Lymph nodes within the D3 area draining the right colon have been mapped in detail, demonstrating nodes surrounding both the superior mesenteric vein and the artery, undoubtedly lying posteriorly [13]. The removal of all D3 lymph nodes can be referred to as D3 extended mesenterectomy. Preoperative awareness of the vascular anatomy by CTA can be used as a road map to prevent and/or control bleeding [14], thus rendering D3 extended mesenterectomy safer. Another concern raised with D3 extended mesenterectomy regards the unavoidable transection of the superior mesenteric nerve plexus with possible alterations in bowel function. A study of patients having right colectomy comparing D3 extended mesenterectomy to D2 lymphadenectomy has shown increased frequency of defecation with no impact upon quality of life [15]. The question whether some form of extended lymph node dissection should be implemented in clinical practice has generated much discussion among surgeons, although not resulting so far in any prospective trial. Lack of training in the demanding dissection in the root of the mesentery of the right colon is likely to be a major obstacle, a phenomenon not unknown from previous debates on improvements in surgical technique, that resulted in better cancer care. On the other hand, skip lymph node metastases were detected in 20% of patients who underwent D3 extended mesenterectomy with upstaging in 4.5% from stage II to stage III (N0 w/ D2 and CME) [16].

25.2.3 Can Robotic Dissection Increase the Rates of Uninvolved Circumferential Resection Margin in Rectal Cancer?

Since 2014, the results of four RCTs have been published: ACOSOG Z6051 [17], ALaCart [18], COLOR II [19], and COREAN [20]. While the primary endpoints were identical for ACOSOG Z6051 and ALaCart (CRM, distal margin, and TME quality), the COLOR II and COREAN trial evaluated local recurrence and 3-year survival. The Z6051 trial enrolled 486 patients in a 1:1 ratio of laparoscopic to open resection. Participating surgeons underwent rigorous credentialing. By protocol design, all patients received neoadjuvant chemoradiation. Successful resection was defined as the achievement of a CRM <1 mm, "complete" and "near complete" TME, and a clear distal margin defined as <5 cm, <2 cm, and <1 mm for upper, mid-, and low rectal lesion. The overall negative CRM rate was 90% in both arms. The rates of negative CRM and complete/near complete TME quality were 88% and 92% and 92% and 95%, respectively, in the laparoscopic and open arms. Successful resection was achieved in 82% of the laparoscopic cases and in 87% of the open counterpart. The authors concluded that "laparoscopic resection … failed to meet the criteria for non-inferiority for pathologic outcomes." Hence "the findings do not support the use of laparoscopic resection in these patients" [17].

The ALaCart trial enrolled 475 patients in a 1:1 ratio. Participating surgeons underwent rigorous credentialing. By protocol design, patients received neoadjuvant chemoradiation based on surgeons' and/or patients' preference. Patients with T4 tumors or involved CRM on preoperative imaging were excluded. The rates of negative CRM and complete/near complete TME were 93% and 97% and 87% and 92%, respectively, in the laparoscopic and open arms. Successful resection was achieved in 82% of the laparoscopic arms and in 89% of the open counterpart. The authors concluded that "Non-inferiority of laparoscopic surgery …was not established." Hence "these findings do not provide sufficient evidence for the routine use of laparoscopic surgery" [18].

The COLOR II included over 1000 patients recruited in a 2:1 ratio. Participating surgeons underwent rigorous credentialing. The negative CRM defined as C2 mm was 90% in both arms, and the rate of complete TME was 84% and 88% in the laparoscopic and open arms, respectively. T3 tumors within 2 mm of the endopelvic fascia were excluded. The locoregional recurrence at 3 years was 5% in both arms. Disease-free and overall survival rates were 75% and 87% for laparoscopic surgery versus 71% and 84% for open surgery. Statistically different rates of CRM involvement were found in the subgroup of patients with cancer of the lower third of the rectum: 9% for laparoscopy and 22% for open surgery. These were associated with 4% and 12% 3-year locoregional recurrence rates, respectively. The authors concluded that "laparoscopic surgery…was associated with rates of locoregional recurrence and disease-free and overall survival similar to those for open surgery" [19].

The COREAN trial enrolled 340 patients in a 1:1 ratio. Participating surgeons underwent rigorous credentialing. The negative CRM defined as C1 mm was 90% in both arms, and the rate of complete TME was 92% and 88% in the laparoscopic and open arms, respectively. All included patients had been clinically diagnosed with cT3N0–2M0 rectal on preoperative imaging. The locoregional recurrence at 3 years was 4.9% (95% CI 2.5–9.6) in open and 2.6% (95% CI 1.0–6.7) in the laparoscopic arm. Disease-free and overall survival rates were 79.2% and 91.7% for laparoscopy versus 72.5% and 90.4% for open surgery. Complete or near complete TME was successfully achieved in 88% of open and 92% of laparoscopic arms. Negative CRM was achieved in 96% of open and 97% of laparoscopic cases. The authors concluded that "laparoscopic resection for locally advanced rectal cancer after preoperative chemoradiotherapy provides similar outcomes … as open resection, thus justifying its use" [20].

A closer look at the four trials reveals a number of serious limitations. The selection of patients with regard to T stage is questionable. COREAN included only T3 lesions, ALaCart excluded T4 and tumors with involved CRM at CT scan, and the COLOR II and ACOSOG trials excluded T4 cancers. The distribution of patients with regard to the selection of only T3 in the COREAN trial and exclusion of tumors with involved CRM at CT scan in the ALaCart trial need to be questioned. Furthermore, neoadjuvant chemoradiation was given to all of the Z6051 and COREAN trial patients, 50% of the ALaCart patients, and less than 60% of the patients enrolled in the COLOR II trial. Only 60% of patients in the COLOR II trial underwent neoadjuvant therapy; this should be questioned especially as the outcomes measured in the trial were recurrence and survival. The percentage of patients with low rectal cancer was 50%, 35%, 28%, and 61% in the Z6051, ALaCart, COLOR II, and COREAN trials, respectively. From the ergonomic perspective, the fulcrum/coning effect will be much greater for lower rectal cancers; the outcomes of this specific subgroup should be of great interest as the dissection comparing laparoscopic and open proctectomy in the deep pelvis is different.

Despite the fact that recent RCTs concluded that laparoscopic resection for rectal cancer is inferior to its open counterpart, a return to the latter is quite unlikely. Therefore, the results of these RCTs are indirectly opening the way to robotic resection for rectal cancer [21]. The main finding of a recent study was that robotic proctectomy resulted in a statistically significantly greater depth of the CRM compared with matched patients treated with open or laparoscopic proctectomy by the same surgeon. Because these were the first 20 consecutive robotic cases (representing the surgeon's learning curve), the most reasonable explanation is that the improved circumferential resection margin was due to the improved ergonomics of the articulating robotic instruments in the confined space of the pelvis. These results were further confirmed in a more recent learning curve study, which, however, revealed the impact of a learning curve on the quality of TME. While the circumferential resection margin was not affected by the surgeons' learning curve, the quality of total mesorectal excision significantly improved during the surgeons' plateau phase. This study confirmed that lack of tactile feedback in robotic surgery entails a learning curve [22].

25.2.4 Surgical Site Infection in Colorectal Surgery

Being the third most common nosocomial infection, surgical site infection (SSI) represents a major source of postoperative morbidity and mortality in colorectal surgery with rates as high as 30% and is responsible for annual costs of up to 10 billion dollars in the USA [23–26]. Despite the identification of SSI as a patient safety priority by the Centers for Medicaid and Medicare Services and the Joint Commission on the Accreditation of Healthcare Organizations and the development of several accountability measures, such as appropriate timing and adequate selection of antibiotics and preoperative glucose control, SSI still remains a significant burden in colorectal surgery. There is controversy in the literature regarding the relative impact of stress-induced hyperglycemia in non-diabetes mellitus (DM) patients. Stress hyperglycemia is defined as acute, transient elevations in blood glucose concentrations occurring during illness [27]. It is a result of a cascade of normal physiologic response to injury leading to the alteration of endogenous hormone production and metabolites, including increased serum cortisol production, insulin resistance, and subsequent hyperglycemia [28]. Stress hyperglycemia was found to be associated with increased risk of SSI in colorectal patients, especially in the absence of pre-existing DM [29, 30]. In 2003, it was suggested that preoperative carbohydrate loading may result in improved insulin sensitivity for as long as 72 h postoperatively [31]. Since then, a number of studies have confirmed benefits of preoperative carbohydrate loading compared to the standard 8-h nil per os (NPO) strategy, however, with little mention of hyperglycemia [32, 33]. Recently, the PROCY study compared preoperative oral intake of 800 mL of water containing 100 g of maltodextrin to 800 mL of water and found no benefit in terms of SSI reduction (16.3% vs 16.0%), although the rate of perioperative hyperglycemia was lower after carbohydrate loading (24.2% vs 57.4%) [34]. A recent observational study reported was that non-DM patients were found to have a postoperative hyperglycemia rate as high as 46% in spite of the implementation of SSI bundle [35]. The authors also reported a positive correlation between stress hyperglycemia and organ/space SSI rates regardless of the DM status. Another recent study suggested that a lower dose of carbohydrate loading coupled with citrulline supplementation might be more effective in reducing the rate of perioperative hyperglycemia to as low as 7% [36].

Another currently unfolding innovation with the potential to reduce SSI rates is the use of a wound protector that combines continuous wound irrigation and barrier protection. Addition of wound irrigation between the barrier and the wound may help to eliminate bacterial contamination that may occur through manipulation of the wound protector device and surgical wound during the operation. In fact, a recent prospective multicenter study reported that the use of such wound protector was associated with a 71% reduction in enteric bacterial contamination (9.5% vs 33.3%, $p < 0.001$) and 66% reduction in overall bacterial contamination (11.9% vs 34.5%, $p < 0.001$) at the protected incision edge versus the exposed incision edge [37].

25.2.5 Intra- Versus Extracorporeal Antiperistaltic Ileocolic Anastomosis

A recent prospective propensity score-matched study reported that intracorporeal ileocolic anastomosis (ICA) reduces incisional SSI rates as compared to its extracorporeal counterpart [38]. Such data seem to point at the fact that fashioning an ICA within a limited laparotomy directly correlates to increased incisional SSI rates. In fact, recent systematic reviews found SSI rates to be significantly lower in patients undergoing intracorporeal ICA with even larger reduction in studies performed after 2012 [39, 40].

One potential disadvantage of intracorporeal ICA lies in the time elapsed between the retrieval of the stapler (used to fashion a side-to-side ICA) and the application of the next stapler closing the enterocolotomy. This may result in organ/space SSI after intracorporeal ICA despite atraumatic bulldogs temporarily delivered on the ileum and colon to prevent spillage [38]. One common feature of intracorporeal and extracorporeal anastomoses is the location of the leak, namely, at the TA (terminal anastomosis) staple line. This point should draw our attention to the fact that the application of a TA stapler to close the enterocolotomy results in a mucosa-everting anastomosis, which may carry higher leak rates when compared to its hand-sewn inverted counterpart [41]. ICA have been most commonly described in the literature to be fashioned as isoperistaltic [42–48]. Other authors reported the ICA to be constructed as antiperistaltic to unalter the rotation of the mesentery with the goal to prevent torsion of the anastomosis [40]. A recent RCT comparing isoperistaltic to antiperistaltic ICA concluded that anastomotic leaks occurred only in the isoperistaltic arm [49]. Although the trial was prematurely terminated due to excess leaks in the isoperistaltic arm, the authors pointed out that the location of the leaks was at the enterocolotomy, which had been hand-sewn closed in a single layer. Oversewing staple lines is a debatable but not uncommon practice. In fact, Widmar et al. reported significantly lower anastomotic leak rates in Crohn's disease patients with stapled oversewn ICA as compared to non-oversewn [50].

25.2.6 Is Transanal TME Victim of a Bum Rap?

Transanal approach to rectal cancer is not novel as it predates the era of laparotomy [51], but transanal TME (taTME) seems to be grabbing the headlines. Obese male patients with tumors of the distal third of the rectum constitute a well-known challenge to low anterior resection with a TME brought into even sharper relief when attempted laparoscopically. There are concerns that such males with a narrow pelvis and a bulky mesorectum may currently be undergoing sphincter-sparing resection with an involved CRM, a poor TME quality, or even an unnecessary abdominoperineal excision (APE). The challenge posed by low rectal cancer is to be distinguished from the issue of tumors located near the dentate line, where transanal intersphincteric resection (ISR) and coloanal anastomosis may be indicated. One of the concerns is whether, unlike transanal ISR, taTME entails a rectal transection inside the pelvis and thereby mandates serious scrutiny due to the potentially increased risk of local recurrence [52]. Nonetheless, it has been claimed recently that transanal TME offers at least three "oncological advantages" [53]: a longer distal resection margin [54], a decreased rate of involved CRM [55], and improved quality of TME [56].

A recent study claimed longer distal resection margin following taTME (2.8 ± 1.8 vs 1.7 ± 1.3 cm; $p < 0.01$). This result was most likely obtained by performing an unnecessary low rectal transection with a coloanal anastomoses on patients with cancer of the mid-rectum. As is widely accepted, a 1.7 cm distal margin would have been adequate even in the case of non-fixed tumors with poor differentiation. In this series of 37 patients who underwent taTME by one surgeon compared to unmatched historical controls operated on by several surgeons in a single institution, a critical appraisal of the data would suggest that taTME was potentially indicated in 11 males with low rectal cancer, of whom 4 were obese and 1 had a large tumor with a bulky mesorectum [54].

A decreased rate of involved CRM following taTME (2 vs 9 cases; $p = 0.025$) was reported in a randomized clinical trial despite no difference in average CRM (7 vs 5 mm; $p = 0.833$). A strength of this study was including only patients with cancer located within the distal 6 cm of the rectum [55]. However, this trial was not registered in a publicly accessible trial database and was underpowered (sample size = 590), and the first patient was randomized in June 2008.

Increased rates of complete TME quality following taTME (24 vs 18; $p < 0.05$) were claimed in a case series by two surgeons. Twenty-five patients with a cancer location ranging from 0 to 16 cm from the anal verge were compared to matched historical controls in a single institution. The only p value reported for TME quality was calculated for the whole series inclusive of patients undergoing APE [56]. A comparison excluding the APE's would have been appropriate as the posterior dissection in APE does not proceed to the anorectal junction and rather stops at the lower sacrum at which point Waldeyer's fascia is divided. It seems appropriate to distinguish the genuine concern for an involved CRM and poor TME quality in obese males undergoing transabdominal TME for low rectal cancer from its extrapolation to the use of taTME for all patients with resectable rectal cancer. In the former we should try to observe the established rules of innovation [56], excluding non-validated metrics [57], and the bias of historical control studies [58]. On the other hand, an unwarranted taTME might at best inflict a repaired rectal perforation and an unnecessary coloanal anastomosis on patients with resectable cancer of the upper rectum and rectosigmoid.

25.2.7 Local Excision for Rectal Cancer

A rigid platform endoscopic transanal approach grabbed the headlines in Europe [59] after over a century had elapsed from the historically first transanal approach [51]. Transanal endoscopic microsurgery (TEM) required a shallow learning curve and a capital budget purchase. The latter factor most likely limited its popularization in the USA given the financial accountability of private institutions requesting sufficient patient volume. Hence, it is not surprising that an American surgeon developed and implemented the concept of soft platform named transanal minimally invasive surgery (TAMIS) [60].

TAMIS is performed by inserting a disposable FDA-approved single-incision port in the anal canal with the patient prone or supine depending on the location of the lesion in the rectum. A pneumorectum is created insufflating CO_2, and laparoscopic instruments are inserted. A retrospective cohort study including 50 patients undergoing TAMIS reported a 4.3% rate of positive margins for malignant tumors and 8% rate for benign tumors [61]. Notwithstanding the opportunities for better visualization, simpler technique and less expensive instrumentation, TAMIS is not flawless. Its limitations include restricted working angles within the confined space of the rectal lumen and external torque in attempt to compensate for the lack of instruments' articulation [62].

It should not be surprising that the abovementioned limitations of laparoscopic instruments created an opportunity for a robotic transanal approach. One of the goals of a robotic soft platform would be to facilitate the suture closure of an anterior rectal wall defect [63]. Clearly, the 360° range of motion of the robotic instruments in the rectal lumen is the key advantage. The reassignment of the robotic arms from left to right and vice versa after instrument crossing and the 3D high-definition visualization allow for instrument manipulation similar to open surgery. Cadaveric studies have shown robotic soft platform to be a precise method for local excision of "pseudolesions" allowing surgeons' unprecedented control of the operative field [62, 64, 65]. The only available clinical data consist of few case reports and one multicenter study including 16 patients only [62, 64–73]. The latter study, however, reported positive margins in 2 of 16 cases (13%) [73]. Alongside with advantages, a robotic soft platform has limitations, such as learning curve and cost.

25.2.8 Pathologic Response After Neoadjuvant Chemoradiation

Restaging after long course of neoadjuvant chemoradiation has been evolving significantly since the historical Swedish RCT first proved its efficacy [74]. A Brazilian study postulated that a complete clinical response could be achieved in selected cases following neoadjuvant chemoradiation [75]. This led to the hypothesis that organ preservation would not jeopardize cure in selected patients with rectal cancer. Complete clinical response has been defined on the basis of the findings at flexible sigmoidoscopy performed during follow-up of such patients, although adequate imaging has not yet been standardized. Timing for restaging seems to be continuously changing in the sense that the longer we wait, the more likely we are to identify a complete clinical response [76]. However, it has been reported that approximately 15% of patients with complete clinical response would achieve complete pathologic response [77]. Along those lines, the safety of the so-called watch-and-wait strategy has been questioned by studies reporting a local recurrence rate of 38% [78]. Nonetheless, organ preservation can be a valid option for patients with prohibitive pre-existing comorbidities that would preclude radical surgery.

25.2.9 Colorectal Polyps

The introduction of endoscopic snaring of colonic polyps has held an unprecedented impact in decreasing the incidence of colon cancer. However, the benefits of polypectomy in the colon may not apply to rectal polyps due to the distinct prognostic value of local staging in rectal cancer. Magnetic resonance imaging (MRI) and positron emission tomography (PET) are of paramount importance for identifying intramural spread of the primary tumor, possible invasion to surrounding structures, and evidence of lymphatic spread. These fine, yet critical, details are a necessity in responsibly evaluating a suspected rectal cancer yet become unfeasible when preceded by snare polypectomy. The reactive lymphadenopathy resulting from snare polypectomy, while a normal physiological inflammatory response, is radiographically indistinguishable from the lymphadenopathy of malignant spread seen in rectal cancer. Differentiating benign reactionary inflammation from malignant lymph nodes on MRI is extremely challenging, especially considering the insidious lymphatic progression seen in rectal malignancies [79]. True lymphatic spread requires neoadjuvant chemotherapy and possible radiotherapy, with proven benefits in controlling the primary tumor as well as minimizing future recurrence risks [80]. Patients with confirmed rectal cancer and indeterminate lymphovascular involvement after snare polypectomy could be exposed to neoadjuvant chemoradiotherapy. Preoperative treatments, such as chemotherapeutic agents and radiation, carry serious adverse effects but are warranted for their benefit in improving survival rates in appropriately staged patients. Exposure to unnecessary radiation therapy would drastically limit treatment options for possible recurrence [81]. Many patients who could meet selection criteria for low-risk procedures, such as TAMIS, will become ineligible as the result of false-positive imaging [81].

All rectal polyps should be referred to PET–MRI imaging followed by cold biopsy of the polyps and without snare polypectomy. Removing the pitfalls of over-staging due to scarring and inflammation from rectal snare polypectomy and avoiding incomplete polyp removal would improve rectal cancer screening and early treatment. Screening colonoscopies have driven the declining incidence of colon cancers, but snaring rectal lesions negatively impacts timely identification of cancerous polyps for appropriate surgical intervention.

With regard to endoscopically unresectable right colon sessile polyps, a recent RCT has shown that laparoscopic-assisted colonoscopic polypectomy (LACP) reduces hospital stay with no difference in morbidity rates compared to laparoscopic right colectomy questioning the rationale for the latter [82].

25.3 Soon Upcoming Innovations

25.3.1 The Impact of Colorectal Cancer Stem Cells on Surgery

The concept of cancer stem cells was initially developed in leukemia in the late 1990s as it became clear that the stochastic growth model (all cancerous cells can proliferate and form new tumors) was not holding true. Dissimilarly, the stem cell growth model showed that only a specific subgroup of cells can proliferate and form new tumors [83]. A decade later, colorectal cancer stem cells were isolated [84]. In order to comprehend the cancer stem cell hypothesis, we must review our knowledge about normal stem cells. In fact, normal stem cells are central to three processes: development, tissue repair, and cancer. One relevant difference between normal differentiated epithelial cells and normal stem cells is the number of mutations required to become cancerous: 6 vs 1–2, respectively. The colorectal cancer stem cell hypothesis entails that cure may not accomplished unless all cancer stem cells are removed. Moreover, en bloc resection of the tumor mass with uninvolved margins would not be necessary if all cancer stem cells could be removed. Although it is known that stem cells are located at the base of the crypts of the colonic mucosa, the exact location of colon cancer stem cells within the bulk of the tumor or in other organs is unknown [85]. We do know, however, that an involved margin after resection for rectal cancer does not always result in local cancer recurrence: a fact in support of the cancer stem cell hypothesis.

25.3.2 Implications of miRNA Dysregulation in Colon Cancer

The most recent population-based study found that despite receiving equal treatment and after controlling for known prognostic factors, African Americans have a 30–50% higher rate of disease-specific mortality than Caucasian Americans [86].

Because one would not expect incidence rates to increase with decreased screening and/or delayed detection, it is highly unlikely that socioeconomic status and dietary factors, factors normally attributed to this phenomenon, are the only determinants of racial cancer disparity. Some attempts to examine the genetic differences contributing to racial differences in colorectal cancer risk have led to analyze the role played by microRNAs (miRNAs), which are frequently dysregulated in cancer and have shown promise as tissue-based markers for prognostication [87]. These small RNAs are able to control gene expression, translational repression, or degradation via specific sites at the 3′-UTR of their target mRNAs. A number of studies have reported differential expression of miRNAs in paired colon cancer tumor and adjacent normal colon sample [88]. miRNAs have also been shown to act either as oncogenes [89] or as tumor suppressors [90]. Thus, the dysregulation of these miRNAs can lead to the development of cancer. In addition, other studies have indicated that miRNAs are involved in tumor migration and invasion, with specific implications that miR-373 and miR-520c are metastasis-promoting miRNAs [91]. As there are many types of miRNAs, an exploratory study was recently carried out to identify candidate miRNAs that could contribute to the biological differences between African Americans and Caucasian Americans. miR-182 was identified to be in tumor tissue and paired adjacent normal colon tissue of African and Caucasian American colon cancer patients. However, miR-182 expression was significantly increased in colon cancer versus adjacent normal tissue and significantly increased in African Americans and versus Caucasian Americans with colon cancer [92]. This observation supports the concept that the expression of miR-182 may contribute to disparities in colon cancer survival and such miRNA should be included in routine testing to better customize therapy.

25.3.3 Colonoscopic Cellular Therapy

The search for a treatment, which targets colorectal cancer cells specifically while preserving normal cells, is a pressing problem. Innovation is focused on demonstrating the feasibility of cellular-based delivery of siRNA to cancer cells resulting in cancer cell apoptosis and reduced tumor size without affecting normal cell function. This innovative approach uses mesenchymal stem cells (MSC) with a specific small interfering RNA (siRNA) directed against the tumor cell protein AKT 1 (serine-/threonine-specific protein kinase or protein kinase B). AKT 1 is upregulated in colorectal cancers [93], and a reduction in AKT activity has been demonstrated to increased apoptosis in tumor cells [94], so this therapy has the potential to provide a central target for cure based by RNA-based therapeutics. In order to be an effective delivery system, MSC must be able to make cell-to-cell connections with cancer cells. It has been previously demonstrated that gap junctions formed by proteins such as connexin 43 provide cell-to-cell communication [95]. Preliminary evidence has demonstrated that human colon cancer cells possess connexin 43 and that MSC and human colon cancer cells make gap junctions, a necessary step for the delivery of siRNA [96]. Preliminary data also provided immunohistochemical evidence of the presence of connexin 43 in human adenocarcinoma ensuring that the MSC-based delivery system can eventually be deployed clinically. The primary advantage of this approach would be the avoidance of the extracellular space as the final common path to cancer cells. In fact, the cellular delivery alternative for siRNA is particularly timely as other delivery systems for siRNA such as viral delivery, attachment to lipid moieties, and hydrodynamic delivery suffer from inefficient delivery and often trigger an immune response [97]. The innovative aspect of this approach is also the colonoscopic delivery of cellular therapy for the treatment of colorectal cancer.

25.3.4 Cold-Inducible RNA-Binding Protein in Colorectal Cancer

Cold-inducible RNA-binding protein (CIRP) is a highly conserved glycine-rich RNA-binding protein (originally identified in the testis as the first mammalian cold shock protein) encoded by the CIRBP gene, which may be induced by hypothermia (32 °C), DNA damage, UV radiation, glucose deprivation, hypoxia, and oxidative stress [98, 99]. CIRP also mediates suppression of cell proliferation by prolonging the G1 phase and contributes to the suppression of apoptosis induced by tumor necrosis factor-α (TNF-α) [100]. An experimental study on 236 human colonic specimens obtained by endoscopy or surgery from patients with ulcerative colitis found significant correlation of CIRP with TNF-α, IL23/IL17, Bcl-2, and stem cell marker expression and explained its role in tumorigenesis, namely, colitis-associated cancer [101]. The authors concluded that suppression and measurement of CIRP expression might be a promising approach for advanced treatment and personalized management of patients with IBD. A recent study evaluating the prognostic value of three RNA-binding proteins, namely, insulin-like growth factor-binding protein 2 (IGFBP2), RNA-binding motif protein 3 (RBM3), and CIRP in colon cancer, reported that the estimated 5-year disease-free survival rate was significantly better for patients with higher expression of RBM3 and CIRP [102]. The authors concluded that RBM3 and CIRP may be useful prognostic biomarkers of colon cancer. Another recent study aiming to develop a new vaccination platform based on CIRP reported that the vaccination led to CD8-dependent tumor rejection in several tumor models when applied in a therapeutic setting. The authors concluded that CIRP-based vaccination strategies could be a valuable clinical tool to include in combinatorial immunotherapeutic strategies in cancer patients [103].

25.4 Conclusions

Although major improvements have been attained in terms of decreasing local recurrence rates, increasing sphincter-saving surgery rates, as well as understanding patient reported outcomes, the fact remains that cure rates for colorectal cancer have been stagnating for decades. A breakthrough may not be expected to derive from the uncritical perpetuation of the same chemoradiation nor from the tedious polemics about the endless variants of minimally invasive surgery but rather from the implementation of translational research into clinical practice. Preoperative imaging able to locate cancer stem cells within the bulk of the tumor, routine testing for miRNA dysregulation and RNA-binding proteins, as well as colonoscopic cellular therapy represent in no particular order examples of future perspectives in value-based care of patients with colorectal cancer.

References

1. Volkmann R. Sammlung Klinischer Vortrage in Verbindung mit deutschen Kliniken. Chirurgie. 1880;29(53):1113–27.
2. Senn N. Enterorrhaphy; its history, technique and present status. JAMA. 1893;21:215–35.
3. Iordache F, Bergamaschi R. Randomized trials in colorectal surgery: a will o' the wisp. Colorectal Dis. 2013;15(8):923–5.
4. Ravitch MM, Steichen FM. A stapling instrument for end-to-end inverting anastomoses in the gastrointestinal tract. Ann Surg. 1979;189(6):791–7.
5. Buess GF. Local excision of tumors of the rectal cavity. Dtsch Med Wochenschr. 1987;112(45):1747–8.
6. Heald RJ, Husband EM, Ryall RD. The mesorectum in rectal cancer surgery—the clue to pelvic recurrence? Br J Surg. 1982;69(10):613–6.
7. Fleshman K, Dargent DJ, Green E, Anvari M, Stryker SK, Beart RW Jr, et al. Laparoscopic colectomy for cancer is not inferior to open surgery based on 5-year data from the COST Study Group trial. Ann Surg. 2007;245:655–62.
8. Swedish Rectal Cancer Trial, Cedermark B, Dahlberg M, Glimelius B, Påhlman L, Rutqvist LE, Wilking N. Improved survival with preoperative radiotherapy in resectable rectal cancer. N Engl J Med. 1997;336(14):980–7.
9. Geng F, Wang Z, Yin H, Yu J, Cao B. Molecular targeted drugs and treatment of colorectal cancer: recent progress and future perspectives. Cancer Biother Radiopharm. 2017;32(5):149–60.
10. Foppa C, Denoya PI, Tarta C, Bergamaschi R. Indocyanine green fluorescent dye during bowel surgery: are the blood supply "guessing days" over? Tech Coloproctol. 2014;18(8):753–8.
11. Hardy KJ. Bowel surgery: some 18th and 19th century experience. ANZ J Surg. 1988;58:335–8.
12. Ignjatovic D, Bergamaschi R. Defining the extent of mesenterectomy in right colectomy: a controversy. Colorectal Dis. 2016;18(7):649.
13. Spasojevic M, Stimec BV, Dyrbekk AP, et al. Lymph node distribution in the d3 area of the right mesocolon: implications for an anatomically correct cancer resection. A postmortem study. Dis Colon Rectum. 2013;56:1381–7.
14. Nesgaard JM, Stimec BV, Bakka AO, Edwin B, Ignjatovic D, RCC Study Group. Navigating the mesentery. A comparative pre- and per-operative visualization of the vascular anatomy. Colorectal Dis. 2015;17:810–8.
15. Thorsen Y, Stimec B, Andersen SN, et al. Bowel function and quality of life after small bowel denervation during right colectomy with extended D3-mesenterectomy. Tech Coloproctol. 2016;20(7):445–53.
16. Liang JT, Lai HS, Huang J, Sun CT. Long-term oncologic results of laparoscopic D3 lymphadenectomy with complete mesocolic excision for right-sided colon cancer with clinically positive lymph nodes. Surg Endosc. 2015;29(8):2394–401.
17. Fleshman J, Branda B, Sargent DJ, et al. Effect of Laparoscopic-assisted resection vs open resection of stage II or III rectal cancer on pathologic outcomes: the ACOSOG Z6051 randomized clinical trial. JAMA. 2015;314(13):1346–55.
18. Stevenson ARL, Solomon MJ, Lumley JW, et al. Effect of laparoscopic-assisted resection vs open resection on pathological outcomes in rectal cancer: the ALaCart randomized clinical trial. JAMA. 2015;314(13):1356–63.

19. Bonjer JH, Deijen CL, Abis GA, et al. A randomized trial of laparoscopic versus open surgery for rectal cancer. N Engl J Med. 2015;372:1324–32.
20. Jeong SY, Park JW, Nam BH, et al. Open versus laparoscopic surgery for mid-rectal or low rectal cancer after neoadjuvant chemoradiotherapy (COREAN trial): survival outcomes of an open-label, non-inferiority, randomized controlled trial. Lancet Oncol. 2014;15(7):767–74.
21. Tou S, Bergamaschi R. Laparoscopic rectal cancer resection: inferior to open or not? Colorectal Dis. 2016;18(3):233.
22. Dyatlov A, Gachabayov M, Lee H, Chudner A, Bergamaschi R. Impact of robotic learning curve on circumferential margin and quality of total mesorectal excision in rectal cancer. P426. Annual Meeting of the American Society of Colon and Rectal Surgeons, Nashville, TN, 22 May 2018.
23. Keenan JE, Speicher PJ, Thacker JK, et al. The preventative surgical site infection bundle in colorectal surgery: an effective approach to surgical site infection reduction and health care cost savings. JAMA Surg. 2014;149(14):1045–52.
24. Tanner J, Khan D, Ball J, et al. Post discharge surveillance to identify colorectal surgical site infection rates and costs. J Hosp Infect. 2009;72(3):242–50.
25. Thompson KM, Oldenburg WA, Deschamps C, et al. Chasing zero: the drive to eliminate surgical site infections. Ann Surg. 2011;254(3):430–6; discussion 436–7.
26. Mahmoud NN, Turpin RS, Yang G, Saunders WB. Impact of surgical site infections on length of stay and costs in selected colorectal procedures. Surg Infect. 2009;10(6):539–44.
27. Dungan KM, Braithwaite SS, Preiser JC. Stress hyperglycemia. Lancet. 2009;373(9677):1798–807.
28. May AK, Kaufmann RM, Collier BR. The place for glycemic control in the surgical patient. Surg Infect. 2011;12(5):405–18.
29. Kwon S, Thompson R, Delinger P, Yanez D, Farrohki E, Flum D. Importance of perioperative glycemic control in general surgery: a report from the Surgical Care and Outcomes Assessment Program. Ann Surg. 2013;257(1):8–14.
30. McConnell YJ, Johnson PM, Porter GA. Surgical site infections following colorectal surgery in patients with diabetes: association with postoperative hyperglycemia. J Gastrointest Surg. 2009;13(3):508–15.
31. Ljungqvist O, Soreide E. Preoperative fasting. Br J Surg. 2003;90(4):400–6.
32. Ramos M, Khalpey Z, Lipsitz S, et al. Relationship of perioperative hyperglycemia and postoperative infections in patients who undergo general and vascular surgery. Ann Surg. 2008;248(4):585–91.
33. Hanazaki K, Maeda H, Okabayashi T. Relationship between perioperative glycemic control and postoperative infections. World J Gastroenterol. 2009;15(33):4122–5.
34. Gianotti L, Biffi R, Sandini M, et al. Preoperative oral carbohydrate load versus placebo in major elective abdominal surgery (PROCY): a randomized, placebo-controlled, multicenter, phase III trial. Ann Surg. 2018;267(4):623–30.
35. Gachabayov M, Senagore AJ, Abbas SK, Yelika SB, You K, Bergamaschi R. Perioperative hyperglycemia: an unmet need within a surgical site infection bundle. Tech Coloproctol. 2018;22(3):201–7.
36. Kielhorn BA, Senagore AJ, Asgeirsson T. The benefits of a low dose complex carbohydrate/citrulline electrolyte solution for preoperative carbohydrate loading: focus on glycemic variability. Am J Surg. 2018;215(3):373–6.
37. Papaconstantinou HT, Ricciardi R, Margolin DA, et al. A novel wound retractor combining continuous irrigation and barrier protection reduces incisional contamination in colorectal surgery. World J Surg. 2018. https://doi.org/10.1007/s00268-018-4568-z.
38. Martinek L, You K, Giuratrabocchetta S, Gachabayov M, Lee K, Bergamaschi R. Does laparoscopic intracorporeal ileocolic anastomosis decreases surgical site infection rate? A propensity score-matched cohort study. Int J Colorectal Dis. 2018;33(3):291–8.
39. Van Oostendorp S, Elfrink A, Borstlap W, et al. Intracorporeal versus extracorporeal anastomosis in right hemicolectomy: a systematic review and meta-analysis. Surg Endosc. 2017;31(1):64–77.

40. Wu Q, Jin C, Hu T, Wei M, Wang Z. Intracorporeal versus extracorporeal anastomosis in laparoscopic right colectomy: a systematic review and meta-analysis. J Laparoendosc Adv Surg Tech A. 2017;27(4):348–57.
41. Stein SA, Bergamaschi R. Extracorporeal versus intracorporeal ileocolic anastomosis. Tech Coloproctol. 2013;17(Suppl 1):S35–9.
42. Jian-Cheng T, Shu-Sheng W, Bo Z, Jian F, Liang Z. Total laparoscopic right hemicolectomy with 3-step stapled intracorporeal isoperistaltic ileocolic anastomosis for colon cancer: an evaluation of short-term outcomes. Medicine (Baltimore). 2016;95(48):e5538.
43. Marchesi F, Pinna F, Percalli L, et al. Totally laparoscopic right colectomy: theoretical and practical advantages over the laparoassisted approach. J Laparoendosc Adv Surg Tech A. 2013;23(5):418–24.
44. Scatizzi M, Kroning KC, Borrelli A, Andan G, Lenzi E, Feroci F. Extracorporeal versus intracorporeal anastomosis after laparoscopic right colectomy for cancer: a case-control study. World J Surg. 2010;34(12):2902–8.
45. Magistro C, Lernia SD, Ferrari G, et al. Totally laparoscopic versus laparoscopic-assisted right colectomy for colon cancer: is there any advantage in short-term outcomes? A prospective comparative assessment in our center. Surg Endosc. 2013;27(7):2613–8.
46. Reggio S, Sciuto A, Cuccurullo D, et al. Single-layer versus double-layer closure of the enterotomy in laparoscopic right hemicolectomy with intracorporeal anastomosis: a single-center study. Tech Coloproctol. 2015;19(12):745–50.
47. Abrisqueta J, Ibanez N, Lujan J, et al. Intracorporeal ileocolic anastomosis in patients with laparoscopic right hemicolectomy. Surg Endosc. 2016;30(1):65–72.
48. Grams J, Tong W, Greenstein AJ, Salky B. Comparison of intracorporeal versus extracorporeal anastomosis in laparoscopic-assisted hemicolectomy. Surg Endosc. 2010;24(8):1886–91.
49. Matsuda A, Miyashita M, Matsumoto S, et al. Isoperistaltic versus antiperistaltic stapled side-to-side anastomosis for colon cancer surgery: a randomized controlled trial. J Surg Res. 2015;196(1):107–12.
50. Widmar M, Cummings DR, Steinhagen E, et al. Oversewing staple lines to prevent anastomotic complications in primary ileocolic resections for Crohn's disease. J Gastrointest Surg. 2015;19(5):911–6.
51. Volkmann R. Concerning rectal cancer and the removal of the rectum. Dis Colon Rectum. 1986;29:679–85.
52. Warren OJ, Solomon MJ. The drive toward transanal total mesorectal excision–science or rhetoric? Dis Colon Rectum. 2015;58:909–10.
53. Rullier E. Transanal mesorectal excision: the new challenge in rectal cancer. Dis Colon Rectum. 2015;58:621–2.
54. Fernandez-Hevia M, Delgado S, Castells A, et al. Transanal total mesorectal excision in rectal cancer: short-term outcomes in comparison with laparoscopic surgery. Ann Surg. 2015;261:221–7.
55. Denost Q, Adam JP, Rullier A, Buscail E, Laurent C, Rullier E. Perineal transanal approach: a new standard for laparoscopic sphincter-saving resection in low rectal cancer, a randomized trial. Ann Surg. 2014;260:993–9.
56. Velthuis S, Nieuwenhuis DH, Ruijter TEG, Cuesta MA, Bonjer HJ, Sietses C. Transanal versus traditional laparoscopic total mesorectal excision for rectal carcinoma. Surg Endosc. 2014;28:3494–9.
57. Wexner SD, Berho M. Transanal TAMIS total mesorectal excision (TME)—a work in progress. Tech Coloproctol. 2014;18:423–5.
58. Abraham NS, Durairaj R, Young JM, Young CJ, Solomon MJ. How does an historic control study of a surgical procedure compare with the "gold standard"? Dis Colon Rectum. 2006;49:1141–8.
59. Buess G, Theiss R, Hutterer F, et al. Transanal endoscopic surgery of the rectum - testing a new method in animal experiments. Leber Magen Darm. 1983;13(2):73–7.
60. Atallah S, Albert M, Larach S. Transanal minimally invasive surgery: a giant leap forward. Surg Endosc. 2010;24:2200–5.

61. Albert M, Atallah S, deBeche-Adams TC, Izfar S, Larach S. Transanal Minimally Invasive Surgery (TAMIS) for local excision of benign neoplasms and early-stage rectal cancer: efficacy and outcomes in the first 50 patients. Dis Colon Rectum. 2013;56:301–7.
62. Atallah S, Albert M, deBeche-Adams TC, Larach S. Robotic transanal minimally invasive surgery in a cadaveric model. Tech Coloproctol. 2011;15:461–4.
63. Popa D, Connolly TM, Barbon C, Bergamaschi R. Design defects can close a study. Colorectal Dis. 2015;17(12):1121–2.
64. Hompes R, Rauh SM, Hagen ME, Mortensen NJ. Preclinical cadaveric study of transanal endoscopic da Vinci surgery. Br J Surg. 2012;99:1144–8.
65. Marks J, Ng S, Mak T. Robotic transanal surgery (RTAS) with utilization of a next-generation single-port system: a cadaveric feasibility study. Tech Coloproctol. 2017;21(7):541–5.
66. Atallah S, Quinteros F, Martin-Perez B, Larach S. Robotic transanal surgery for local excision of rectal neoplasms. J Robot Surg. 2014;8:193–4.
67. Atallah S, Parra-Davila E, deBeche-Adams T, Albert M, Larach S. Excision of a rectal neoplasm using robotic transanal surgery (RTS): a description of the technique. Tech Coloproctol. 2012;16:389–92.
68. Buchs NC, Pugin F, Volonte F, Hagen ME, Morel P, Ris F. Robotic transanal endoscopic microsurgery: technical details for the lateral approach. Dis Colon Rectum. 2013;56:1194–8.
69. Erenler I, Aytac E, Bilgin IA, Baca B, Hamzaoglu I, Karahasanoglu T. Robotic transanal minimally invasive surgery (R-TAMIS) with the da Vinci Xi system – a video vignette. Colorectal Dis. 2017;19(4):401.
70. Harr JN, Obias V. Robotic-assisted transanal excision of a large rectal mass – a video vignette. Colorectal Dis. 2016;18(1):107–8.
71. Laird R, Obias VJ. Robotic transanal fistula repair – a video vignette. Colorectal Dis. 2015;17(1):90.
72. Stack ME, Umanskiy K. Robotic-assisted transanal repair of a rectovaginal fistula. J Gastrointest Surg. 2016;20(12):2106.
73. Hompes R, Rauh SM, Ris F, Tuynman JB, Mortensen NJ. Robotic transanal minimally invasive surgery for local excision of rectal neoplasms. Br J Surg. 2014;101:578–81.
74. Initial report from a Swedish multicentre study examining the role of preoperative irradiation in the treatment of patients with resectable rectal carcinoma. Swedish Rectal Cancer Trial. Br J Surg. 1993;80(10):1333–6.
75. Habr-Gama A, Perez RO, Nadalin W, et al. Operative versus nonoperative treatment for stage 0 distal rectal cancer following chemoradiation therapy: long-term results. Ann Surg. 2004;240(4):711–7; discussion 717–8.
76. Vailati BB, Habr-Gama A, Mattacheo AE, São Julião GP, Perez RO. Quality of life in patients with rectal cancer after chemoradiation: watch-and-wait policy versus standard resection-are we comparing apples to oranges? Dis Colon Rectum. 2018;61(3):e21.
77. Guillem JG, Chessin DB, Shia J, et al. Clinical examination following preoperative chemoradiation for rectal cancer is not a reliable surrogate end point. J Clin Oncol. 2005;23(15):3475–9.
78. Renehan AG, Malcomson L, Emsley R, et al. Watch-and-wait approach versus surgical resection after chemoradiotherapy for patients with rectal cancer (the OnCoRe project): a propensity-score matched cohort analysis. Lancet Oncol. 2016;17(2):174–83.
79. Torkzad MR, Påhlman L, Glimelius B. Magnetic resonance imaging (MRI) in rectal cancer: a comprehensive review. Insights Imaging. 2010;1:245–67.
80. Tytherleigh MG, Warren BF. Management of early rectal cancer. Br J Surg. 2008;95:409–23.
81. Nicholls RJ, Zinicola R, Binda GA. Indications for colorectal resection for adenoma before and after polypectomy. Tech Coloproctol. 2004;8:s291–4.
82. Lascarides C, Buscaglia JM, Denoya PI, Nagula S, Bucobo JC, Bergamaschi R. Laparoscopic right colectomy vs laparoscopic-assisted colonoscopic polypectomy for endoscopically unresectable polyps: a randomized controlled trial. Colorectal Dis. 2016;18(11):1050–6.
83. Bonnet D, Dick JE. Human acute myeloid leukemia is organized as a hierarchy that originates from a primitive hematopoietic cell. Nat Med. 1997;3:730–7.

84. Ricci-Vitiani L, Lombardi DG, Pilozzi E, et al. Identification and expansion of human colon-cancer-initiating cells. Nature. 2007;445(7123):111–5.
85. Yeung TM, Mortensen NJ. Colorectal cancer stem cells. Dis Colon Rectum. 2009;52:1788–96.
86. Clegg LX, Li FP, Hankey BF, Chu K, Edwards BK. Cancer survival among US whites and minorities: a SEER (Surveillance, Epidemiology, and End Results) Program population-based study. Arch Intern Med. 2002;162:1985–93.
87. Croce CM. Causes and consequences of microRNA dysregulation in cancer. Nat Rev Genet. 2009;10:704–14.
88. Schetter AJ, Leung SY, Sohn JJ, et al. MicroRNA expression profiles associated with prognosis and therapeutic outcome in colon adenocarcinoma. JAMA. 2008;299:425–36.
89. He L, Thomson JM, Hemann MT, et al. A microRNA polycistron as a potential human oncogene. Nature. 2005;435:828–33.
90. Shell S, Park SM, Radjabi AR, et al. Let-7 expression defines two differentiation stages of cancer. Proc Natl Acad Sci U S A. 2007;104:11400–5.
91. Huang Q, Gumireddy K, Schrier M, et al. The microRNAs miR-373 and miR-520c promote tumour invasion and metastasis. Nat Cell Biol. 2008;10:202–10.
92. Li E, Ji P, Ouyang N, et al. Differential expression of miRNA in colon cancer between African and Caucasian Americans: implications for cancer racial health disparities. Int J Oncol. 2014;45(2):587–94.
93. Parsons D, Wang TL, Samuels Y, et al. Colorectal cancer: mutations in a signaling pathway. Nature. 2005;436:792.
94. Jing H, Zhou X, Dong X, et al. Abrogation of Akt signaling by isobavachalcone contributes to its anti-proliferative effects towards human cancer cells. Cancer Lett. 2010;294:167–77.
95. Valiunas V, Polosina Y, Miller H, et al. Connexin-specific cell-to-cell transfer of short interfering RNA by gap junctions. J Physiol. 2005;568:459–68.
96. Vivanco I, Sawyers CL. The phosphatidylinositol 3-Kinase AKT pathway in human cancer. Nat Rev Cancer. 2002;2(7):489–501.
97. Kim DH, Rossi JJ. Strategies for silencing human disease using RNA interference. Nat Rev Genet. 2007;8:173.
98. Nishiyama H, Itoh K, Kaneko Y, Kishishita M, Yoshida O, Fujita J. A glycine-rich RNA-binding protein mediating cold-inducible suppression of mammalian cell growth. J Cell Biol. 1997;137:899–908.
99. Wellmann S, Buhrer C, Moderegger E, et al. Oxygen-regulated expression of the RNA-binding proteins RBM3 and CIRP by a HIF-1-independent mechanism. J Cell Sci. 2004;117:1785–94.
100. Sakurai T, Itoh K, Higashitsuji H, et al. Cirp protects against tumor necrosis factor-alpha-induced apoptosis via activation of extracellular signal-regulated kinase. Biochim Biophys Acta. 2006;1763:290–5.
101. Sakurai T, Kashida H, Watanabe T, et al. Stress response protein cirp links inflammation and tumorigenesis in colitis-associated cancer. Cancer Res. 2014;74(21):6119–28.
102. Jang HH, Lee HN, Kim SY, Hong S, Lee WS. Expression of RNA-binding motif protein 3 (RBM3) and cold-inducible RNA-binding protein (CIRP) is associated with improved clinical outcome in patients with colon cancer. Anticancer Res. 2017;37(4):1779–85.
103. Villanueva L, Silva L, Llopiz D, et al. The Toll like receptor 4 ligand cold-inducible RNA-binding protein as vaccination platform against cancer. Oncoimmunology. 2017;7(4):e1409321.

Training Curriculum for Colorectal Cancer Surgery

26

Mickael Chevallay, Giulio C. Vitali, Nicolas C. Buchs, and Frederic Ris

26.1 Introduction

Trend to centralize patients within center of excellence urges the surgeons to acquire a certain level of expertise. The past self-taught way is no longer possible, and acquisition of skills should be conducted in supervised training programs. Surgeons used to acquire the skills by performing a large number of operations without any feedback or overlooking from colleague, and he/she could only count on himself/herself to improve. The aim of the training is to offer safety and good outcomes during the learning curve of complex cases, notably in colorectal surgery. Surgeons cannot gain experience at the expense of patient safety, and structured program might overcome the lengthy learning curve. With the development of technology, many tools are available for the trainee. Several skills can be acquired and practiced outside the operating room, in a safer environment than on a real patient, where the consequences of a mistake are less deleterious. Simulation training outside the operating room has become a vital part of laparoscopic training, by shortening the learning curves. From the virtual reality to the cadaveric training until the final step with independent intervention on a real patient, we review in this chapter the pathway of training in colorectal surgery.

26.2 The English Example: National Training Program

The emergence of new techniques introduces a potential problem: there are more people willing to learn than teacher. In the early 1990s [1], laparoscopic colectomy was an evolving technique whose oncologic safety had not been yet proved. Now, it

M. Chevallay · G. C. Vitali · N. C. Buchs · F. Ris (✉)
Department of Visceral Surgery, Geneva University Hospitals and medical school, Geneva, Switzerland
e-mail: frederic.ris@hcuge.ch

N. de'Angelis et al. (eds.), *Emergency Surgical Management of Colorectal Cancer*, Hot Topics in Acute Care Surgery and Trauma,
https://doi.org/10.1007/978-3-030-06225-5_26

is applicable to the majority of colorectal resections, including those for malignant disease. In spite of the benefits of laparoscopy, its widespread use might have come up against the quality of the teaching. Such risks can potentially mitigate the associated benefits of minimally invasive colorectal surgery.

In 2006, laparoscopic approach was recommended in the United Kingdom to selected patients undergoing colorectal surgery by the UK National Institute for Health and Care Excellence (NICE) [2]. At that time, only 5% of colorectal surgeons were trained in this technique. The steep learning curve, associated with an increased risk of complications, slowed down the uptake of the technique. In 2007, a National Training Program (NTP) for Laparoscopic Colorectal Surgery in England [3] was initiated. Its aim was to provide hands-on training to established colorectal surgeons in England. The program was a multicenter educational scheme (ten training centers) with the aim to shorten the learning curve while minimizing patient morbidity and mortality rates. The NTP provided a stepwise competency-based training. This pathway included candidate selection (delegates), a preclinical phase (course), a clinical phase (supervised operating), and a structured sign-off process followed by post-sign-off independent audited practice.

Since its implementation, the percentage of colorectal resections performed laparoscopically in England increases from 8.8% in 2007 to 61% in 2013 [4], without sacrificing the short- and long-term outcomes. Therefore, this was a proof of concept that an educational program can spread a complex surgical technique in a structured way. To assure that the training has been effective, a post-sign-off audit was proposed by the NTP. This helped the surgeons to assure a long-term feedback and to ensure the quality of the specialized surgery offered. Each program could therefore be inspired by this model. The NTP, on the other hand, focused on the techniques in the operating room. Several basic and advanced skills should be acquired before.

26.3 Virtual Reality

Computer-generated simulators have been used for many years in the training of pilots. Aviation was one of the first industries to use simulation. The philosophy was to create an environment as similar to the real one as possible. The pilots find themselves sitting within a cockpit, experiencing the same forces and audiovisual stimuli as in a real plane. However, the last 15 years have seen numerous attempts to introduce virtual reality imaging into clinical medicine. The term virtual reality (VR) refers to a computer-generated representation of an environment that allows sensory interaction, thus giving the impression of actually being present. However, despite its introduction to surgery in 1993 by Satava [5], acceptance of the VR training approach has been slow. It was previously thought that training on a simulator simply improved a surgeon's ability to operate on a simulator, but there is now a growing body of evidence that shows that VR simulator training can lead to improved performance in the real environment of the operating room. Virtual reality simulators have the advantage to provide automatic and instantaneous measures of performance: length of time, completion of the procedure, number of movements, etc. These metrics can serve to monitor progress while learning a technical skill. It comprises basic tasks, suturing tasks, procedural tasks or modules, and full procedures that range from basic to advanced laparoscopic surgery.

Virtual reality training might reduce the long learning curves in the operating room, especially in a society where working-hour limitation has become the rule.

The authors of a meta-analysis [6] including six trials have reported the superiority of VR training compared to no training at all, in terms of lower operative times, fewer errors, higher scores in validated performance scores, and higher overall accuracy. They concluded that VR training appears to decrease the operating time and to improve the operative performance of surgical trainees with limited laparoscopic experience when compared with no training. However, agreement among studies regarding the superiority of more expensive VR systems to the less expensive box trainers is not uniform. VR systems provide objective performance assessment metrics, thus permitting the monitoring of trainees' performances over time and elimination of preceptor-based assessment and its cost. While 30–60 cases in real patients are required for a novice to achieve an experienced level, with virtual reality, most studies showed that novice surgeons reached expert proficiency after ten trials in basic skills [7]. The aim of a non-operative logbook is to acquire a basic level of proficiency before entering the operating room and to reduce the learning curve.

Disadvantages of VR systems compared to both cadaveric and animal models include higher cost, lack of consideration of anatomic variations, poor tissue replication and tactile feedback, and lack of unexpected situations that are only present in live surgery.

26.4 Anatomic Training: Animal and Cadaveric Station

The virtual reality will not replace the realism of cadaveric tissue or animal models. They will serve as an intermediate step between the virtual training and operating room training. The feeling of tissues or structures and recognition of anatomical structures are crucial to understand an intervention. Knowledge of basic anatomy and mastery of every aspect of the procedure are essential to cope with any unusual deviation. The VR cannot mimic all these parameters. Training on animal or human structures is therefore mandatory using either animal organs or whole animal or cadaver.

26.4.1 Ex Vivo Animal

Most of porcine organs are very similar to those of the human. They can therefore be used to simulate parts of an intervention, either for open or laparoscopic approach (Fig. 26.1). For example, transanal stapling requires knowledge of the material as well as tactile sensation to avoid any complications in real situation. This part can be re-created by the use of a box trainer. Two trainees with one supervisor can try

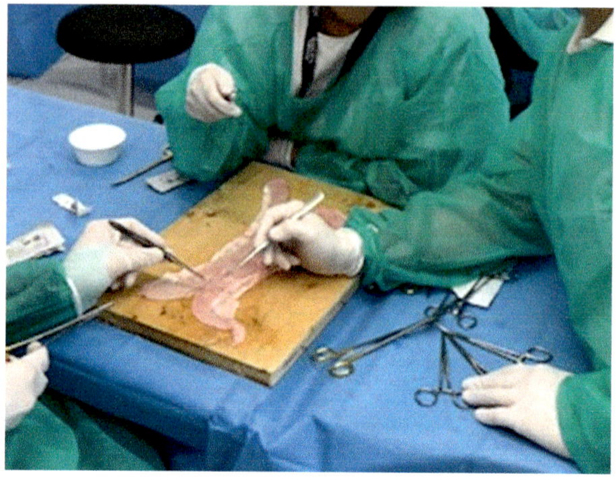

Fig. 26.1 Ex vivo animal model with young trainees performing intestinal anastomosis

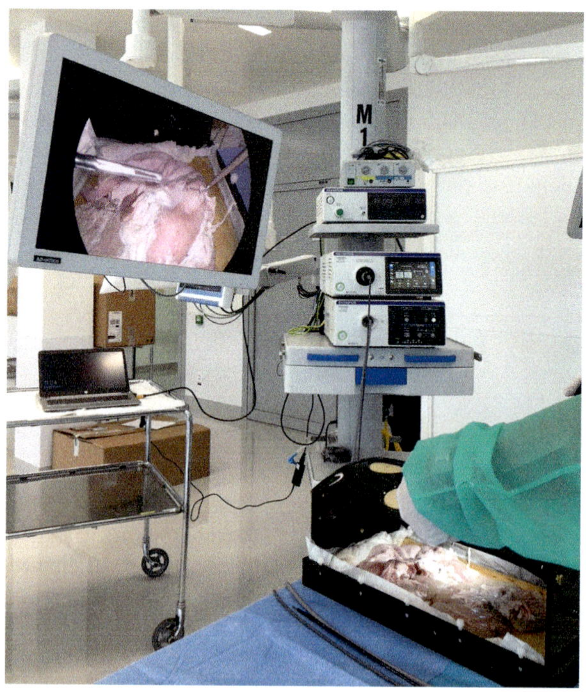

Fig. 26.2 Laparoscopic suture practice within a box trainer with porcine model

the stapling process with direct feedback. Limitations of a box trainer (Fig. 26.2) are the absence of bleeding and the lack of management of space (e.g., no other organs can obstruct the view). The organs on the other hand are cheap and easy to obtain (no obvious ethical problems).

A meta-analysis with eight trials [8] could not conclude with the actual evidence if laparoscopic box model training reduces mortality or morbidity. It seems that box trainer improves technical skills compared with standard surgical training in trainees, but more studies and evidences are required.

Finally, porcine rectum and anus can be used as a good practical exercise when performing the recent transanal total mesorectal excision (taTME). Especially, the purse-string part (which remains not only crucial but difficult also) can be trained with an ex vivo porcine model, and repeated indefinitely until proficiency is achieved.

26.4.2 Animal Model

The first description of an animal model as educational tools in colorectal surgery was made in 1994 by Böhm et al. [9]. They described several porcine and canine models. The advantage of the animal model is the ease of access and the simulation of bleeding. The preclinical performance of intraperitoneal bowel mobilization and anastomosis, dissection of mesentery, and control of bleeding can only be practiced and perfected in live animal models. The surgeon can learn to handle intraperitoneal organs atraumatically, to achieve hemostasis, to dissect mesentery with lymphadenectomy and high-tie ligation of major vessels, and to accomplish a variety of intraperitoneal anastomoses. Acquisition of these skills is essential in the quest to perform successful laparoscopic colorectal surgery. These skills cannot be learned in inanimate training models. However, the anatomical planes are crucial for an understanding of the procedure. Therefore, the value of an animal model with a different anatomy is questionable. Operation on live animals is limited by ethics committees, which could limit their use.

26.4.3 Cadaveric Training

Cadaveric training appears to be superior, in terms of reality and learning effect. One systematic review found that cadaveric training was superior to VR training, in terms of improved skills, such as dissection, retraction, suturing, hand–eye coordination, and decreased times to task completion [10]. Two studies comparing the ProMIS simulator to cadaveric training for conventional and hand-assisted laparoscopic colectomy reported that simulator training was more suitable for trainees earlier in their learning curves, while cadaveric training was associated with a greater degree of difficulty and was more appropriate for more experienced trainees [11, 12]. VR training should be followed by cadaveric training to optimally achieve learning curve reduction. Operating on human cadavers is generally superior, and one meta-analysis found that trainees were more satisfied after cadaveric courses than after animal courses [13]. Cadaveric training models are considered superior to animal models due to their more accurate anatomy, port placement, and the use of instruments. This constitutes an overall training experience far closer to real operative conditions than any other training modalities. Creating pneumoperitoneum is an additional challenge for formalin-fixed cadaveric models, since their distention is limited. Other fixation process, for example, the Thiel soft-fix embalming method, allows to obtain a tissue elasticity level close to reality. Most of the time, courses are conducted on fresh (e.g., defrost) cadavers. Animal models are also less expensive with an approximate cost of $550 for a single training session, compared to $2550 for a cadaver lab [14]. In total, the limitations of cadaveric training are the cost, ethical concern, availability, and tissue compliance.

26.5 Real Practice: Patients

The transition to practice on patients is the final stage of learning. The trainees should have past all the previous steps with satisfactory evaluations. Surgery is often compared to aviation in learning skills. As a pilot cannot correct his abilities after a crash, surgery requires an optimal level of mastery before dealing with human life. It is unethical to increase the rate of negative outcomes during the learning phase. By selecting the cases, one could limit the risks of complication by adapting the complexity of the patients according to the surgeon's level. BMI, type of resection, and diagnostic are crucial factors that can predict the risk of complications, conversion, and complexity of cases. During the learning curve, appropriate case selection is crucial to reduce postoperative morbidity and mortality rates. In addition, appropriate case selection may assist in reducing competition for cases among trainees. Based on this concept, easier procedures are assigned to junior trainees, while more complex procedures are undertaken by senior trainees (Fig. 26.3). One study developed and validated a risk prediction score based on the

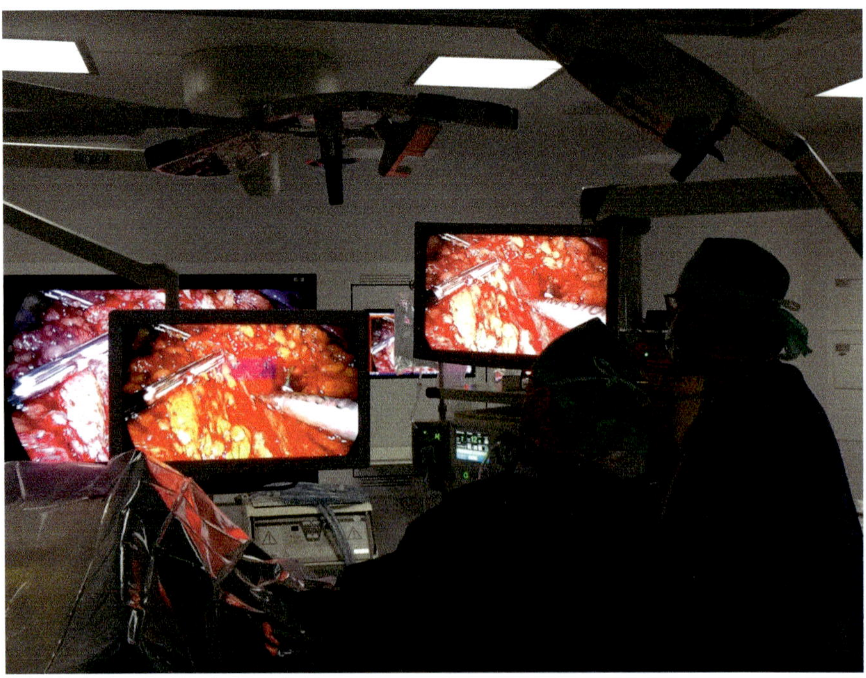

Fig. 26.3 Live surgery with expert surgeon training a resident in left hemicolectomy

UK's NTP, including higher body mass index (BMI), American Society of Anesthesiologists (ASA) score of 3 or 4, male sex, prior abdominal surgery, and type of resection, with high-risk cases (score > 6) being associated with greater dependency of trainees on their trainers, thereby contributing to higher training quality [15]. The risk prediction score developed by the NTP appears to be the most suitable tool for case selection. The higher the score, the higher was the rate of post-operative complications and reoperation rates. With regard to oncologic procedures, another study suggested that cases associated with female sex, low BMI, sigmoid location, superficial tumor depth, and small tumor size are more suitable for junior trainees [16].

The number of procedures needed to gain proficiency in laparoscopic colorectal surgery is reported to be in between 88 and 152 [17]. The limited number of cases put a pressure on the trainees as he/she needs to find the case load in order to become independent. Doing a part of the intervention allows several trainees to benefit from one patient. This modular training system was initially introduced in minimally invasive prostatectomy and is now applied to colorectal surgery. Laparoscopic surgery is more difficult to teach based on the traditional companionage model, since the trainer is not able to control directly the trainee as in open surgery.

One study [18] splits the intervention in three modules for the purpose of training:

1. Patient setup and positioning, creation of a pneumoperitonuem, port placement, displacement of small bowel from the operative field, isolation and division of vessels, and medial to lateral dissection.
2. Lateral mobilization, flexure mobilization, intracorporeal or extracorporeal bowel division, specimen extraction, and anastomosis.
3. This module included pelvic dissection (TME) for rectal resection.

It was possible to provide at least one module of training during 98% of all laparoscopic colorectal resections. The authors concluded that a single surgeon was able to train four senior colorectal trainees for independent laparoscopic practice in 23 months. They did not experienced any compromise of clinical outcomes compared to other series.

Advantages of modular training include a reduced learning curve, simultaneous training of multiple trainees, effective training even during difficult cases, adequate time for skill consolidation, and encouragement of focused cognitive preparation.

In order to improve, several performance assessment tools have been developed and validated to assess the technical competency. They can provide objective tools for tracking the trainees' progress. One study found that by the end of their specialized training, colorectal surgeons were not comfortable in performing the more complex components of LCS demonstrating that traditional assessment paradigms, such as minimum case requirements, may not ensure proficiency in all procedural steps [19]. One performance assessment tool, the Colorectal Objective Structured Assessment of Technical Skills (COSATS), has been used by the American Board of Colon and Rectal Surgery for board certification purposes [20, 21]. It assesses many parameters, such as tissue and instrument handling, time to completion, and procedural knowledge. Other validated tools exist and have been validated: the Observational Clinical Human Reliability Analysis (OCHRA) tool, which measures errors and near misses [22], the Global Assessment Scale (GAS), and the Laparoscopic Colorectal Assessment Tool (L-CAT) [23]. The last two are used in the NTP to assess the trainee performance for each procedural part. The main drawback associated with these performance assessment tools is the need for an assessor, as well as the lack of objective evaluation of nontechnical skills, such as teamwork, decision-making, communication, and leadership. In the future, automated tools will emerge to objectively evaluate trainees. Investigator bias can be avoided and reliance on reproducible parameters.

Operations performed by trainees have been perceived to have poorer results than those done by experienced surgeons. Moreover, the operating surgeon was previously considered as an independent determiner of surgical outcome. Surgery must be of the same quality no matter if the case has been selected for teaching purpose. A meta-analysis [24] of 19 studies concluded that there was no difference in leak rate and postoperative adverse events and no difference in the rate of R0 resection. Although supervised trainees had significantly longer laparoscopic operating times, the mean difference was only 10 min. The results of this study revealed that, when a modular-based training system is combined with case selection, no increase in adverse events is observed, and laparoscopic colorectal resections can be safely undertaken with the trainee as the lead surgeon. Nevertheless, supervision should be performed by an expert surgeon in the field of colorectal surgery.

Surgical technique is best learned through repetition, and the more frequent the trainee can participate, the more likely he will progress.

26.6 Robotic Surgery in Colorectal

Robotic approach can potentially have several advantages over laparoscopy: better depth vision, optics with three-dimensional vision, tremor filtration, less limitation of movement with endowrist instrument, and improved surgeon ergonomic. In the narrow pelvis, rectal surgery benefits the most of stable camera and 360° movement. As robotic technology tends to gain acceptance, it should be introduced early in the surgical cursus. The trainee willing to learn robotic procedures should first participate to courses where he/she can learn not only the technique but also to deal with a new technology [25]: operating room setup, trocar placement, patient positioning, and manipulation of the console. Then, he/she can apply these principles on live patient. In a survey conducted among the colon and rectal surgeons in 2017, 80% of the colon and rectal surgery residents over 3 years participated in a robotic training course. However, only 11% of the residents did more than 20 cases in their institution [26]. The inability to gain access to the robot and the mentor still in learning curve were the principal explanations [27]. The introduction of more and more robotics programs will reduce these limitations.

A systematic review concerning the learning curve of robotic in general surgery found nine articles specific to colorectal surgery. Each studies used time to determine the learning curve. The authors concluded that between 15 and 25 cases were needed to overcome the initial learning curve [28].

Laparoscopic experience is not essential to access robotic surgery. One report from Ireland [29] compared two surgeons, one with laparoscopic training and one without experience. They compared their robotic cases and found no differences in short-term outcomes. They concluded that a background in minimally invasive colorectal surgery is not essential prior to starting a robotic training. The experience could be gained in parallel rather than sequentially.

With which procedure to start? Right hemicolectomy seems to be the best initial experience with robotic. According to the authors [30], this procedure has several advantages to initiate a learning phase on the robot (full robotic procedure, linear docking, multi-quadrant surgery, and one vascular dissection with lymphadenectomy) and includes double intestinal resection and intracorporeal anastomosis. These key points identify right colectomy as useful operation for surgeons that are facing this new approach. On the other hand, rectopexy seems the perfect candidate to start with robotic rectal dissection and is usually the first step in any robotic rectal experience.

26.7 New Technique in Colorectal Surgery: Transanal Total Mesorectal Excision (TaTME)

Surgery is in constant improvement to perfect existing techniques. For rectal cancer, a major step was the introduction of total mesorectal excision (TME) proposed by Heald in 1982 [31]. From this advance, new technique araised with the most promising being the rectal mobilization using a transanal approach (TaTME). Its acquisition should be structured and established. An expert consensus in 2017 sets the basis for a structured training for TaTME. Evidence from previous surgical training suggest that proctoring can shorten the learning curve and reduce major complications. An expert consensus concluded that to learn the TaTME approach, a minimum of 30 laparoscopic rectal cases and completion of training and accreditation in laparoscopic colorectal surgery are required [32]. They also set the prerequisite basis for being a mentor: at least 5 years in the surgical specialty, 30 TaTME cases performed independently, and 2 papers per year as an academic output.

In conclusion, the structured TaTME training curriculum is simplifed as:

- Self-learning (live case observation, VR, published literature)
- Cadaver workshop
- Proctorship (for initial five to ten cases with feedback from proctor)
- Independent practice (collection into registry, audit of outcomes)

Several cadaveric workshops exists. Four in Oxford and two in Chicago were studied by a survey. Forty-seven cases of TaTME were performed with improvement of the TME specimen quality between the first and second case. Eighty-one percent of the surgeons who participated continued to applicate this procedure in their local hospitals [33].

The Saint-Gallen expert consensus [34] offers a guidance to implementation of this technique. The consensus concluded that a safe and successful introduction and development of TaTME require adequate training. A course participation prior to performing any TaTME cases is advised. The presence of a proctor with an expert surgeon is strongly advised. The overall learning curve is more than 20 cases.

A new technique follows a well-defined tract: first the surgeon should learn its principles and applications during a theoritical course and a cadaveric workshop. Then, when performing it for the first time, he/she should be counseled and guided by a proctor until he/she is independent. And finally, to maintain a surgery with the same quality, he/she should participate in audit and give feedback to responsible organizations.

26.8 Conclusion

The path from general surgeon to an expert in colorectal surgery is long and with some pitfalls. Restriction on working hours, reduction of surgical indications, and the emergence of new technologies make more difficult to acquire the experience required. A clear training curriculum for all steps seems to be the answer to these difficulties. We propose in Fig. 26.4 an example for trainee supervision and a support in their progress.

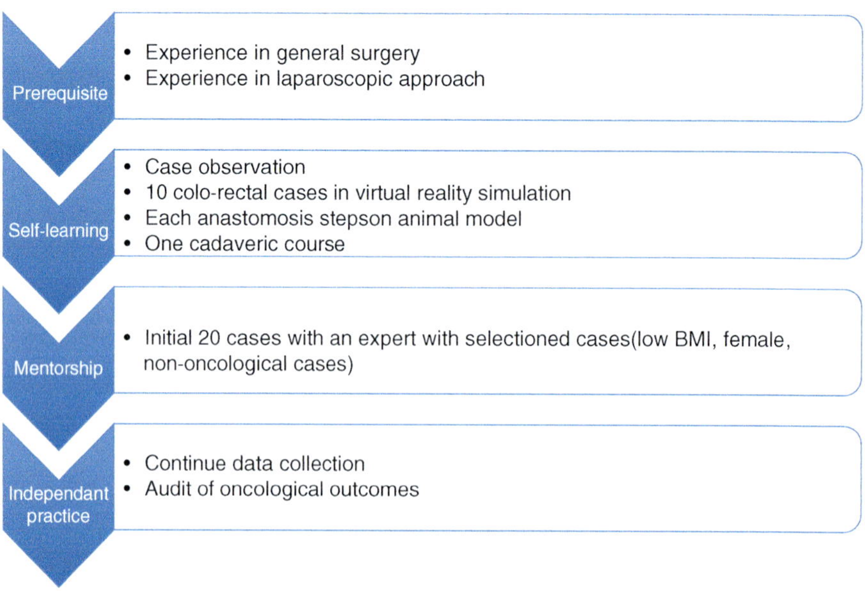

Fig. 26.4 Example of training curriculum in colorectal surgery

References

1. Jacobs M, Verdeja JC, Goldstein HS. Minimally invasive colon resection (laparoscopic colectomy). Surg Laparosc Endosc. 1991;1:144–50.
2. National Institute for Health and Care Excellence (NICE). Laparoscopic surgery for colorectal cancer. NICE technology appraisal guidance TA105. 2006. http://www.nice.org.uk/guidance/ta10.
3. www.lapco.nhs.uk/about-the-programme.php.
4. Health and Social Care Information Centre. National Bowel Cancer Audit Progress Report. Tripartite Colorectal Meeting, Birmingham. 2014. http://www.hscic.gov.uk/bowel.
5. Satava RM. Virtual reality surgical simulator. The first steps. Surg Endosc. 1993;7:203.
6. Nagendran M, Gurusamy KS, Aggarwal R, Loizidou M, Davidson BR. Virtual reality training for surgical trainees in laparoscopic surgery. Cochrane Database Syst Rev. 2013;(8):CD006575.
7. Grantcharov TP, Funch-Jensen P. Can everyone achieve proficiency with the laparoscopic technique? Learning curve patterns in technical skills acquisition. Am J Surg. 2009;197(4):447–9.
8. Gurusamy KS, Nagendran M, Toon CD, Davidson BR. Laparoscopic surgical box model training for surgical trainees with limited prior laparoscopic experience. Cochrane Database Syst Rev. 2014;(3):CD010478. https://doi.org/10.1002/14651858.CD010478.pub2.
9. Böhm B, Milsom JW. Animal models as educational tools in laparoscopic colorectal surgery. Surg Endosc. 1994;8(6):707–13.
10. Willaert W, Van De Putte D, Van Renterghem K, Van Nieuwenhove Y, Ceelen W, Pattyn P. Training models in laparoscopy: a systematic review comparing their effectiveness in learning surgical skills. Acta Chir Belg. 2013;113:77–95.
11. Leblanc F, Champagne BJ, Augestad KM, et al. A comparison of human cadaver and augmented reality simulator models for straight laparoscopic colorectal skills acquisition training. J Am Coll Surg. 2010;211:250–5.
12. Leblanc F, Senagore AJ, Ellis CN, et al. Hand-assisted laparoscopic sigmoid colectomy skills acquisition: augmented reality simulator versus human cadaver training models. J Surg Educ. 2010;67:200–4.
13. Miskovic D, Wyles SM, Ni M, Darzi AW, Hanna GB. Systematic review on mentoring and simulation in laparoscopic colorectal surgery. Ann Surg. 2010;252:943–51.
14. Ansell J, Goddard S, Gupta V, Warren N, Williams G, Haray P, Appleton B, Phillips S, Torkington J. A new ex vivo animal simulation model for skills training in laparoscopic colorectal surgery. Bull R Coll Surgeons Engl. 2014;96(4):122–4.
15. Mackenzie H, Miskovic D, Ni M, et al. Risk prediction score in laparoscopic colorectal surgery training. Ann Surg. 2015;261:338–44.
16. Ogiso S, Yamaguchi T, Fukuda M, et al. Laparoscopic resection for sigmoid and rectosigmoid colon cancer performed by trainees: impact on short-term outcomes and selection of suitable patients. Int J Colorectal Dis. 2012;27:1215–22.
17. Miskovic D, Ni M, Wyles SM, Tekkis P, Hanna GB. Learning curve and case selection in laparoscopic colorectal surgery: systematic review and international multicenter analysis of 4852 cases. Dis Colon Rectum. 2012;55(12):1300–10. (learning Curve).
18. Hemandas A, Flashman K, Farrow J, et al. Modular training in laparoscopic colorectal surgery maximizes training opportunities without clinical compromise. World J Surg. 2011;35:409–14.
19. Mackenzie H, Miskovic D, Ni M, et al. Clinical and educational proficiency gain of supervised laparoscopic colorectal surgical trainees. Surg Endosc. 2013;27:2704–11. https://doi.org/10.1007/s00464-013-2806-x.
20. de Montbrun S, Roberts PL, Satterthwaite L, MacRae H. Implementing and evaluating a national certification technical skills examination. Ann Surg. 2016;264:1–6. https://doi.org/10.1097/SLA.0000000000001620.
21. de Montbrun SL, Roberts PL, Lowry AC, et al. A novel approach to assessing technical competence of colorectal surgery residents: the development and evaluation of the Colorectal

Objective Structured Assessment of Technical Skill (COSATS). Ann Surg. 2013;258:1001–6. https://doi.org/10.1097/SLA.0b013e31829b32b8.
22. Miskovic D, Ni M, Wyles SM, Parvaiz A, Hanna GB. Observational clinical human reliability analysis (OCHRA) for competency assessment in laparoscopic colorectal surgery at the specialist level. Surg Endosc. 2012;26:796–803. https://doi.org/10.1007/s00464-011-1955-z.
23. Hemandas A, Flashman KG, Farrow J, O'Leary DP, Parvaiz A. Modular training in laparoscopic colorectal surgery maximizes training opportunities without clinical compromise. World J Surg. 2011;35:409–14. https://doi.org/10.1007/s00268-010-0837-1.
24. Kelly M, Bhangu A, Singh P. Systematic review and meta-analysis of trainee- versus expert surgeon-performed colorectal resection. Br J Surg. 2014;101:750–9.
25. Buchs NC. Training in robotic general surgery: the next challenge. Adv Robot Autom. 2012;1:1.
26. Disbrow DE, Pannell SM, Shanker BA, et al. The effect of formal robotic residency training on the adoption of minimally invasive surgery by young colorectal surgeons. J Surg Educ. 2018;75(3):767–78.
27. Buchs NC, Pugin F, Volonté F, et al. Learning tools and simulation in robotic surgery: state of the art. World J Surg. 2013;37(12):2812–9.
28. Pernar LIM, Robertson FC, Tavakkoli A, et al. An appraisal of the learning curve in robotic general surgery. Surg Endosc. 2017;31(11):4583–96.
29. Sian TS, Tierney GM, Park H, et al. Robotic colorectal surgery: previous laparoscopic colorectal experience is not essential. J Robot Surg. 2018;12(2):271–5.
30. Raimondi P, Marchegiani F, Cieri M, et al. Is right colectomy a complete learning procedure for a robotic surgical program? J Robot Surg. 2018;12(1):147–55.
31. Heald RJ, Husband EM, Ryall RDH, et al. The mesorectum in rectal cancer surgery, the clue to pelvic recurrence? Br J Surg. 1982;69(10):613–6.
32. Francis N, Penna M, Mackenzie H, et al. Consensus on structured training curriculum for transanal total mesorectal excision (TaTME). Surg Endosc. 2017;31(7):2711–9.
33. Penna M, Whiteford M, Hompes R, et al. Developing and assessing a cadaveric training model for transanal total mesorectal excision: initial experience in the UK and USA. Colorectal Dis. 2017;19(5):476–84.
34. Adamina M, Buchs NC, Penna M, et al. St.Gallen consensus on safe implementation of transanal total mesorectal excision. Surg Endosc. 2018;32(3):1091–103.

Emergency Colorectal Surgery Checklists and Technical Considerations

27

Pietro Genova, Solafah Abdalla, Francesco Brunetti, and Nicola de'Angelis

27.1 General Overview on Checklists in Surgery

The number of surgical operations performed every year all over the world is estimated at 234 million [1]. Some studies carried out in industrialized countries showed a perioperative mortality rate for inpatient surgery of 0.4–0.8%, whereas the rate of major complications was 3–17% [2–4]. These estimations have been considered likely to be higher in developing countries [5–8]. Moreover, three quarters of in-hospital adverse events might be related to surgery [9–12], and at least half of all surgical complications could be avoidable [2, 4, 9–12]. It follows that safety within the operating room (OR) represents an important public health concern, and that any effort should be done to avoid preventable morbidity related to surgery.

In this context, the World Health Organization (WHO) launched in 2008 the Surgical Safety Checklist (SSC), a control procedure dividing the perioperative period into three phases and identifying within each phase some main steps to be checked through one by one, with the general objective of increasing the safety of surgical patients and preventing avoidable complications worldwide [13]. Notably, ten essential objectives for safe surgery were identified: (1) correct site surgery, (2) provision of safe anaesthesia, (3) management of airway problems, (4) management of haemorrhage, (5) avoiding known allergies, (6) minimizing the risk of surgical site infection, (7) preventing the retention of swabs and instruments, (8) accurate

P. Genova (✉) · F. Brunetti · N. de'Angelis
Department of Digestive, Hepatobiliary and Hepatic Transplantation Surgery, Henri Mondor University Hospital, Assistance Publique—Hôpitaux de Paris (AP-HP), Université Paris Est—Créteil (UPEC), Créteil, France

S. Abdalla
Department of General and Digestive Surgery, Bicêtre University Hospital, Assistance Publique—Hôpitaux de Paris (AP-HP), Université Paris—Saclay, Paris, France

N. de'Angelis et al. (eds.), *Emergency Surgical Management of Colorectal Cancer*, Hot Topics in Acute Care Surgery and Trauma,
https://doi.org/10.1007/978-3-030-06225-5_27

identification of specimens, (9) effective communication within the surgical team, and (10) routine surveillance of surgical outcomes [14].

In 2009, Haynes et al. [3] carried out a prospective study which demonstrated that the checklist implementation was associated with a significant reduction of mortality and morbidity rates among patients undergoing noncardiac surgery. The institutional sites selected represented the diverse set of socioeconomic environments in which the WHO operates. Overall, postoperative complications decreased by 36% on average, a similar amount for mortality rate, and the checklist proved to be neither costly nor lengthy. In particular, the overall rate of complications fell from 11.0% to 7.0% ($p < 0.001$), and the total in-hospital mortality rate decreased from 1.5% to 0.8% ($p = 0.003$). The overall rates of surgical site infection (SSI) and unplanned reoperation also declined significantly ($p < 0.001$ and $p = 0.047$, respectively). Moreover, results concerning mortality and complications were independent from the institutional site, suggesting that the checklist program could improve the safety of surgical patients worldwide.

Over the years, several studies confirmed the association between the use of the WHO Surgical Safety Checklist and a significant reduction in mortality and morbidity rates, including two meta-analyses published in 2014 and another meta-analysis published in 2018 [9, 15]. Notably, Bergs et al. [9] demonstrated a risk ratio of 0.59 for any complications (95% CI, 0.47–0.74), 0.77 for mortality (95% CI, 0.60–0.98) and 0.57 for SSI (95% CI, 0.41–0.79). A strong correlation between the significant decrease in postoperative complications and the adherence to the checklist was also reported ($Q = 0.82$, $p = 0.042$). Similar results were provided by Abbott et al. [15], who showed a significant association between checklist use, reduced mortality (OR 0.75, 0.62–0.92, $p < 0.01$) and reduced incidence of postoperative complications (OR 0.73, 0.61–0.88, $p < 0.01$). And although no significant reduction in mortality rate could be found by Gillespie et al. [16], in the same study the checklist use was associated with a significant reduction in any complications rate (RR, 0.63; 95% CI, 0.58–0.72; $p < 0.0001$), wound infection rate (RR, 0.54; 95% CI, 0.40–0.72; $p = 0.0001$) and blood loss (RR, 0.56; 95% CI, 0.45–0.70; $p = 0.0001$). No advantages, neither in mortality nor in morbidity rates, were found in orthopaedic surgery [17].

The mechanisms responsible for the improvement of surgical outcomes after checklist implementation are not completely clear, probably multifactorial, partly due to ameliorated individual and institutional perioperative practices and better communication among surgical team members [3, 18–22]. Concerning ameliorated practices, many examples can be given: teams are stimulated to confirm orally patient's identity and surgical site, which is often not done; the administration of antibiotics within the operating room is encouraged, since delays are more frequent in preoperative wards, and confirmation of their appropriate use is provided, increasing the adherence to recommendations [3, 22]. A better communication between surgical team members is also stimulated, with preoperative briefings and postoperative debriefings, which have already shown to improve safety processes and attitudes [3, 18–20, 22].

By September 2014, the WHO registered 4132 institutions who had expressed their interest in using the checklist and 1790 institutions which were actively using the checklist in at least one operating theatre [23]. However, although most of the studies evaluating the impact of checklists on surgical outcomes refer to WHO SSC, some studies demonstrated similar benefits by using other types of surgical checklists [24], and other programmes are currently tested and evaluated in several countries and institutions [21, 25].

In conclusion, it must be noted that several studies have evaluated the compliance to the correct implementation of surgical checklists among OR teams, founding that they are often only partially followed and opening a debate on the best way to ensure their adequate integration within routine health processes [18, 26–28].

27.2 Historical Reference: From Aviation to Operating Rooms

The WHO SSC was adapted from the field of aeronautics, where checklists represent a common practice since many decades. An interesting article by S. W. Harden [29] spices up this apparently dry subject with a curious historical reference.

The use of checklists in aviation was developed after an air crash occurring in 1935 and involving one of the most experienced American pilots of that time. At Wright Air Field in Dayton, Ohio, the US Army Air Corps held a flight competition for airplane manufacturers vying to build its new-generation long-range bomber. The very favoured test plane was the Boeing's Model 299, which could fly faster and twice as far as previous bombers, and carry five times as many bombs as requested by the Army. The competition was almost a mere formality. Moreover, the pilot operating the airplane was Major Ployer Peter Hill, chief of the US Army Air Corps flight testing chief, few aviators being more experienced than him at that time. But unexpectedly, after taking off and climbing to 300 ft, the airplane stalled and crashed in a big explosion. Two of the five crew members died, including Hill. The following investigation revealed no mechanical fail and concluded that the air crash was due to a pilot error. Substantially more complex than previous aircrafts, the new plane required the pilot to attend to many different and complex tasks. While doing that, he forgot to release a mechanism on the elevator and rudder controls: "too much airplane for one man to fly", as a newspaper wrote. Nevertheless, the new airplane was judged to be reliable, but its functioning was considered too complicated to be left to the memory of any pilot, however expert. A checklist with step-by-step checks for take-off, flight, landing and taxying was created for pilots, and thanks to it, they went on to fly the Model 299 a total of 1.8 million miles without accidents. The aircraft was ultimately dubbed B-17, the Army ordering almost 13,000. It was commonly named "Flying Fortress" and provided allied forces a decisive air advantage in WW2, enabling US devastating bombing campaign across Nazi Germany.

In a sense, the WHO came to the same conclusion of the plane crash investigation team: even highly skilled OR teams need tools to help them prevent avoidable complications and achieve optimal results. Hence, a checklist for surgical operations was drawn up.

27.3 Surgical Checklists in Emergency

Emergency colorectal surgery is associated with higher risk of both mortality and morbidity compared to scheduled settings, with death and complications rates estimated at 10–25% and 30–50%, respectively, according to Western studies [30–33]. In this context, the exacerbated acuity of the pathological condition and time pressure may contribute to critical omissions and errors, further increasing the already high risks for the patients [22].

In emergency settings, a possible concern could originate from believing that the use of a checklist would interrupt the workflow and cause significant delays, increasing risks for patients [22, 34, 35]. Nonetheless, delays determining higher risks for patients are measured in hours rather than in minutes, and a brief perioperative checklist may avert errors that are common in emergency surgery [22]. In 2010, Weiser et al. [22] prospectively evaluated the occurrence of major complications and death during a period of up to 30 days from emergency surgery before and after SSC implementation. The overall complications rate decreased from 18.4% to 11.7% (p = 0.0001). The in-hospital death rate decreased from 3.7% to 1.4% (p = 0.0067). Moreover, the rate of surgical site infections fell from 11.2% to 6.6% (p = 0.0008), and the rate of estimated blood loss greater than 500 mL declined from 20.2% to 13.2% (p = 0.0001). Results concerning death and complications were independent from the institutional site. In this study, colorectal surgery represented 15.6% of the 842 emergency operations performed without surgical checklist and 22.2% of the 908 emergent surgical procedures carried on with. The same study could not conclude on the checklist utility in extreme emergency, such as active arterial bleeding with hemodynamic instability, such cases being uncommon in the series considered. However, the authors suggested that surgical teams should exercise judgment as to whether pausing for a checklist is a danger in such extreme cases. The WHO Surgical Safety Checklist in operations requiring intervention within 24 h of assessment was associated with significant reductions in complications and mortality rate and substantial improvements in safety practices in eight diverse facilities around the world.

27.4 How the Surgical Checklist Works

In order to describe the structure and functioning of a surgical checklist, the present chapter refers to the implementation manual of the WHO Surgical Safety Checklist published in 2009 [14]. The WHO SSC is shown in Fig. 27.1.

Generally, the responsible for checking the boxes on the list should be a single person. This designated checklist coordinator is often a circulating nurse, but it can be any professional participating in the operation.

In the checklist, the operation is divided into three phases, each one corresponding to a specific time period in the normal flow of a surgical procedure:

1. Before induction of anaesthesia (sign in)

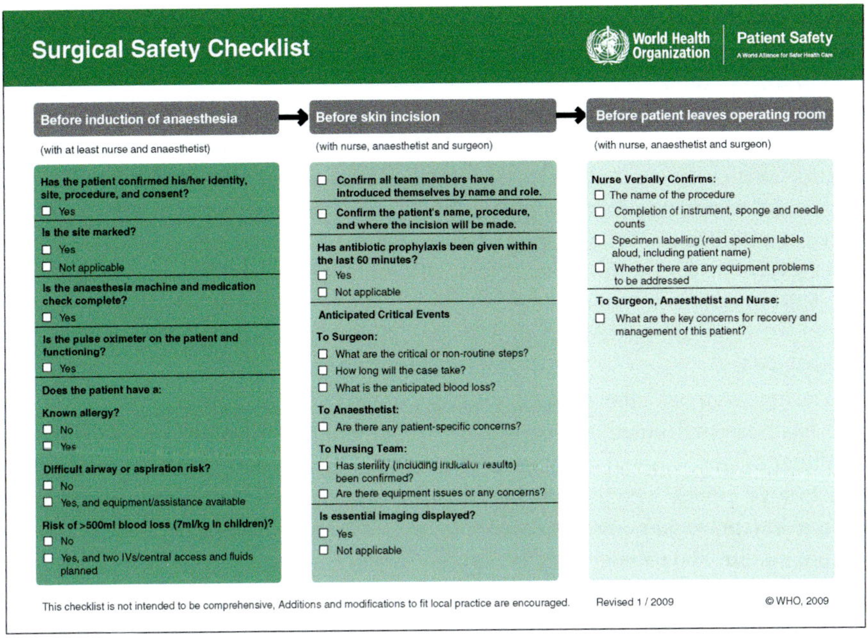

Surgical Safety Checklist

World Health Organization | Patient Safety — A World Alliance for Safer Health Care

Before induction of anaesthesia (with at least nurse and anaesthetist)

Has the patient confirmed his/her identity, site, procedure, and consent?
- ☐ Yes

Is the site marked?
- ☐ Yes
- ☐ Not applicable

Is the anaesthesia machine and medication check complete?
- ☐ Yes

Is the pulse oximeter on the patient and functioning?
- ☐ Yes

Does the patient have a:

Known allergy?
- ☐ No
- ☐ Yes

Difficult airway or aspiration risk?
- ☐ No
- ☐ Yes, and equipment/assistance available

Risk of >500ml blood loss (7ml/kg in children)?
- ☐ No
- ☐ Yes, and two IVs/central access and fluids planned

Before skin incision (with nurse, anaesthetist and surgeon)

- ☐ **Confirm all team members have introduced themselves by name and role.**
- ☐ **Confirm the patient's name, procedure, and where the incision will be made.**

Has antibiotic prophylaxis been given within the last 60 minutes?
- ☐ Yes
- ☐ Not applicable

Anticipated Critical Events

To Surgeon:
- ☐ What are the critical or non-routine steps?
- ☐ How long will the case take?
- ☐ What is the anticipated blood loss?

To Anaesthetist:
- ☐ Are there any patient-specific concerns?

To Nursing Team:
- ☐ Has sterility (including indicator results) been confirmed?
- ☐ Are there equipment issues or any concerns?

Is essential imaging displayed?
- ☐ Yes
- ☐ Not applicable

Before patient leaves operating room (with nurse, anaesthetist and surgeon)

Nurse Verbally Confirms:
- ☐ The name of the procedure
- ☐ Completion of instrument, sponge and needle counts
- ☐ Specimen labelling (read specimen labels aloud, including patient name)
- ☐ Whether there are any equipment problems to be addressed

To Surgeon, Anaesthetist and Nurse:
- ☐ What are the key concerns for recovery and management of this patient?

This checklist is not intended to be comprehensive, Additions and modifications to fit local practice are encouraged. Revised 1 / 2009 © WHO, 2009

Fig. 27.1 World Health Organization (WHO) Surgical Safety Checklist (SSC)

2. After induction and before surgical incision (time out)
3. During or immediately after wound closure but before removing the patient from the OR (sign out)

For each phase, the checklist coordinator should be permitted to confirm that the team has completed its tasks before proceeding further. After OR teams become familiar with the checklist steps, they can integrate the checks into their familiar work patterns and verbalize the completion of each step without the explicit intervention of a checklist coordinator. Each team should try to incorporate the use of the checklist into its work with maximum efficiency and minimum disruption while aiming to accomplish the steps effectively.

Nearly all the steps should be checked verbally with the appropriate personnel to ensure that the key actions have been performed.

During "sign in", before induction of anaesthesia, the checklist coordinator should verbally review with the patient (when possible) that his or her identity has been confirmed, that the procedure and operative site are correct and that consent for surgery has been given. The checklist responsible should visually confirm that the surgical site has been marked (if appropriate) and that a pulse oximeter has been place on the patient and it is functioning. The same coordinator should also verbally review with the anaesthesia personnel the patient's risk of blood loss, airway difficulty and allergic reaction and whether a full anaesthesia safety check has been completed. Ideally the surgeon should be present for "sign in", as he or she the surgeon could have a clearer idea of eventual blood loss, allergies or other complicating factors. However, the surgeon's presence is not essential for completing this part of the checklist.

During "time out", after induction and before surgical incision, each team member should introduce himself or herself by name and role, but the team could simply confirm that everyone in the room is known to each other. Immediately before skin incision, the operating room members should pause in order to confirm out loud that they are performing the correct operation on the correct patient and site and then should verbally review the critical elements of their plans for the operation using the checklist questions for guidance. They should also confirm that prophylactic antibiotics have been administered within the previous 60 min and that essential imaging is displayed.

During "sign out", the team members should review together what type of operation has been performed, the completion of sponge and instrument counts and the labelling of any surgical specimen. They should also review any equipment malfunction or issues which would need to be addressed. Finally, the team should review key plans and concerns regarding postoperative management and recovery before moving the patient from the operating room.

The availability of a single person to lead the checklist process is very important for its success. In the complex setting of an operating room, any of the steps might be overlooked during the fast preoperative, intraoperative or postoperative preparations, especially in case of an emergency. Hence, designating a single person to confirm the completion of each checklist step could ensure that safety steps are not omitted in the rush to move forward with the next phase of the operation. For this reason, the checklist process should be led by a single coordinator until team members are familiar with the steps involved. However, a possible disadvantage of a single person leading the checklist is that an antagonistic relationship might be established with other operating team members. The checklist coordinator should prevent the team from progressing to the next phase of the operation until each step is checked, irritating other team members. Therefore, hospitals might carefully consider which staff member is most suitable for this role. As mentioned above, it is often played by a circulating nurse, although any health professional can coordinate the checklist process.

27.5 Technical Considerations

Although emergency represents a condition where fast decisions and actions are demanded, it is always useful to provide a multidisciplinary approach to acute surgical settings, trying to involve all specialists concerned.

Notably, emergency room doctors are called to provide all useful information about patient's history and conditions, in order to let the anaesthesia and reanimation team assess the emergency degree and the suitability to postpone surgery and focus on clinical stabilization.

It is very important to evaluate preoperative imaging carefully, especially together with a radiologist, focusing on the factors which could lead the surgeon to modify his surgical strategy, with the aim to minimise perioperative unexpected findings: site and size of the tumour, involvement of surrounding structures, colonic or rectal perforation, intra-abdominal liquid and its composition according to its density, important vascular lesions, presence and extent of ischemic injuries.

In order to achieve best results, it is proved to be very important to have good communication with OR nurses as well.

27.5.1 Operating Room Set-Up [36–39]

27.5.1.1 Emergency Open Surgery

Right Colectomy (Fig. 27.2)

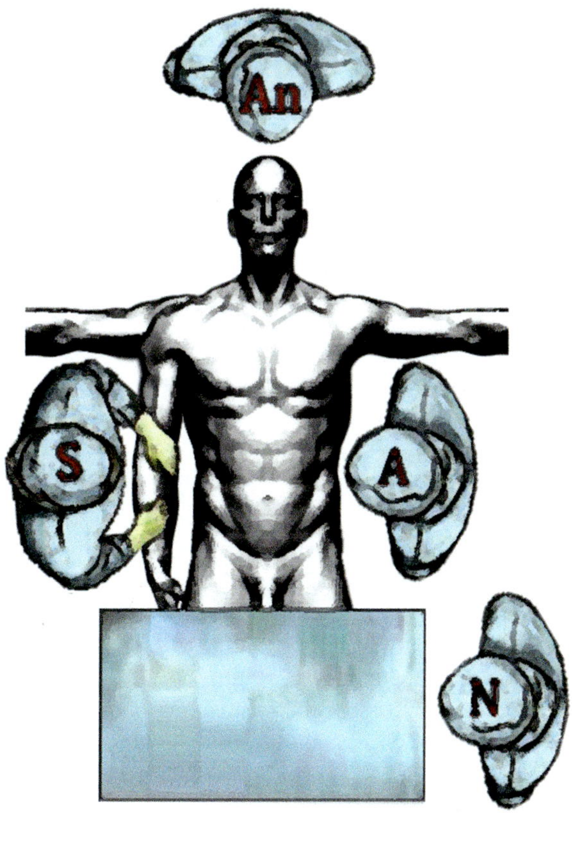

Fig. 27.2 Open right colectomy set-up: *An* anaesthesia team, *S* surgeon, *A* assistant, *N* nurse. Left or both arms abducted

Patient positioning

1. In supine position
2. Left arm or both arms abducted
3. Drawing up surgical landmarks
4. Surgical table accessories for adequate retracting installed (above patient's right shoulder)
5. Nasogastric tube
6. Urinary catheter
7. Left-tilting

Surgical team and equipment

1. Surgeon on patient's right
2. First assistant on patient's left
3. Second assistant on surgeon's left, when needed
4. Scrub nurse on first assistant's left

Midline supra- and sub-umbilical laparotomy, to be extended cranially and caudally according to surgical needs. This set-up could be used.

Left Colectomy, Low Anterior Resection, Hartmann's Procedure, Subtotal and Total Colectomy (Fig. 27.3)

Patient positioning

1. In modified lithotomy position
2. Right arm or both arms abducted
3. Buttocks at the table edge
4. Legs in stirrups, thighs parallel to abdominal wall
5. Drawing up surgical landmarks
6. Surgical table accessories for adequate retracting installed (above patient's left shoulder and above or between legs)
7. Nasogastric tube
8. Urinary catheter
9. Digital rectal exam
10. Right-tilting
11. Trendelenburg for steps in middle and lower quadrants
12. Reverse Trendelenburg in upper quadrant step

Surgical team and equipment

1. Surgeon on patient's left (on patient's right for left colic angle and left colon mobilization; variable according to needs and preferences)
2. First assistant on patient's right, always opposite to the surgeon
3. Second assistant between patient's legs
4. Scrub nurse on surgeon's left

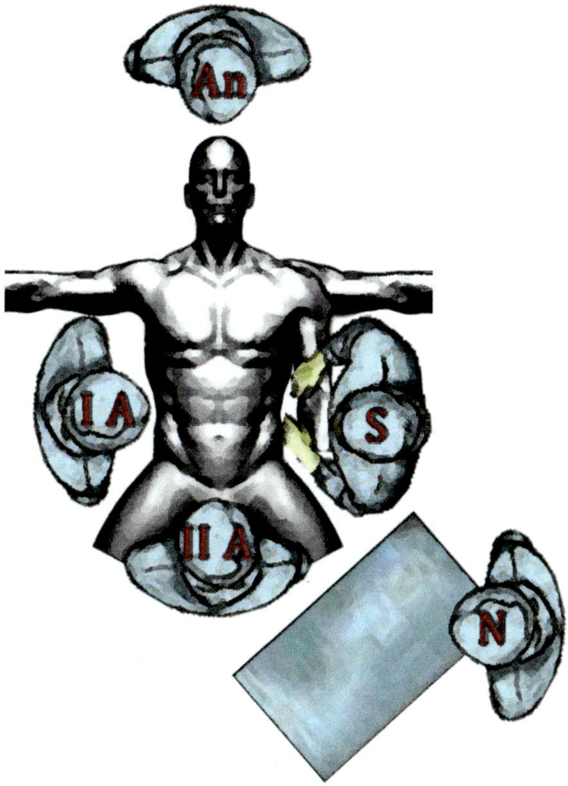

Fig. 27.3 Open left colectomy set-up: *An* anaesthesia team, *S* surgeon, *IA* first assistant, *IIA* second Assistant, *N* nurse. Right or both arms abducted

Lower midline laparotomy or xipho-pubic laparotomy according to lesion site and extent.

27.5.1.2 Laparoscopic Surgery

Equipment

Grasping, dissection and suturing instruments

1. 30° laparoscope
2. Atraumatic fenestrated graspers (3)
3. Dissectors (one large and one small right-angled dissectors, one Maryland)
4. Clip applier (1)
5. Scissors (1)
6. Needle holder (1)

Energy devices

1. Bipolar coagulation forceps (1)
2. Radiofrequency or ultrasound devices for haemostatic dissection (1)

Staplers

1. Laparoscopic linear stapler 45–60 (reloads for vascular and medium/thick tissues)
2. Laparoscopic circular stapler 28–30 (for surgery involving left colon and rectum)

Always prepare for a fast and safe conversion to open surgery if needed.

Right Colectomy (Fig. 27.4)

Patient positioning

1. In modified lithotomy position
2. Right arm abducted
3. Buttocks at the table edge
4. Legs in stirrups, thighs parallel to abdominal wall
5. Drawing surgical landmarks
6. Nasogastric tube
7. Urinary catheter
8. Left-tilting
9. Trendelenburg for middle and lower quadrants
10. Reverse Trendelenburg for upper quadrants

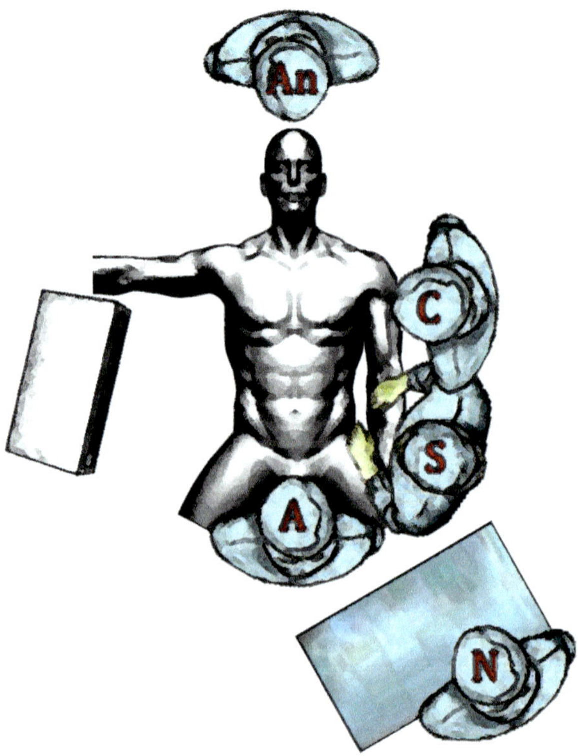

Fig. 27.4 Laparoscopic right colectomy set-up: *An* anaesthesia team, *S* surgeon, *C* camera operator, *A* assistant, *N* nurse. Monitor in front of the surgeon

Surgical team and equipment

1. Surgeon on patient's left
2. Camera operator on surgeon's right
3. Assistant between patient's legs
4. Scrub nurse on surgeon's left
5. Monitor on patient's right, in front of the surgeon
6. Energy devices platform on patient's right

In case of extracorporeal anastomosis, a midline supra- and sub-umbilical laparotomy is usually performed and used to remove the specimen. In case of intracorporeal anastomosis, the specimen can be removed through a Pfannenstiel laparotomy.

Left Colectomy, Low Anterior Resection, Hartmann's Procedure, Subtotal and Total Colectomy (Fig. 27.5)

Patient positioning

1. In modified lithotomy position
2. Left arm abducted
3. Buttocks at the table edge

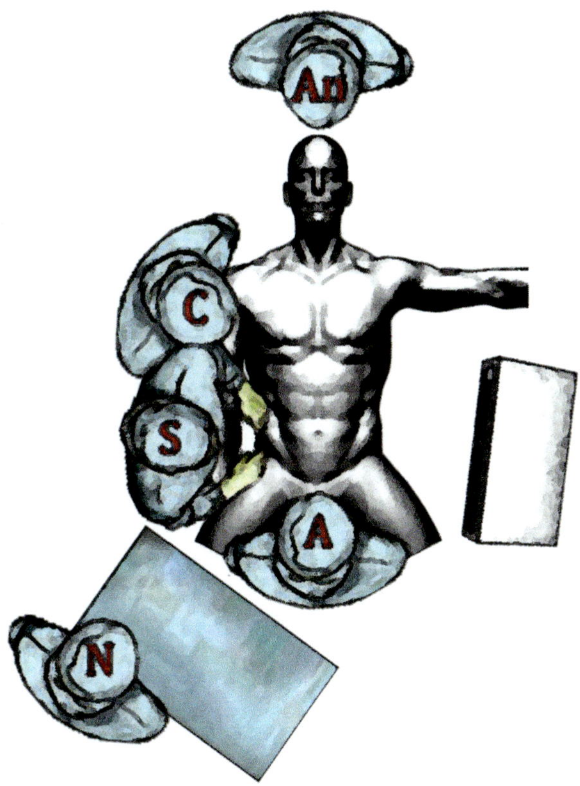

Fig. 27.5 Laparoscopic left colectomy set-up: *An* anaesthesia team, *S* surgeon, *C* camera operator, *A* assistant, *N* nurse. Monitor in front of the surgeon

4. Legs in stirrups, thighs parallel to abdominal wall
5. Drawing surgical landmarks
6. Nasogastric tube
7. Urinary catheter
8. Digital rectal exam
9. Right-tilting
10. Trendelenburg for middle and lower quadrants
11. Reverse Trendelenburg for upper quadrants

Surgical team and equipment
1. Surgeon on patient's right
2. Camera operator on patient's right, on surgeon's left
3. Assistant between patient's legs
4. Scrub nurse on surgeon's right
5. Monitor on patient's left, in front of the surgeon
6. Energy device platform on patient's left

A Pfannenstiel laparotomy is usually performed for extracorporeal anastomosis and specimen removal.

27.5.2 Port Placement [37, 40–43]

27.5.2.1 Right Colectomy (Fig. 27.6)

1. 12 mm umbilical port (camera)
   Supraumbilical incision

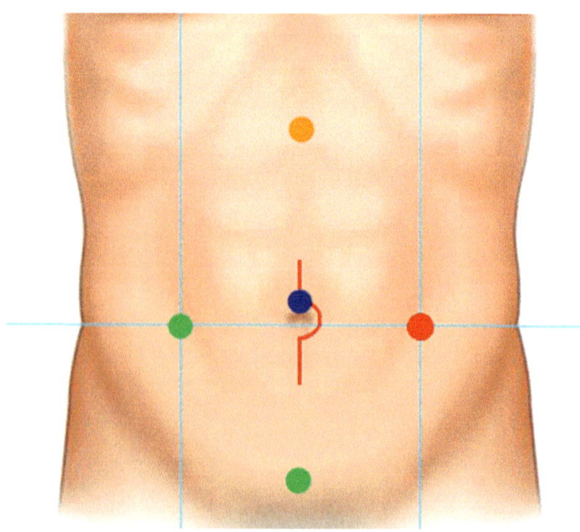

Fig. 27.6 Laparoscopic right colectomy ports placement: blue = 12 mm camera port, red = 12 mm port for surgeon's working right hand, green = 5 mm port, yellow = optional 5 mm port. Specimen removed from a midline supra- and sub-umbilical laparotomy (red line)

2. 12 mm left lumbar port (right hand working)
   At the umbilical level, on left midclavicular line
3. 5 mm suprapubic port (left hand working)
   Two finger breadth cranially from the pubis
4. 5 mm right lumbar port (assistant)
   At the umbilical level, on right midclavicular line
5. 5 mm epigastric port (optional)
   It can be useful in case of difficult exposure

27.5.2.2 Left Colectomy, Low Anterior Resection, Hartmann's Procedure (Fig. 27.7)

1. 12 mm umbilical port (camera)
   Supraumbilical incision
2. 5 mm right lumbar port (left hand working)
   At the umbilical level, on the right midclavicular line
3. 12 mm right iliac port (right hand working)
   Four finger breadth caudally from the previous
4. 5 mm suprapubic port (assistant)
   Two finger breadth cranially from the pubis
5. 5 mm left lumbar port (assistant)
   At the umbilical level, on the left midclavicular line

27.5.2.3 Subtotal and Total Colectomy (Fig. 27.8)

1. 12 mm umbilical port (camera)
   Supraumbilical incision
2. 12 mm right iliac port
   Four finger breadth caudally from camera port, on right midclavicular line

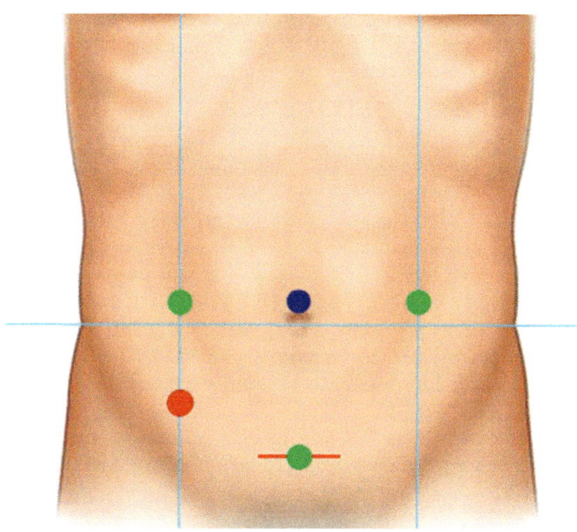

Fig. 27.7 Laparoscopic left colectomy ports placement: blue = 12 mm camera port, red = 12 mm port for surgeon's working right hand, green = 5 mm port. Specimen removed from a Pfannenstiel laparotomy (red line)

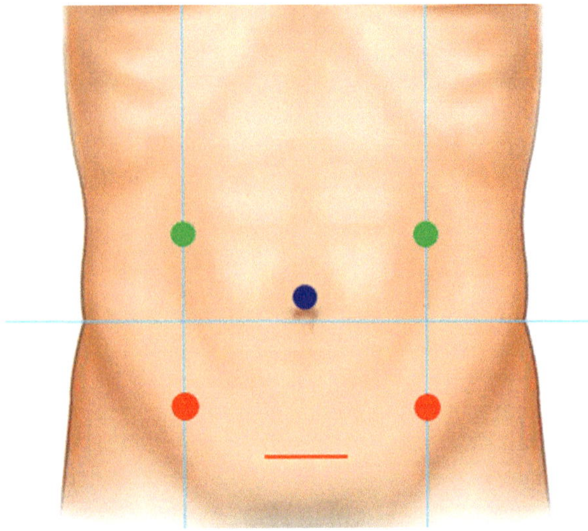

Fig. 27.8 Laparoscopic subtotal or total colectomy ports placement: blue = 12 mm camera port, red = 12 mm port, green = 5 mm port. Specimen removed from a Pfannenstiel laparotomy (red line)

3. 5 mm right hypochondrium port
   Four finger breadth cranially from camera port, on the right midclavicular line
4. 12 mm left iliac port
   Four finger breadth caudally from camera port, on the left midclavicular line
5. 5 mm left hypochondrium port
   Four finger breadth cranially from camera port, on the left midclavicular line

To be noted: all operating room set-ups reported above reflect authors' preferences. Indeed, equipment, patient's and surgical team members' position, surgical incision and port placement are generally quite variable in colorectal surgery. Decisions are conditioned by patient's habitus, surgeon's personal preferences, medical school habits and surgical steps carried out within the operation.

References

1. Weiser TG, Regenbogen SE, Thompson KD, et al. An estimation of the global volume of surgery: a modelling strategy based on available data. Lancet. 2008;372(9633):139–44.
2. Gawande AA, Thomas EJ, Zinner MJ, Brennan TA. The incidence and nature of surgical adverse events in Colorado and Utah in 1992. Surgery. 1999;126(1):66–75.
3. Haynes AB, Weiser TG, Berry WR, et al. A surgical safety checklist to reduce morbidity and mortality in a global population. N Engl J Med. 2009;360(5):491–9.
4. Kable AK, Gibberd RW, Spigelman AD. Adverse events in surgical patients in Australia. Int J Qual Health Care. 2002;14(4):269–76.
5. McConkey SJ. Case series of acute abdominal surgery in rural Sierra Leone. World J Surg. 2002;26(4):509–13.
6. Bickler SW, Sanno-Duanda B. Epidemiology of paediatric surgical admissions to a government referral hospital in the Gambia. Bull World Health Organ. 2000;78(11):1330–6.

7. Yii MK, Ng KJ. Risk-adjusted surgical audit with the POSSUM scoring system in a developing country. Physiological and Operative Severity Score for the enUmeration of Mortality and morbidity. Br J Surg. 2002;89(1):110–3.
8. Ouro-Bang'na Maman AF, Tomta K, Ahouangbevi S, Chobli M. Deaths associated with anaesthesia in Togo, West Africa. Trop Doct. 2005;35(4):220–2.
9. Bergs J, Hellings J, Cleemput I, et al. Systematic review and meta-analysis of the effect of the World Health Organization surgical safety checklist on postoperative complications. Br J Surg. 2014;101(3):150–8.
10. de Vries EN, Ramrattan MA, Smorenburg SM, Gouma DJ, Boermeester MA. The incidence and nature of in-hospital adverse events: a systematic review. Qual Saf Health Care. 2008;17:216–23.
11. Pearse RM, Moreno RP, Bauer P, et al. Mortality after surgery in Europe: a 7 day cohort study. Lancet. 2012;380(9847):1059–65.
12. Zegers M, de Bruijne MC, de Keizer B, et al. The incidence, root-causes, and outcomes of adverse events in surgical units: implication for potential prevention strategies. Patient Saf Surg. 2011;5:13.
13. World Health Organization & WHO Patient Safety. Implementation manual: WHO surgical safety checklist. 1st ed. Geneva: World Health Organization; 2008. http://www.who.int/iris/handle/10665/70046.
14. WHO. WHO Guidelines for safe surgery 2009. Safe surgery saves lives. http://whqlibdoc.who.int/publications/2009/9789241598552_eng.pdf. Accessed 15 May 2018.
15. Abbott TEF, Ahmad T, Phull MK, et al. The surgical safety checklist and patient outcomes after surgery: a prospective observational cohort study, systematic review and meta-analysis. Br J Anaesth. 2018;120(1):146–55.
16. Gillespie BM, Chaboyer W, Thalib L, John M, Fairweather N, Slater K. Effect of using a safety checklist on patient complications after surgery: a systematic review and meta-analysis. Anesthesiology. 2014;120(6):1380–9.
17. Sewell M, Adebibe M, Jayakumar P, et al. Use of the WHO surgical safety checklist in trauma and orthopaedic patients. Int Orthop. 2011;35(6):897–901.
18. Conley DM, Singer SJ, Edmondson L, Berry WR, Gawande AA. Effective surgical safety checklist implementation. J Am Coll Surg. 2011;212(5):873–9.
19. Lingard L, Regehr G, Orser B, et al. Evaluation of a preoperative checklist and team briefing among surgeons, nurses, and anesthesiologists to reduce failures in communication. Arch Surg. 2008;143(1):12–17; discussion 18.
20. Pugel AE, Simianu VV, Flum DR, Patchen Dellinger E. Use of the surgical safety checklist to improve communication and reduce complications. J Infect Public Health. 2015;8(3):219–25.
21. Treadwell JR, Lucas S, Tsou AY. Surgical checklists: a systematic review of impacts and implementation. BMJ Qual Saf. 2014;23(4):299–318.
22. Weiser TG, Haynes AB, Dziekan G, et al. Effect of a 19-item surgical safety checklist during urgent operations in a global patient population. Ann Surg. 2010;251(5):976–80.
23. Woodman N, Walker I. World Health Organization surgical safety checklist; 2016.
24. de Vries EN, Prins HA, Crolla RM, et al. Effect of a comprehensive surgical safety system on patient outcomes. N Engl J Med. 2010;363(20):1928–37.
25. Walker IA, Reshamwalla S, Wilson IH. Surgical safety checklists: do they improve outcomes? Br J Anaesth. 2012;109(1):47–54.
26. Levy SM, Senter CE, Hawkins RB, et al. Implementing a surgical checklist: more than checking a box. Surgery. 2012;152(3):331–6.
27. Poon SJ, Zuckerman SL, Mainthia R, et al. Methodology and bias in assessing compliance with a surgical safety checklist. Jt Comm J Qual Patient Saf. 2013;39(2):77–82.
28. Russ S, Rout S, Caris J, et al. Measuring variation in use of the WHO surgical safety checklist in the operating room: a multicenter prospective cross-sectional study. J Am Coll Surg. 2015;220(1):1–11 e14.

29. Harden SW. The birth of the checklist.
30. Aydin HN, Tekkis PP, Remzi FH, Constantinides V, Fazio VW. Evaluation of the risk of a non-restorative resection for the treatment of diverticular disease: the Cleveland Clinic diverticular disease propensity score. Dis Colon Rectum. 2006;49(5):629–39.
31. Han EC, Ryoo SB, Park BK, et al. Surgical outcomes and prognostic factors of emergency surgery for colonic perforation: would fecal contamination increase morbidity and mortality? Int J Colorectal Dis. 2015;30(11):1495–504.
32. Isbister WH, Prasad J. Emergency large bowel surgery: a 15-year audit. Int J Colorectal Dis. 1997;12(5):285–90.
33. Kim CN. Emergent colorectal surgery: what should be considered? Ann Coloproctol. 2016;32(4):124–5.
34. Bickell NA, Aufses AH Jr, Rojas M, Bodian C. How time affects the risk of rupture in appendicitis. J Am Coll Surg. 2006;202(3):401–6.
35. Gustilo RB, Merkow RL, Templeman D. The management of open fractures. J Bone Joint Surg Am. 1990;72(2):299–304.
36. Encyclopédie Médico-Chirurgicale (EMC). Techniques Chirurgicales - Appareil Digestif. Paris: Elsevier; 1970.
37. Dulucq J-L, Wintringer P, Périssat J. Tips and techniques in laparoscopic surgery. New York: Springer; 2005.
38. Valleur P. Chirurgie du tube digestif bas. Paris: Elsevier; 2005.
39. Young-Fadok TM. Colorectal resections: patient positioning and operating room setup. In: Whelan RL, Fleshman JW, Fowler DL, editors. The sages manual. New York: Springer; 2006. p. 150–62.
40. Ferzli GS, Fingerhut A. Trocar placement for laparoscopic abdominal procedures: a simple standardized method. J Am Coll Surg. 2004;198(1):163–73.
41. Croce E, Olmi S, Azzola M, Russo R, Di Bonifacio M. Laparoscopic colectomy: indications, standardized technique and results after 6 years experience. Hepato-Gastroenterology. 2000;47(33):683–91.
42. Laparoscopically assisted colectomy is as safe and effective as open colectomy in people with colon cancer Abstracted from: Nelson H, Sargent D, Wieand HS, et al., for the Clinical Outcomes of Surgical Therapy Study Group. A comparison of laparoscopically assisted and open colectomy for colon cancer. N Engl J Med. 2004;350:2050–9. Cancer Treat Rev. 2004;30(8):707–9.
43. de'Angelis N, Lizzi V, Azoulay D, Brunetti F. Robotic versus laparoscopic right colectomy for colon cancer: analysis of the initial simultaneous learning curve of a surgical fellow. J Laparoendosc Adv Surg Tech A. 2016;26(11):882–92.

Clinical Cases on Colorectal Cancer Emergency

28

Solafah Abdalla, Pietro Genova, and Christophe Penna

28.1 Case Study No. 1

You have to manage in the emergency room a 75-year-old man with a medical history of pulmonary embolism 4 months ago and currently treated with warfarin. He has no history of abdominal surgery. He consults for diffuse abdominal pain, cessation of flatus and stools for 4 days, and fever of 38.7 °C and chills for 24 h. He vomited once 24 h ago. He also experienced asthenia and recent weight loss of 7 kg over the past 6 months not attributable to diet or exercise. He complains with progressively aggravating alternation of diarrhea and constipation for 3 months. He finally remembers that he noticed several times in the last months the presence of red blood in the stools, about which he did not worried because he thought it came from the hemorrhoids.

Vital Signs: Blood pressure, 86/45 mmHg; pulse, 117 bpm; respiratory rate, 22 breaths/min; temperature, 38.6 °C; sats, 97% on room air; weight, 73 kg; height, 179 cm.

Physical Examination: Sclerae is anicteric with pale conjunctiva. The abdomen is distended and tympanic. You hear no intra-abdominal rumbling noise. There is no inguinal, crural, or umbilical herniation. There is no palpable adenopathy. Cardiac and pulmonary auscultation are unremarkable.

Question 1:

Physical examination suggests the diagnosis of colonic obstructive syndrome. How do you complete your physical examination?

S. Abdalla (✉) · C. Penna
Department of Digestive Surgery and Surgical Oncology, Bicêtre Hospital, Assistance Publique Hôpitaux de Paris, Université Paris-Sud, Le Kremlin Bicêtre, France

P. Genova
Department of General and Oncological Surgery, Azienda Ospedaliera Universitaria Policlinico Paolo Giaccone, Palermo, PA, Italy

N. de'Angelis et al. (eds.), *Emergency Surgical Management of Colorectal Cancer*, Hot Topics in Acute Care Surgery and Trauma,
https://doi.org/10.1007/978-3-030-06225-5_28

The completion of your physical examination shows:

His last colonoscopy was performed 10 years ago and several benign polyps were removed.

The patient presents clammy skin on the knees. Palpation of the abdomen shows an elective tenderness on the right flank and right iliac fossa and pain without tenderness in the left iliac fossa. Examination of the anal margin and digital rectal exam reveals the presence of grade II hemorrhoids, the absence of stool in the rectum, the absence of intrarectal mass, and the absence of blood on the finger cot.

Laboratory findings at the emergency room:

White blood cell (WBC) count	12,700 cells/mm^3
Hemoglobin	9.3 g/dL
Hematocrit	51%
Mean corpuscular volume	70 μm^3
Platelet count	500,000/μL
Sodium	145 mEq/L
Potassium	4.2 mEq/L
Urea nitrogen	10 mmol/L
Creatinine	150 μmol/L (1.70 mg/dL)
Creatinine clearance (MDRD)	67 mL/min/1.73 m^2
C-reactive protein (CRP)	45 mg/L
International normalized ratio	4.2

Question 2:

What is your interpretation of the laboratory findings?

Question 3:

What imaging exam do you ask to make the diagnosis? In what time frame? What precautionary measures do you take?

Question 4:

What is your interpretation of this imaging exam (Figs. 28.1, 28.2, 28.3, 28.4, and 28.5)?

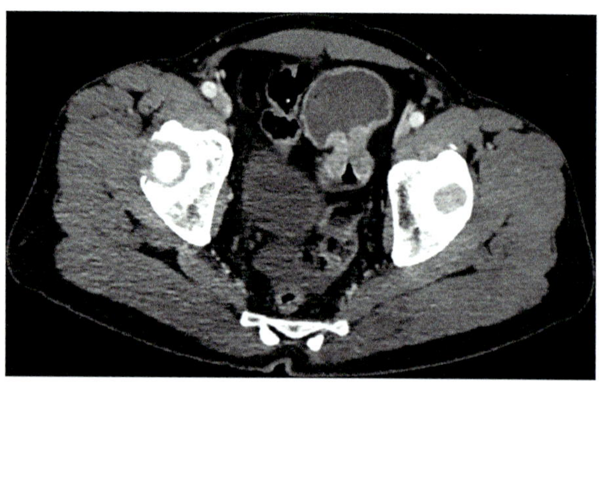

Fig. 28.1 Abdominal CT scan with contrast, portal phase, cross-sectional view

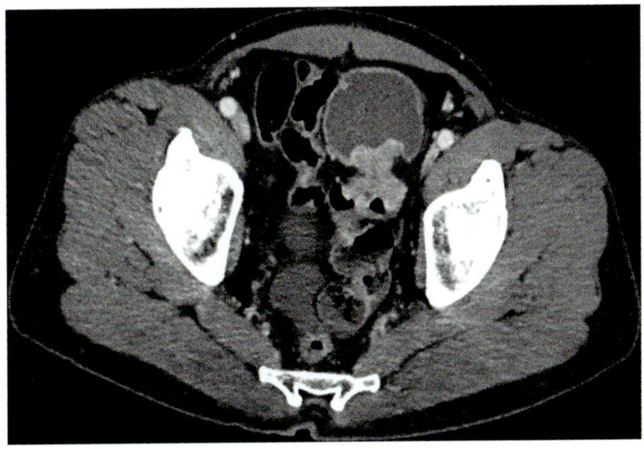

Fig. 28.2 Abdominal CT scan with contrast, portal phase, cross-sectional view

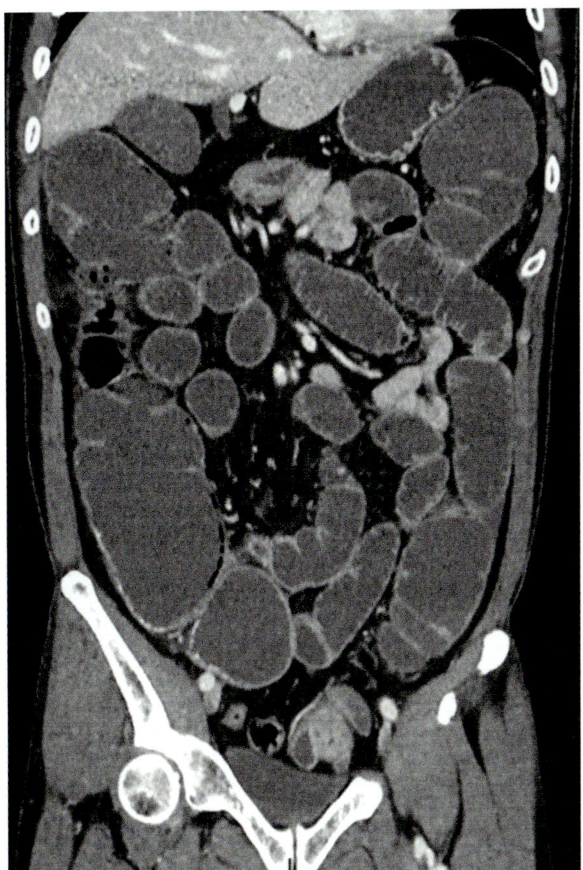

Fig. 28.3 Abdominal CT scan with contrast, portal phase, coronal view

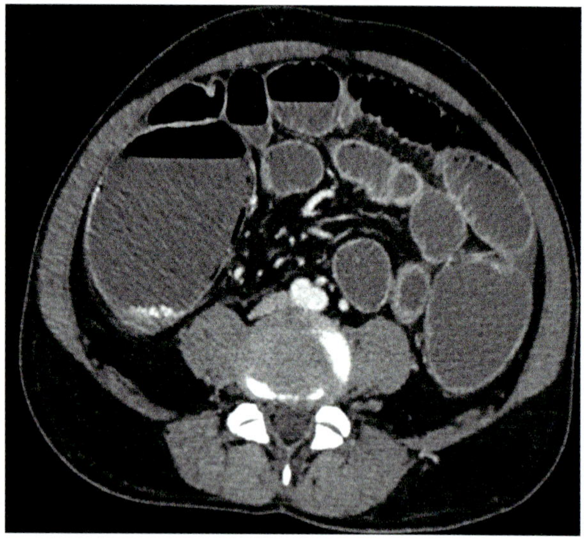

Fig. 28.4 Abdominal CT scan with contrast, portal phase, cross-sectional view

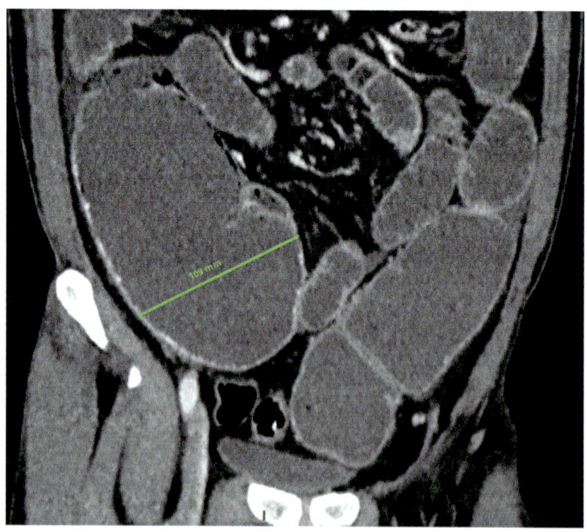

Fig. 28.5 Abdominal CT scan with contrast, portal phase, coronal view

Question 5:
What is your final diagnosis?
Question 6:
What is your etiologic emergency treatment?

A. Isolated non-operative treatment: nasogastric tube aspiration
B. Endoscopic self-expandable metal colonic stent placement
C. Surgical treatment: proximal loop left colostomy

D. Surgical treatment: proctectomy with Hartmann's procedure and left colostomy
E. Surgical treatment: total coloproctectomy with terminal ileostomy
F. Surgical treatment: total colectomy with ileorectal anastomosis ± derivation ileostomy

Question 7:

Is there an indication for an endoscopic placement of a self-expandable metallic colonic stent to treat the occlusion? Why?

Question 8:

Describe the general the steps of your treatment.

Question 9:

You chose a surgical treatment. Operative findings are shown in Figs. 28.6 and 28.7. Identify the two main operative findings (black star and black arrow), and describe the steps of the surgical treatment.

At the fifth postoperative day, the patient has not had any flatus or stools yet. Physical examination shows abdominal distension but no tenderness. There is no wound complication. Rectal digital exam shows the absence of stools in the rectum. The anastomosis is too high to be reached. Nasogastric tube aspiration output is 1900 mL/day of digestive liquid.

Question 10:

What is your diagnosis?

Question 11:

In this case, before concluding with a functional etiology, what are the two diagnoses that you have to eliminate?

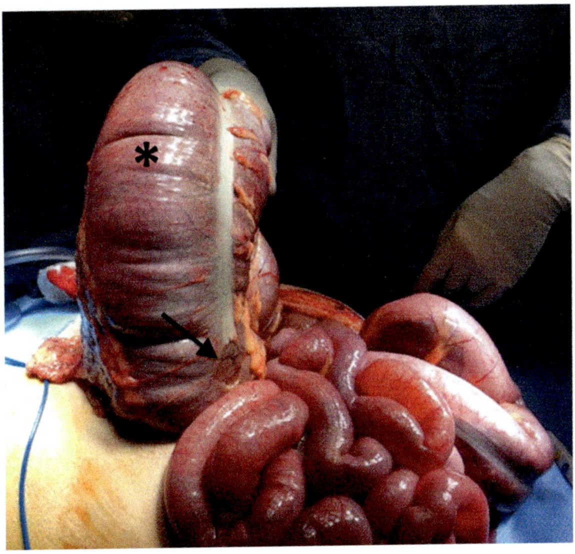

Fig. 28.6 Intra-operative findings

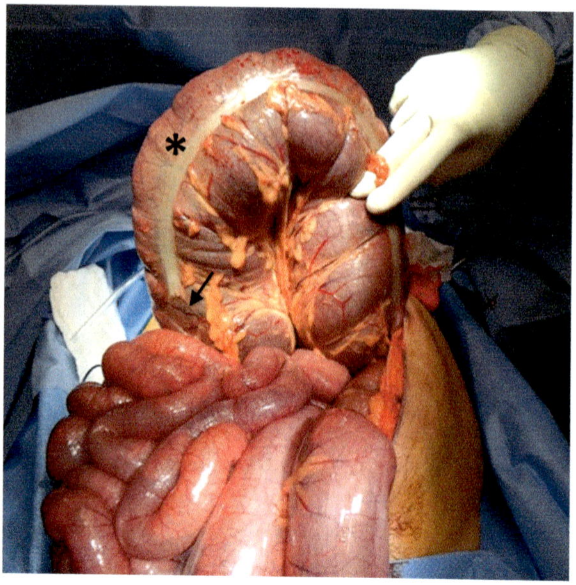

Fig. 28.7 Intra-operative findings

Question 12:

What most frequent underlying causes of this condition do you suspect?

Question 13:

What complementary exams do you ask to determine the cause of this condition?

28.2 Answers: Case Study No. 1

Question 1:

Physical examination suggests the diagnosis of colonic obstructive syndrome. How do you complete your physical examination?

Answer 1:

Other clinical signs of dehydration and hypovolemic shock

- Thirst
- Less frequent urination
- Confusion
- Clammy skin
- Freshness of his hands and feet

Clinical gravity signs of the obstructive syndrome

- Pain on the right flank and right iliac fossa indicating critical distension of the cecum
- Clinical signs of digestive perforation and peritonitis: abdominal tenderness or abdominal guarding

Etiology of the colonic obstruction

Fecaloma? colorectal cancer? diverticular stenosis?

- Medical history of diverticulitis
- Time of the last colonoscopy and results
- Digital rectal exam: intrarectal mass, fecaloma, hemorrhoids, bleeding

Question 2:
What is your interpretation of the laboratory findings?
Answer 2:

- Acute kidney failure (elevated creatininemia, creatinine clearance <90 mL/min) caused by dehydration (hypernatremia, hematocrit >50%, increased urea nitrogen) without biological criteria for hemodialysis (no threatening hyperkaliemia)
- Biological inflammatory syndrome (elevated white blood cell count and C-reactive protein)
- Microcytic anemia (hemoglobin <13 g/dL, decreased mean corpuscular volume)

Question 3:
What imaging exam do you ask to make the diagnosis? In what time frame? What precautionary measures do you take?
Answer 3:

- Abdominal IV CT scan
- In emergency
- After having put a nasogastric tube
- Rapid intravenous hydration before and particularly after the IV CT scan to prevent the aggravation of the kidney failure

Another possible answer: thoracic and abdominal IV CT scan. With the previous diagnosis of pulmonary embolism, the thoracic slices would be useful to look for lung metastases and recurrence of pulmonary embolism.

Question 4:
What is your interpretation of this imaging exam (Figs. 28.1, 28.2, 28.3, 28.4, and 28.5)?
Answer 4:

- Apple core stenosing mass of the sigmoid colon (red star in Figs. 28.8 and 28.9)
- Dilatation of the whole upstream colon (red crosses in Figs. 28.10, 28.11, and 28.12)
- Cecum diameter at 109 mm (Fig. 28.12)
- Parietal pneumatosis of the cecum (red arrows in Figs. 28.10 and 28.11)
- Dilatation of the small bowel (red circles in Figs. 28.10, 28.11, and 28.12) and incompetence of the ileocecal valve

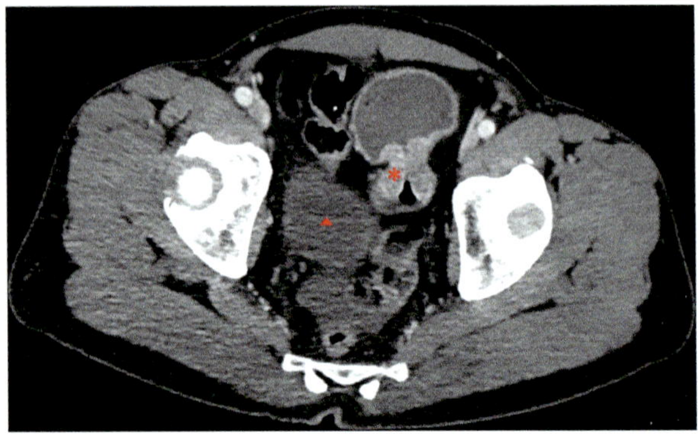

Fig. 28.8 Abdominal CT scan with contrast, portal phase, cross-sectional view

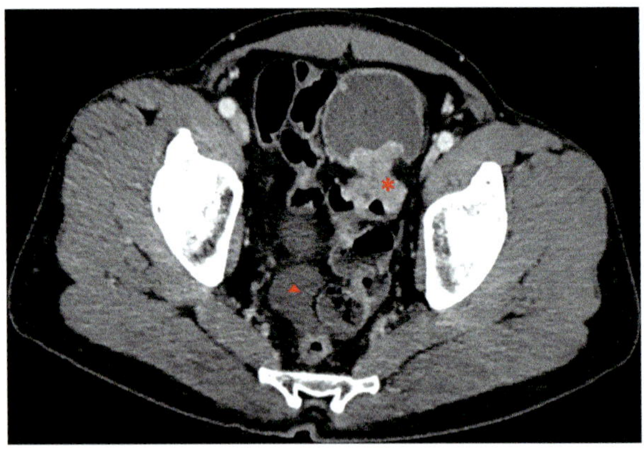

Fig. 28.9 Abdominal CT scan with contrast, portal phase, cross-sectional view

- Moderate intra-abdominal effusion (red triangle in Figs. 28.8 and 28.9)
- Absence of pneumoperitoneum
- Absence of peritoneal carcinomatosis
- Absence of hepatic metastases

Question 5:
What is your final diagnosis?
Answer 5:

Nonmetastatic stenosing tumor of the sigmoid colon with signs of parietal suffering of the cecum without digestive perforation, associated with acute renal failure by dehydration

Question 6:
What is your etiologic emergency treatment?
Answer 6:

A. ~~Isolated non-operative treatment: nasogastric tube aspiration~~
B. ~~Endoscopic self-expandable metal colonic stent placement~~

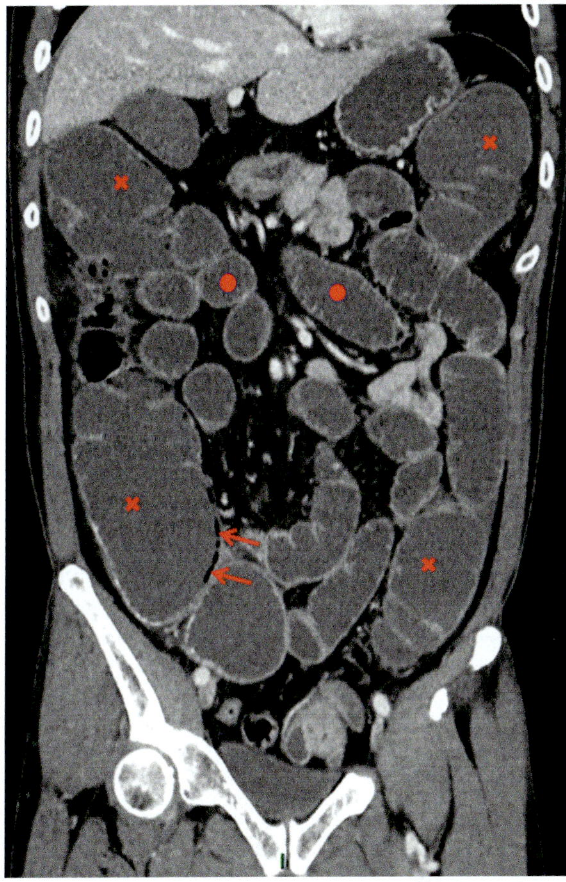

Fig. 28.10 Abdominal CT scan with contrast, portal phase, coronal view

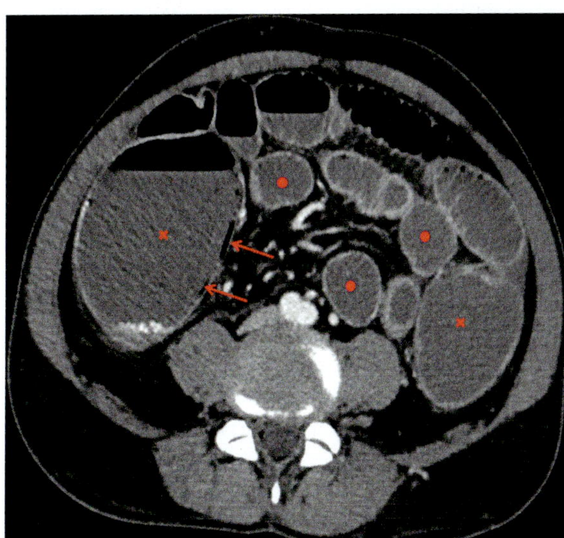

Fig. 28.11 Abdominal CT scan with contrast, portal phase, cross-sectional view

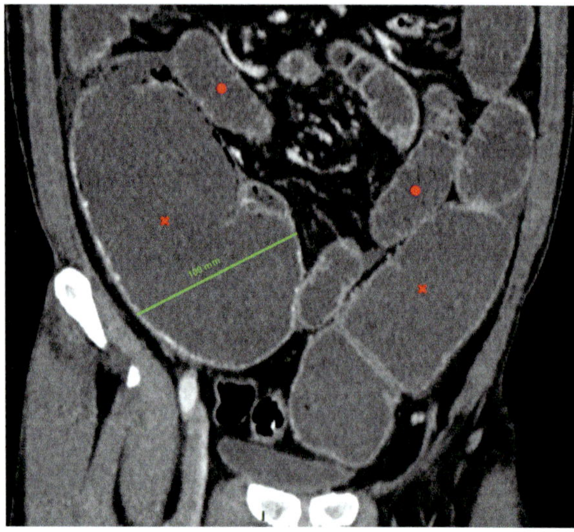

Fig. 28.12 Abdominal CT scan with contrast, portal phase, coronal view

C. ~~Surgical treatment: proximal loop left colostomy~~
D. ~~Surgical treatment: proctectomy with Hartman's procedure and left colostomy~~
E. ~~Surgical treatment: total coloproctectomy with terminal ileostomy~~
F. Surgical treatment: total colectomy with ileorectal anastomosis ± derivation ileostomy

Answer F is true.

The suspicion of cecal ischemia requires a surgical exploration and eventually a treatment (resection). Therefore, answers A, B, and C are non-valid.

Answers D, E, and F are valid. However, in this case, total coloproctectomy with terminal ileostomy (answer E) should not be performed as the first-line surgical treatment because of high postoperative morbidity and poor quality of life. After exploration, and only in the absence of ischemia of the caecum and transverse colon, proctectomy with Hartmann's procedure and left colostomy (answer D) could be a licit alternative, but with a 50% risk of definitive colostomy. In this case, the best surgical treatment is total colectomy with ileorectal anastomosis, with derivation ileostomy (answer F) depending on the level and quality of the colorectal anastomosis.

Question 7:

Is there an indication for an endoscopic placement of a self-expandable metallic colonic stent to treat the occlusion? Why?

Answer 7:

No. Several studies showed that, in large bowel obstruction by adenocarcinoma, the placement of a self-expandable metallic stent was associated with a risk of tumor spread (in addition to the risk of failure or perforation) and decreased survival rates [1, 2]. Moreover, in this case, endoscopic stenting is contraindicated because the cecum is nearly perforated and colonic insufflation could lead to colonic perforation and peritonitis. The colonic stent can be discussed in palliative situations or when the general medical state of the patient does not allow general anesthesia and surgery [3].

Question 8:

Describe the steps of your pre-operative treatment.

Answer 8:

- In emergency
- Information of the patient:
  - Management in emergency
  - Probable cancer of the colon
  - Risk of temporary colostomy
  - Risk of postoperative morbidity and mortality
  - Risk of intraoperative bleeding
  - Possible postoperative stay in the intensive care unit
- Intravenous fluid replacement with normal saline solution to treat the hypovolemic shock and acute renal failure
- Probabilistic antibiotherapy depending on the local protocol: e.g., amoxicillin + clavulanic acid
- Antagonization of the antivitamin K treatment (warfarin):
  - Intravenous vitamin K
  - ±Prothrombin complex
- Order two units of blood in case of emergent transfusion necessity
- Intravenous antalgic and antispasmodic treatment
- Intravenous antiacid treatment

Question 9:

You chose a surgical treatment. Operative findings are shown in Figs. 28.6 and 28.7. Identify the two main operative findings (star and arrow) and describe the steps of the surgical treatment.

Answer 9:

Operative findings:

- Black star: major colonic dilatation
- Black arrow: diastatic dilaceration

Steps of the surgical treatment:

Patient installation

- Supine position, legs apart
- Nasogastric tube
- Urinary catheter
- Two peripheral venous catheters

Surgical approach

- Median laparotomy beginning from above the umbilicus to the pubis
- Laparoscopic approach is also a valid option

Surgical treatment

- Emergency surgical treatment
- Curative treatment
- Treatment of the obstructive syndrome and of the cancer
- Exploration of the abdominal cavity:
  - Collect peritoneal fluid for cytological and bacteriological analysis.
  - Nature of the peritoneal fluid: serous? bloody? purulent? stercoral?
  - Search for peritoneal carcinomatosis and liver metastasis.
- Tumor:
  - Localization: sigmoid colon
  - Invasion of the adjacent organs (ureter, bladder, small bowel)
- Viability of the upstream colon:
  - Dilatation
  - Cecal parietal thickness
  - Area of necrosis
  - Diastatic perforation
- Procedure performed:
  - Carcinological total colectomy.
  - Section of the mesenteric inferior artery 1 cm after its origin for optimal lymph node dissection.
  - 5 cm margin under the inferior pole of the tumor.
  - Partial mesorectal excision.
  - Send the resected sample for pathological analysis.
  - Mechanical high or middle ileorectal anastomosis.
  - No diversion ileostomy.
  - Pelvic drainage optional.

Question 10:
What is your diagnosis?
Answer 10:
Postoperative ileus
Question 11:
In this case, before concluding with a functional etiology, what are the two diagnoses that you have to eliminate?

Answer 11:
Mechanical obstruction:

- Ileorectal anastomosis stenosis
- Adhesive small bowel obstruction

Question 12:
What most frequent underlying causes of this condition do you suspect?
Answer 12:

- Intraperitoneal sepsis: intraperitoneal abscess, ileorectal anastomosis leakage
- Electrolyte abnormalities: hypokalemia, hyponatremia, hypomagnesaemia
- Use of medications that are produce ileus: opiates

Question 13:
What complementary exams do you ask to determine the cause of this condition?
Answer 13:

- Laboratory exams: blood ionogram looking for electrolyte abnormalities
- Abdominal IV CT scan opacification through rectal route looking for intraperitoneal complications: mechanical obstruction (ileorectal anastomosis stenosis, adhesive obstruction), abscess, ileorectal anastomosis leakage

28.3 Case Study No. 2

You are asked about your opinion in the oncology day hospital for a 65-year-old male patient. He is currently under neoadjuvant chemotherapy for a locally advanced right colic cancer associated with synchronous liver metastases. The colon cancer was until now asymptomatic, and the liver metastases were initially considered as borderline for resection. He has already received three courses of FOLFIRI (irinotecan, folinic acid, 5-fluorouracil) and bevacizumab and was admitted today to receive the fourth course. He received the third course 15 days ago.

The patient has no other medical history. He complains of acute abdominal pain and 39 °C fever for 24 h. He also had one episode of bloody diarrhea last week. Your physical examination shows that the vital signs are normal, temperature is 38.7 °C. Abdominal physical examination shows an elective tenderness in the right iliac fossa. The abdomen is not distended, and there is no transit disorder. Rectal digital examination is within normal limits. Karnofsky performance status is 80%; weight, 55 kg; height, 180 cm; and body mass index, 17 kg/m^2.

Laboratory findings are the following:

White blood cell (WBC) count	12,500 cells/mm^3
Hemoglobin	12.5 g/dL
Hematocrit	51%
Mean corpuscular volume	55 μm^3
Platelet count	250,000/μL
Sodium	137 mEq/L
Potassium	4.2 mEq/L
Urea nitrogen	3 mmol/L
Creatinine	65 μmol/L (0.74 mg/dL)
Creatinine clearance (MDRD)	81 mL/min/1.73 m^2
C-reactive protein (CRP)	90 mg/L
Proteins	75 g/L
Albumin	25 g/L
Prealbumin	0.111 g/L
AST	150 IU/L
ALT	167 IU/L
Alkaline phosphatase	70 IU/L
Gamma GT	150 IU/L
Total bilirubin	34 μmol/L (2.0 mg/dL)
Conjugated bilirubin	13.6 μmol/L (0.8 mg/dL)

Question 1:

In case of metastatic colon cancer, what are the indications of the resection of the primitive tumor?

Question 2:

What is the percentage of complication risk of an unresected primitive colonic tumor during chemotherapy associated with biotherapy?

Question 3:

What is the risk of emergency colectomy for local complications of a colonic primitive tumor under chemotherapy and biotherapy?

Question 4:

What are the most frequent complications related to the primitive colonic tumor occurring under chemotherapy and biotherapy (bevacizumab in particular)?

Question 5:

In this case, what imaging exam do you ask to make the diagnosis? In what time line?

Question 6:

What is your interpretation of the images of this exam (Figs. 28.13, 28.14, 28.15, and 28.16)?

Question 7:

What is your final diagnosis?

Question 8:

What is your initial management of this patient?

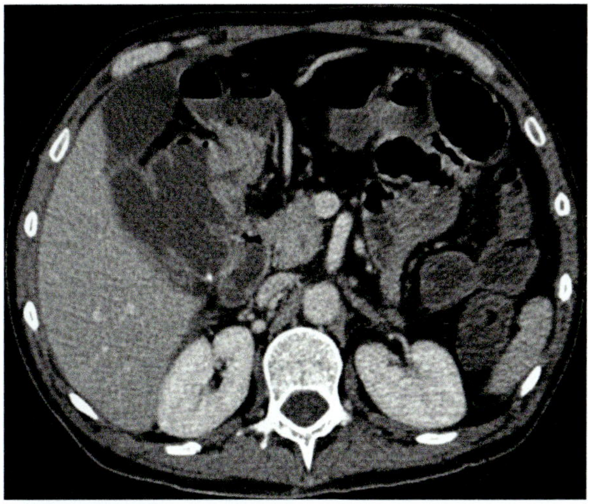

Fig. 28.13 Abdominal CT scan with contrast, portal phase, cross-sectional view

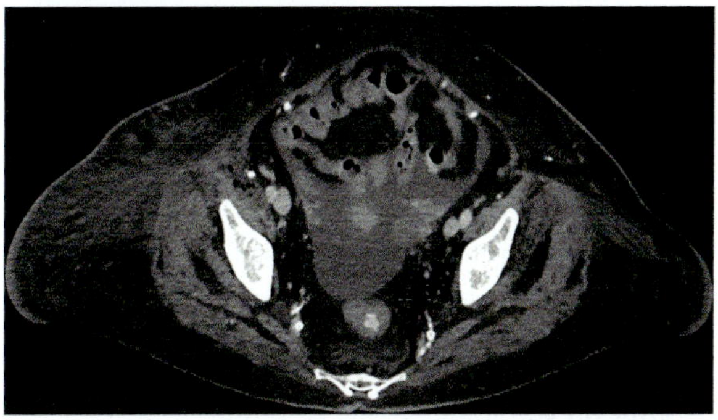

Fig. 28.14 Abdominal CT scan with contrast, portal phase, cross-sectional view

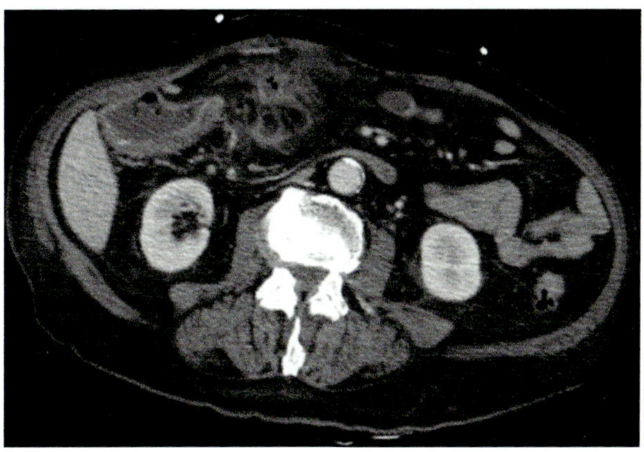

Fig. 28.15 Abdominal CT scan with contrast, portal phase, cross-sectional view

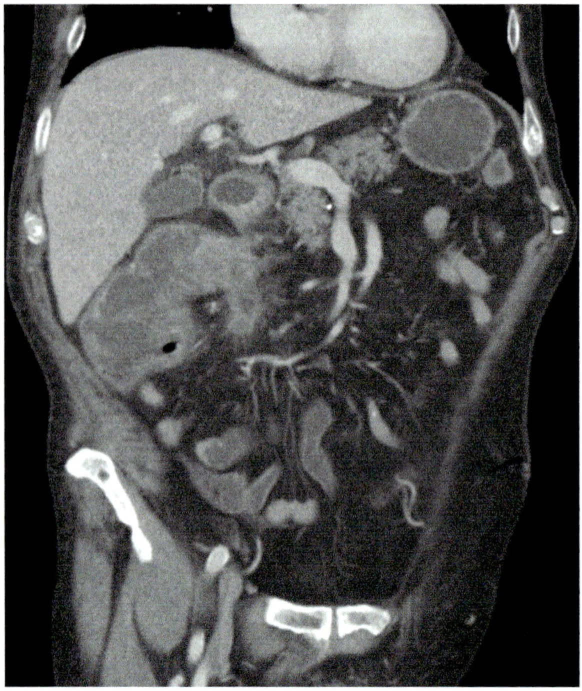

Fig. 28.16 Abdominal CT scan with contrast, portal phase, coronal view

After 72 h of the initial treatment, abdominal pain is persisting along with the right iliac fossa tenderness and fever. Laboratory findings show an increase of the biological inflammatory syndrome.

Question 9:

How do you manage this situation?

A. You plan a complementary abdominal IV CT scan in emergency.
B. You plan an emergency colonoscopy.
C. You pursue the initial medical treatment.
D. You broaden the antibiotherapy.
E. You decide to resume chemotherapy and biotherapy.

The CT scan shows a pericecal 55 × 62 mm abscess. There is also an increase of the intraperitoneal effusion and an increase of the pericecal pneumoperitoneum.

The radiologist calls you to tell you that the abscess is accessible to a percutaneous drainage and that he is available to drain it in emergency.

Question 10:

What is your answer to the radiologist?

Question 11:

Describe your specific treatment.

Question 12:

What is the percentage of definitive stoma associated with emergency surgery for a complication related to a primitive colonic cancer under chemotherapy and biotherapy?

At the fifth postoperative day, the patient presents an abundant serous effusion from the median laparotomy abdominal scar.

Question 13:

What diagnosis do you suspect?

Question 14:

Describe the management of this complication.

28.4 Answers: Case Study No. 2

Question 1:

In case of metastatic colon cancer, what are the indications of the resection of the primitive tumor?

Answer 1:

In cases of metastatic colon cancer, the resection of the colonic tumor is indicated when the colon cancer is symptomatic: sub-obstructive or obstructive tumor, tumoral hemorrhage, and tumoral abscess or perforation. It is also discussed when the metastases are resectable (i.e., colectomy followed by chemotherapy and then resection of metastases).

Question 2:

What is the percentage of complication risk of an unresected primitive colonic tumor during chemotherapy associated with biotherapy?

Answer 2:

The complication risk is 15–25% [4–6].

Question 3:

What is the risk of emergency colectomy for local complications of a colonic primitive tumor under chemotherapy and biotherapy?

Answer 3:

The risk of emergency colectomy for local complications of a colonic primitive tumor under chemotherapy and biotherapy is 7–16% [4–7].

Question 4:

What are the most frequent complications related to the primitive colonic tumor occurring under chemotherapy and biotherapy (bevacizumab in particular)?

Answer 4:

Colonic obstruction, tumoral hemorrhage, and digestive perforation [8, 9]

Question 5:

In this case, what imaging exam do you ask to make the diagnosis? In what time line?

Answer 5:

Abdominal IV CT scan, in emergency

Question 6:

What is your interpretation of the images of this exam (Figs. 28.13, 28.14, 28.15, and 28.16)?

Answer 6:

The imaging exam shows the following:

- Parietal thickening of the right colon (red star in Fig. 28.17)
- Infiltration of the right mesocolonic fat and reaction ileitis (red cross in Fig. 28.18)

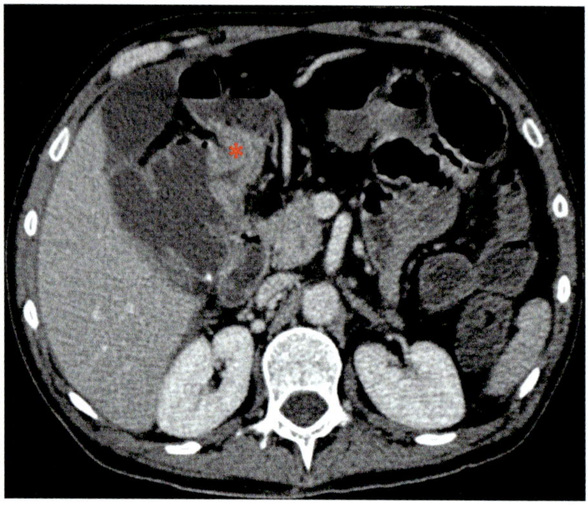

Fig. 28.17 Abdominal CT scan with contrast, portal phase, cross-sectional view

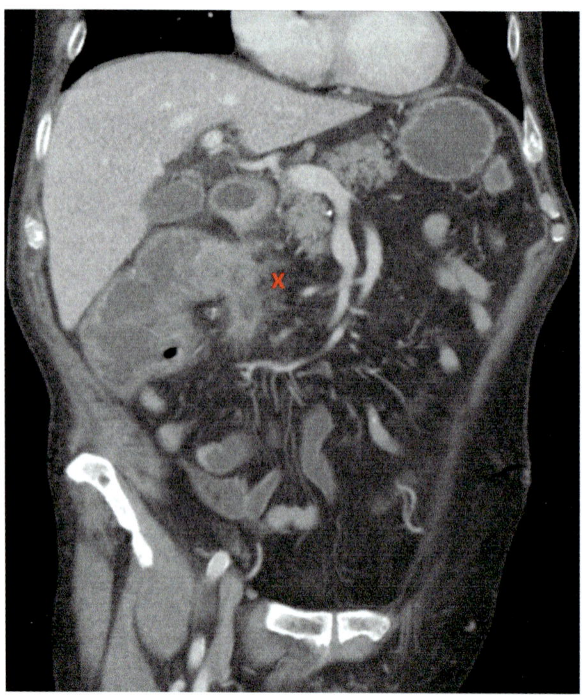

Fig. 28.18 Abdominal CT scan with contrast, portal phase, coronal view

- Pelvic effusion (red triangle in Fig. 28.19)
- Localized extraluminal gas within the pericecal fat without free pneumoperitoneum (red arrow in Fig. 28.20)

Question 7:
What is your final diagnosis?
Answer 7:
Infected right colonic cancer with localized microperforation
Question 8:
What is your initial management of this patient?
Answer 8:

- In emergency
- Hospitalization in the general surgery department
- Initial medical treatment
- Patient under fasting condition
- Intravenous antibiotherapy effective against gram-negative and anaerobic bacteria
- Suspension of the chemotherapy

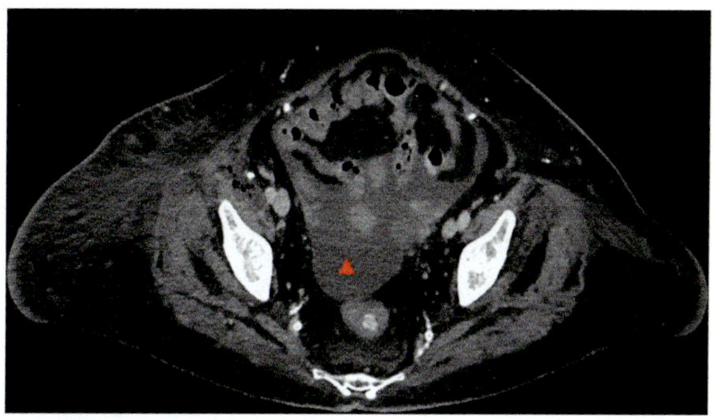

Fig. 28.19 Abdominal CT scan with contrast, portal phase, cross-sectional view

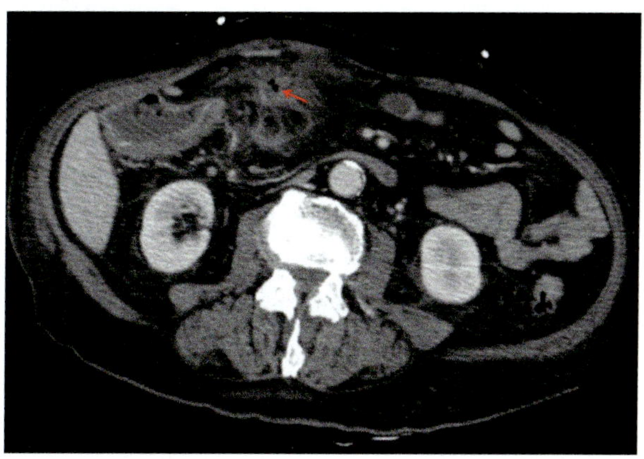

Fig. 28.20 Abdominal CT scan with contrast, portal phase, cross-sectional view

Question 9:
How do you manage this situation?

A. You plan a complementary abdominal IV CT scan in emergency
B. ~~You plan an emergency colonoscopy~~
C. ~~You pursue the initial medical treatment~~
D. You broaden the antibiotherapy
E. ~~You decide to resume chemotherapy and biotherapy~~

Answer 9:
A and D
In this case, the CT scan is necessary to reevaluate efficiency of the medical treatment and to check for complications. If invasive treatment is indicated, CT scan allows to decide whether radiological or surgical treatment is optimal.
Question 10:
What is your answer to the radiologist?
Answer 10:
In this case, apart from the peritumoral abscess, there are radiologic signs of localized peritonitis. Percutaneous drainage of the abscess will not be sufficient to treat the intra-abdominal sepsis.
Question 11:
Describe your specific treatment.
Answer 11:

- Emergency surgical treatment.
- Surgical approach: periumbilical median laparotomy.
- Complete exploration of the abdomen: effusion sample for bacteriological exam, localization of the abscess, check for peritoneal carcinomatosis.
- Surgical drainage of the abscess.
- Oncological right colectomy.
- Ileocolonic anastomosis is contraindicated: there is a localized peritonitis and the patient is under bevacizumab treatment.
- Ileocolostomy in the right iliac fossa.
- Abundant intra-abdominal lavage.
- Drainage of the abdomen.

Question 12:
What is the percentage of definitive stoma associated with emergency surgery for a complication related to a primitive colonic cancer under chemotherapy and biotherapy?
Answer 12:
There is a 30% risk of definitive stoma after this type of surgery [5]. However, this series includes Hartmann's procedures, and the risk is probably inferior after ileocolostomy.

Question 13:
What diagnosis do you suspect?
Answer 13:
Covered evisceration

Patients treated with biotherapies and particularly with bevacizumab have an increased risk of abdominal wall complications related to retarded wound healing. Generally, the delay between the last administration of bevacizumab and planned surgery should be 6–8 weeks, and bevacizumab administration can be resumed 28 days after surgery [10, 11]. When emergency surgery is required, the benefit/risk balance should be carefully evaluated, and the surgeon should be informed of the increased postoperative complications rate.

In cases of early postoperative evisceration, it is also of utter importance to look for the cause: intra-abdominal septic complication, intra-abdominal abscess digestive fistula, etc.

Question 14:
Describe the management of this complication:

- Emergency surgical treatment.
- There is no need to perform complementary imaging exam.
- Under general anesthesia.
- Opening of the cutaneous scar.
- Control the presence of aponeurotic disunion.
- Sample the serous effusion for bacteriological exam.
- If an aponeurotic disunion is objectified, complete opening of the median laparotomy.
- Exploration of the abdominal cavity to look for intra-abdominal septic complication.
- Intra-abdominal positioning of a resorbable mesh (optional).
- Careful aponeurotic closure of the median laparotomy with separated stitches.
- Skin closure.

28.5 Case Study No. 3

You have to manage in the emergency room a 55-year-old man who consults for abdominal pain and nausea. He is treated with beta blockers for high blood pressure. At the age of 36 years old, he was operated for appendectomy. He noticed an aggravation of his usual constipation and abdominal pain which used to decrease after the emission of stools. He hasn't had flatus nor stools for 2 days and has had several episodes of fecaloid vomiting for the last 24 h. Physical examination shows abdominal distension. You hear no intra-abdominal rumbling noise. There is no inguinal, crural, or umbilical herniation. There is no palpable adenopathy. Cardiac and pulmonary auscultation are unremarkable.

Question 1:

What important clinical sign do you look for at the physical examination?

Question 2:

You suspect a digestive obstructive syndrome. What is the first therapeutic measure you take?

Question 3:

Among the following imaging exams, what exam do you choose? (several are possible)

A. Abdominal IV CT scan ± opacification through rectal route
B. Pelvic MRI
C. Colonoscopy after bowel preparation
D. Videocapsula
E. Abdominal ultrasound

Question 4:

What do you search on this exam?

The imaging exam shows apple core stenosing mass of the high rectum with a dilatation of the whole upstream colon and dilatation of the small bowel. The ileocecal valve is incompetent and the stomach is full. There is no intra-abdominal effusion, no pneumoperitoneum, no colonic parietal pneumatosis, and no peritoneal carcinomatosis. There is also a 40 mm hypodense lesion evoking a liver metastasis of the segment III.

Question 5:

What is your final diagnosis?

Question 6:

What emergency therapeutic options can you propose?

A. Non-operative treatment: nasogastric tube aspiration
B. Endoscopic self-expandable metal colonic stent placement
C. Surgical treatment: proximal loop left colostomy
D. Surgical treatment: proctectomy with Hartmann's procedure and left colostomy
E. Surgical treatment: total coloproctectomy with terminal ileostomy
F. Surgical treatment: total colectomy with ileorectal anastomosis ± derivation ileostomy
G. Surgical treatment: rectosigmoid resection with colorectal anastomosis ± derivation ileostomy and liver tumorectomy
H. Surgical treatment: resection of the rectal tumor after intraoperative colonic irrigation with anastomosis, with or without a diverting ileostomy depending on the level and quality of the colorectal anastomosis

Question 7:

Describe the steps of your emergency treatment

Question 8:
How do you conduct the further management of the patient?

The extension work-up shows that the tumor is limited to the upper rectum, without any other metastases. You perform the oncologic rectosigmoid resection with middle colorectal anastomosis. Postoperative course is uneventful. The tumor is graded pT3N1M0 and adjuvant therapy is required. The following 3-year follow-up of this patient is uneventful, and the patient is lost sight for 5 years.

During one of your shifts at the emergency room, once again, you have to manage this patient. He is admitted for severe loss of body weight and condition. Karnofsky performance status is 60%. He feels exhausted and very thirsty. He has not had flatus nor stools for 3 days. He presented several episodes of vomiting. He also complains of shortness of breath every time he lays down. Physical examination shows a distended abdomen with the presence of bilateral flank dullness. Digital rectal exam shows the absence of fecaloma.

Vital Signs: Blood pressure, 90/45 mmHg; pulse, 122 bpm; respiratory rate, 22 breaths/min; temperature, 36.6 °C; sats, 97% on room air; weight, 55 kg; height, 170 cm; body mass index, 17.3 kg/m^2

Laboratory findings at the emergency room:

White blood cell (WBC) count	9700 cells/mm^3
Hemoglobin	12.3 g/dL
Hematocrit	52%
Mean corpuscular volume	65 μm^3
Platelet count	500,000/μL
Sodium	147 mEq/L
Potassium	4.2 mEq/L
Urea nitrogen	11 mmol/L
Creatinine	160 μmol/L (1.70 mg/dL)
Creatinine clearance (MDRD)	40.5 mL/min/1.73 m^2
C-reactive protein (CRP)	42 mg/L

Question 10:
What is the most likely diagnosis?

A. Adhesive small bowel obstruction
B. Obstructive peritoneal carcinomatosis
C. Anastomotic tumoral recurrence
D. Anastomotic stenosis
E. Recurrence of a colon cancer

Question 9:
What is the specific medical treatment of this condition?
Question 10:
In the event of failure of the medical treatment, what are the possible other alternatives?

28.6 Answers: Case Study No. 3

Question 1:

What important clinical sign do you look for at the physical examination?

Answer 1:

Spontaneous or provoked pain in the right flank or right iliac fossa. The presence of this physical sign is a marker of critical distension or suffering of the cecum and should push for rapid management.

Question 2:

You suspect a digestive obstructive syndrome. What is the first therapeutic measure you take?

Answer 2:

The patient has vomited several times. To prevent from the risk of inhalation, you put a nasogastric tube for gentle digestive aspiration. This measure should be performed as soon as the diagnosis of small bowel or colonic obstructive syndrome is raised and before the imaging confirmation.

Question 3:

Among the following imaging exams, what exam do you choose? (several are possible)

A. Abdominal IV CT scan ± opacification through rectal route
B. ~~Pelvic MRI~~
C. ~~Colonoscopy after bowel preparation~~
D. ~~Videocapsula~~
E. ~~Abdominal ultrasound~~

Answer 3:

Answer A

Question 4:

What do you search on this exam?

Answer 4:

- The cause of the colonic obstruction: volvulus, tumor, fecaloma
- Signs of colonic suffering or perforation: pneumoperitoneum, parietal pneumatosis, peritoneal effusion, cecum diameter >10 cm
- Liver metastasis, peritoneal carcinomatosis

Question 5:

What is your final diagnosis?

Answer 5:

Colonic obstructive syndrome originating from a tumoral stenosis of the upper rectum with an isolated and resectable liver metastasis in the segment III

Question 6:
What emergency therapeutic options can you propose?

A. ~~Non-operative treatment: nasogastric tube aspiration~~
B. ~~Endoscopic self-expandable metal colonic stent placement~~
C. Surgical treatment: proximal loop left colostomy
D. Surgical treatment: proctectomy with Hartmann's procedure and left colostomy
E. ~~Surgical treatment: total coloproctectomy with terminal ileostomy~~
F. ~~Surgical treatment: total colectomy with ileorectal anastomosis ± derivation ileostomy~~
G. ~~Surgical treatment: rectosigmoid resection with colorectal anastomosis ± derivation ileostomy and liver tumorectomy~~
H. Surgical treatment: resection of the rectal tumor after intraoperative colonic irrigation with anastomosis, with or without a diverting ileostomy depending on the level and quality of the colorectal anastomosis

Answer 6:

Answer A: False. Nasogastric tube aspiration is not sufficient to treat the organic colonic obstruction. It only prevents the patient from inhalation.

Answer B: False. In this case, the patient is in good medical condition and can undergo general anesthesia and surgery. Moreover, the liver metastasis is unique and resectable. The objective of the treatment is therefore curative and not palliative. There is no indication for self-expandable colonic metallic stent [12].

Answer C: True. There is no clinical and radiological sign of colonic or small bowel suffering or perforation. The first aim of the treatment is to treat the colonic obstruction to prevent diastatic perforation. This can be achieved by upstream colostomy. The resection of the tumor will be performed later. The main advantages of this option are a short operative time and the possibility to complete the staging of the tumor before the second step of proctectomy or neoadjuvant therapy.

Answer D: True. If this procedure is licit in this case, it is not the best option to choose. The advantage of this operation is to allow an oncologic resection of the rectum during the first operation without any possibility of postoperative leakage. However, there is a risk of suboptimal lymphadenectomy due to technical difficulties during operation because of a dilated colon and a risk of definitive stoma in up to 50% of the patients [13, 14]. Hartmann's procedure should probably be restricted to elderly patients with underlying comorbidities and high American Society of Anesthesiologists (ASA) score and advanced obstruction with proximal distention in whom Hartmann's procedure is considered to be a definitive curative procedure.

Answers E, F: False. There is no indication for emergency total colectomy with or without anastomosis since there's no suffering of the upstream colon.

Answer G: False. Emergency treatment should focus on the treatment of the colonic obstruction. There is no emergency to treat the liver metastasis. Moreover, further liver MRI should be first performed to stage the tumor, and look for other liver metastasis and determine the most efficient adjuvant oncological treatment to perform.

Answer H: True. Although no recommendations have been established, single-stage primary resection of the rectal cancer and colorectal or anal anastomosis after intraoperative colonic irrigation with temporary ileostomy can also be proposed. This option allows to treat the obstruction and the rectal cancer with less morbidity at the ileostoma closure. However, this option has several drawbacks: firstly, performing a colorectal or a coloanal anastomosis in a dilated and unprepared large bowel exposes the patient to a high risk of leakage. Secondly, intraoperative colonic irrigation also includes risks as a longer operative time and a fecal spillage in the abdominal cavity which can increase the occurrence of an anastomotic leakage. Only selected patients with only partial intestinal obstruction and minor large bowel dilation can be proposed for such strategy.

Question 7:

Describe the steps of your emergency treatment.

Answer 7:

- In emergency
- Information of the patient:
  - Management in emergency
  - Probable cancer of the colon with resectable liver metastasis
  - Temporary colostomy
  - Risk of postoperative morbidity and mortality
  - Risk of intraoperative bleeding
  - Possible postoperative stay in the intensive care unit
- Nasogastric aspiration
- Intravenous fluid replacement with normal saline solution
- Intravenous antalgic and antispasmodic treatment
- Intravenous antiacid treatment

Patient installation
- Supine position, legs apart
- Urinary catheter
- Two peripheral venous catheters

Surgical treatment
- Periumbilical median laparotomy.
- This type of incision is preferable to a left transverse median for further rectosigmoid resection.
- In this case, laparoscopic approach is not safe: the small bowel and the colon are dilated and fragile; there is a risk of digestive lesion or perforation at the insertion of the trocars and at the manipulation of the digestive loops.
- Exploration of the abdominal cavity:
  - Collect peritoneal fluid for cytological and bacteriological analysis.
  - Nature of the peritoneal fluid: serous? bloody? purulent? stercoral?

  - Search for peritoneal carcinomatosis and liver metastasis.
  - Localization of the tumor: high rectum.
- Viability of the upstream colon:
  - Dilatation
  - Cecal parietal thickness
  - Area of necrosis
  - Diastatic perforation
- Procedure performed:
  - Identification of the distal part of the sigmoid loop just above the tumor
  - Lateral colostomy fashioning

Question 8:
How do you carry on the further management of the patient?
Answer 8:

In order to accurately stage the tumor, it is necessary to perform a colonoscopy through the stoma and through the rectal route. The objective is to explore the rest of the colon to check for another tumor localization and to perform biopsies of the tumor.

Concerning the extension staging, it is necessary to perform a liver MRI to check for additional liver metastases and a thoracic CT scan to look for pulmonary metastases. The dosage of the ACE tumoral markers is relevant as a baseline for the follow-up.

Question 9:
What is the most likely diagnosis?
Answer 9:

A. ~~Adhesive small bowel obstruction~~
B. Obstructive peritoneal carcinomatosis
C. ~~Anastomotic tumoral recurrence~~
D. ~~Anastomotic stenosis~~
E. ~~Recurrence of a colon cancer~~

Answer B

All the diagnoses are plausible and have to be raised in a patient with a medical history of surgery for colon cancer. However, the severe loss of body weight and condition and the ascites are strongly suggestive of peritoneal carcinomatosis.

Question 10:
What is the specific medical treatment of this condition?
Answer 10:

- Nasogastric tube aspiration
- Intravenous hydration
- Parenteral nutrition
- Analgesic treatment
- Antispasmodic treatment: scopolamine butylbromide (antiperistaltic and antisecretory effects)
- Antiemetic treatment

- Antisecretory treatment: subcutaneous or continuous intravenous administration of octreotide
- Intravenous corticotherapy

Question 11:

In the event of failure of the medical treatment, what are the possible other alternatives?

Answer 11:

- Endoscopic self-expandable metal colonic stent placement
- Percutaneous endoscopic or radiological or open surgical decompressive gastrostomy
- Surgical diverting ileostomy or internal bypass
- Surgical resection of the obstructive nodule of peritoneal carcinomatosis

28.7 Case Study No. 4

You have to manage in the emergency room an 80-year-old woman with a medical history of right femoral hernia operated 30 years ago. She also has had pelvic static disorders for years with episodic fecal and urinary incontinence. Her last colonoscopy was performed 7 years ago. She recalls that several benign polyps were resected. She complaints of an increase of her waist circumference (she recently had to wear bigger pants) and noticed blood in her stools twice in the last few weeks. Within the last month, she experienced unusual constipation and tenesmus. In the last 48 h, she had diffuse abdominal pain, cessation of flatus and stools, and 38.9 °C fever. She did not vomit but is extremely queasy.

Question 1:

What complementary clinical signs do you check in your physical examination?

The completion of your physical examination shows the following:

Blood pressure, 110/75 mmHg; pulse, 117 bpm; absence of other clinical signs of shock. There is no hernia. Abdominal palpation shows diffuse abdominal tenderness especially in the right flank. Digital rectal exam is painful and reveals mucosal rectal prolapse, the absence of stool in the rectum, absence of palpable rectal mass, and the presence of blood trails on the finger cot.

Laboratory findings at the emergency room are the following:

White blood cell (WBC) count	17,700 cells/mm^3
Hemoglobin	10.5 g/dL
Hematocrit	51%
Mean corpuscular volume	55 μm^3
Platelet count	500,000/μL
Sodium	145 mEq/L
Potassium	4.2 mEq/L
Urea nitrogen	3 mmol/L
Creatinine	65 μmol/L (0.74 mg/dL)
Creatinine clearance (MDRD)	81 mL/min/1.73 m^2
C-reactive protein (CRP)	253 mg/L

Question 2:

What diagnosis do you suspect?

Question 3:

What imaging exam do you ask to confirm the diagnosis and in what time frame?

Question 4:

What signs do you look for on this imaging exam?

Your final diagnosis is peritonitis secondary to a diastatic perforation of the caecum above an obstructing tumor of the high rectum.

Question 5:

Among the following options, which surgical treatment you consider optimal?

A. Total colectomy with low ileorectal anastomosis, no diverting ileostomy
B. Total colectomy with low ileorectal anastomosis and diverting ileostomy
C. Total colectomy with terminal ileostomy and stapling of the rectal stump
D. Right colectomy with ileocolostomy, followed within 7–10 days by a rectosigmoid resection with colorectal anastomosis ± associated with ileocolonic stoma closure

Question 6:

How do you assess the nutritional status of this patient?

Question 7:

The patient has severe protein energy malnutrition. How do you plan to optimize his nutritional status postoperatively?

28.8 Answers: Case Study No. 4

Question 1:

What complementary clinical signs do you check in your physical examination?

Answer 1:

Clinical signs of septic/hypovolemic shock

- Tachycardia
- Hypotension
- Oliguria
- Clammy skin
- Thirst

Clinical signs indicating the etiology of the digestive obstructive syndrome

- Examination of the herniation holes, recurrence of the right femoral hernia
- Digital rectal exam: intrarectal mass, fecaloma, bleeding

Clinical gravity signs of the obstructive syndrome

- Pain on the right flank and right iliac fossa indicating critical distension of the cecum
- Clinical signs of digestive perforation and peritonitis: abdominal tenderness or abdominal guarding

Question 2:

What diagnosis do you suspect?

Answer 2:

Peritonitis secondary to a diastatic perforation of the cecum above a stenosing tumor of the colon or the high rectum

Question 3:

What imaging exam do you ask to confirm the diagnosis and in what time frame?

Answer 3:

- In emergency
- Abdominal IV CT scan

You suspect colonic perforation: colonoscopy is contraindicated.

In this case of suspicion of colonic obstruction and perforation, oral contrast enema is contraindicated.

Question 4:

What signs do you look for on this imaging exam?

Answer 4:

Signs of digestive perforation

- Pneumoperitoneum (*pneumoperitoneum is inconstant, and its presence depends on the localisazion of the perofration on the caecum*)

Localization of the digestive perforation

- Dilatation of cecum with a cecum diameter >10 cm
- Signs of cecal parietal lesions: thickening of the cecal wall, parietal pneumatosis of the cecum, ischemic lack of parietal enhancement of the cecum
- Competence of the ileocecal valve

Signs of peritonitis

- Intra-abdominal effusion
- Pericecal infiltrated peritoneal layers

Etiology of the occlusive syndrome

- Colonic obstructive syndrome
- Circumferential apple core stenosing mass of the high rectum and dilatation of the whole upstream colon

- Mesorectal adenopathies
- Stercoral stasis of the whole upfront colon

The perforation of the anterior wall of the cecum leads to a massive pneumoperitoneum and therefore to an easy diagnosis. On the contrary, a little breach on the posterior wall of the cecum leads to a partially covered perforation. This results in a limited peritoneal inflammatory site with a pneumoperitoneum of low abundance that can even be absent. These limited areas of pericecal peritoneal inflammation can be mistaken with appendicitis or periappendicular abscesses.

Question 5:

Among the following options, which surgical treatment you consider optimal?

A. ~~Total colectomy with low ileorectal anastomosis, no diverting ileostomy~~
B. ~~Total colectomy with low ileorectal anastomosis and diverting ileostomy~~
C. ~~Total colectomy with terminal ileostomy and stapling of the rectal stump~~
D. Right colectomy with ileocolostomy, followed within 7–10 days by a rectosigmoid resection with colorectal anastomosis ± associated with ileocolonic stoma closure

Answer 5:

A. *False*. In scheduled surgery as well as in emergency surgery, low colorectal or ileorectal anastomoses are at high risks of anastomotic leakages. In cases of limited intra-abdominal infections, if the decision to perform the anastomosis is made, diverting ileo- or colostomy is mandatory to decrease the incidence and gravity of the anastomotic leakage [15].
B. *False*. In cases of limited intra-abdominal sepsis or in localized peritonitis, when the colonic perforation is managed early, it is legitimate to perform total colectomy with ileorectal anastomosis and diverting ileostomy. However, in this case study, there is a generalized peritonitis which precludes this intervention, due to the high risk of postoperative anastomotic leakage, morbidity, and reintervention. Moreover, functional results of middle ileorectal anastomosis is poor at this age, especially when the patient presents pre-existing pelvic static disorders [16, 17].
C. *False*. In the conditions of generalized peritonitis in this case study, total colectomy with terminal ileostomy and stapling of the rectal stump allows to control the intra-abdominal sepsis and treat the rectal tumor. However, morbidity of terminal ileotomy in the elderly is high. The restoration of the digestive continuity can be discussed 3–6 months after the first intervention, depending on the general state of the patient and the quality of the expected functional results. Indeed, in this woman with anterior fecal and urinary incontinence, a poor functional result is expected.
D. *True*. The first step of this treatment is right colectomy with ileocolostomy to treat the colonic perforation. Secondly, after 7–10 days, the second step consists of treating the primitive rectal tumor with rectosigmoid resection and middle

colorectal anastomosis. Depending on the general condition of the patient, nutritional status, and the quality and level of the colorectal anastomosis, two options are possible: (1) if the patient presents malnutrition and the anastomosis is at risk of anastomotic leakage, the aim is to keep the ileocolostomy to divert the fecal stream and to protect the colorectal anastomosis. Ileocolostomy closure would be performed 8 weeks later. (2) Perform ileocolostomy closure and ileocolonic anastomosis within the same intervention if the patient has normal nutritional status.

Question 6:
How do you assess the nutritional status of this patient?
Answer 6:

Clinical examination

- Ingesta assessment
- Height
- Current weight
- Usual weight
- Percentage of the weight loss and date of the beginning of the weight loss
- Body mass index (BMI): weight (kg)/height^2 (m)
- Lean body mass: tricipital skinfold thickness and mid-arm muscle circumference

Mini Nutritional Assessment form [18] is a useful tool to collect these informations. Each item is labeled with a score. The final score indicates the nutritional status of the patient: normal nutritional status (24–30 points), at risk of malnutrition (17–23.5 points), and malnourished (less than 17 points).

Biological markers (Table 28.1)

- Albuminemia
- Pre-albuminemia (transthyretin)

Multiparametrical index

- Nutritional risk index (NRI) (Buzby index): NRI = 1519 × albuminemia (g/L) + 0.417 × (current weight/usual weight) × 100 (Table 28.2).

Table 28.1 Grades of malnutrition according to the levels of albumin and pre-albumin

	Albumin	Pre-albumin
Half-life	21 days	2 days
Normal range	35–50 g/L	0.25–0.35 g/L
Moderate malnutrition	30–35 g/L	0.15–0.25 g/L
Severe malnutrition	<30 g/L	<0.15 g/L

Table 28.2 Grades of malnutrition according to the nutritional risk index

	NRI (%)
Normal nutritional status	>97.5
Moderate malnutrition	83.5–97.5
Severe malnutrition	<83.5

Question 7:

The patient has severe protein energy malnutrition. How do you plan to optimize his nutritional status postoperatively?

Answer 7:

- Oral feeding as soon as possible in the absence of postoperative bowel obstruction or ileus
- Systematic nutritional assistance:
  - Enteral nutrition assistance: hyperproteinated solute 25–30 kcal/kg/day including 1.2–1.5 g of proteins/kg
  - Parenteral nutrition assistance: 25–30 kcal/kg/day including 0.20–0.25 g/kg/day nitrogen + electrolytes (50–100 mmol NaCl/24 h + 40–80 mmol KCl/24 h)
- In cases of postoperative complications: glutamine IV 0.3 g/kg/day without exceeding 21 days of treatment
- Immunonutrition IMPACT®: oral or enteral 1000 mL/day

References

1. Maruthachalam K, Lash GE, Shenton BK, et al. Tumour cell dissemination following endoscopic stent insertion. Br J Surg. 2007;94:1151–4.
2. Sabbagh C, Browet F, Diouf M, et al. Is stenting as "a bridge to surgery" an oncologically safe strategy for the management of acute, left-sided, malignant, colonic obstruction? A comparative study with a propensity score analysis. Ann Surg. 2013;258:107–15.
3. van Hooft JE, van Halsema EE, Vanbiervliet G, et al. Self-expandable metal stents for obstructing colonic and extracolonic cancer: European Society of Gastrointestinal Endoscopy (ESGE) clinical guideline. Endoscopy. 2014;46:990–1053.
4. Poultsides GA, Servais EL, Saltz LB, et al. Outcome of primary tumor in patients with synchronous stage IV colorectal cancer receiving combination chemotherapy without surgery as initial treatment. J Clin Oncol. 2009;27:3379–84.
5. McCahill LE, Yothers G, Sharif S, et al. Primary mFOLFOX6 plus bevacizumab without resection of the primary tumor for patients presenting with surgically unresectable metastatic colon cancer and an intact asymptomatic colon cancer: definitive analysis of NSABP trial C-10. J Clin Oncol. 2012;30:3223–8.
6. Suárez J, Marín G, Vera R, et al. Complications from the primary tumour are not related with survival in patients with synchronous stage IV colorectal cancer receiving chemotherapy without primary tumour resection. Int J Colorectal Dis. 2015;30:1357–63.
7. Karoui M, Roudot-Thoraval F, Mesli F, et al. Primary colectomy in patients with stage IV colon cancer and unresectable distant metastases improves overall survival: results of a multicentric study. Dis Colon Rectum. 2011;54:930–8.
8. Seo GJ, Park JW, Yoo SB, Kim SY, Choi HS, Chang HJ, et al. Intestinal complications after palliative treatment for asymptomatic patients with unresectable stage IV colorectal cancer. J Surg Oncol. 2010;102:94–9.

9. Ferrand F, Malka D, Bourredjem A, et al. Impact of primary tumour resection on survival of patients with colorectal cancer and synchronous metastases treated by chemotherapy: results from the multicenter, randomised trial Fédération Francophone de Cancérologie Digestive 9601. Eur J Cancer. 2013;49:90–7.
10. Ellis LM, Curley SA, Grothey A. Surgical resection after downsizing of colorectal liver metastasis in the era of bevacizumab. J Clin Oncol. 2005;23:4853–5.
11. Hurwitz H, Fehrenbacher L, Novotny W, Cartwright T, Hainsworth J, Heim W, et al. Bevacizumab plus irinotecan, fluorouracil, and leucovorin for metastatic colorectal cancer. N Engl J Med. 2004;350:2335–42.
12. van Hooft JE, van Halsema EE, Vanbiervliet G, et al. Self-expandable metal stents for obstructing colonic and extracolonic cancer: European Society of Gastrointestinal Endoscopy (ESGE) clinical guideline. Endoscopy. 2014;46:990–1053.
13. Desai DC, Brennan EJ, Reilly JF, et al. The utility of the Hartmann procedure. Am J Surg. 1998;175:152–4.
14. Zorcolo L, Covotta L, Carlomagno N, et al. Safety of primary anastomosis in emergency colorectal surgery. Colorectal Dis. 2003;5:262–9.
15. Bakker IS, Grossmann I, Henneman D, et al. Risk factors for anastomotic leakage and leak-related mortality after colonic cancer surgery in a nationwide audit. Br J Surg. 2014;101:424–32.
16. Peeters KCMJ, van de Velde CJH, Leer JWH, et al. Late side effects of short-course preoperative radiotherapy combined with total mesorectal excision for rectal cancer: increased bowel dysfunction in irradiated patients--a Dutch colorectal cancer group study. J Clin Oncol. 2005;23:6199–206.
17. Trenti L, Galvez A, Biondo S, et al. Quality of life and anterior resection syndrome after surgery for mid to low rectal cancer: a cross-sectional study. Eur J Surg Oncol. 2018;44:1031–9.
18. Kaiser MJ, Bauer JM, Ramsch C, et al. Validation of the Mini Nutritional Assessment short-form (MNA-SF): a practical tool for identification of nutritional status. J Nutr Health Aging. 2009;13:782–8.

Printed by Printforce, the Netherlands